THE
LOW-FAT
SUPERMARKET

Judith Scharman Smith, M.S., R.D.
Scott D. Smith, M.D.

THE LOW-FAT SUPERMARKET

Judith Scharman Smith, M.S., R.D.
Scott D. Smith, M.D.

STARBURST PUBLISHERS

P.O. Box 4123, Lancaster, Pennsylvania 17604

To schedule Author appearances write:
Author Appearances, Starburst Promotions, P.O. Box 4123
Lancaster, Pennsylvania 17604 or call (717) 293-0939

Credits:
Cover art by Bill Dussinger

We, The Publisher and Author, declare that to the best of our knowledge all
material (quoted or not) contained herein is accurate, and we shall not be held
liable for the same.

THE LOW-FAT SUPERMARKET

First Printing, February 1993

ISBN: 0-914984-44-6
Library of Congress Catalog Number 92-81392

Printed in the United States of America

Acknowledgement

To Our Parents

Disclaimer

The Authors and Publisher take no responsibility for any possible consequence of use of the material in this book. The publisher advises the reader to check with his or her physician before beginning any dietary program or therapy. This book does not take the place of a physician's recommendation for diet modification.

The nutritional values in this book are a compilation of statistics submitted by manufacturers and obtained from published government data and product labels. Sincere efforts were made to be as accurate and current as possible at the time of data collection. However, since product formulations change and published data are revised from time to time, some nutritional values may not be current.

Note To The Health Professional Reader

This book can be a great quick reference for the health professional. In addition to providing specific low-fat product information, its easy-to-understand explanations and helpful shopping tips can enhance patient education. Since new products are continually being introduced, another useful reference is Leni Reed's Supermarket Savvy™ Newsletter. Used in conjunction with this book, you will have a thorough and up-to-date reference to help patients make positive lifestyle changes.

Table Of Contents

Foreword

The average supermarket has over 25,000 products to choose from (including food and non-food items) and the average shopper certainly takes no more than an hour to decide what to put into his or her cart . . . and what to leave in the store. With so little time to make so many important decisions, the *Low-Fat Supermarket* can be a big help. Simply by flipping through its pages, you can zero in on the best products for a low-fat diet. And, the products are all listed by brand-name.

In addition, the text of the book clearly explains:

☞ The basics of a healthy diet,

☞ How to read the fine print on product labels . . . so you won't be misled by the bold print. Also, what to expect of the proposed new nutrition labels.

☞ How to select lower fat foods in fast food restaurants.

Because this book is an excellent guide for choosing low-fat foods, it's a valuable resource to anyone who wants to lose weight or lower his or her cholesterol.

Just be sure to take it to the store with you!

Happy and healthy eating!

Leni Reed, M.P.H., R.D.
Supermarket Savvy®

CLARIFYING THE FAT CONFUSION
CHAPTER 1

The benefits of a low-fat diet have become more and more evident over the past several years. Reducing fat intake can help you control your weight, lower your cholesterol level and improve your overall health. With a basic understanding of dietary fat and a few simple tools to assist you in low-fat shopping and cooking, following a low-fat diet can be easy. Without these resources consumers can be forced to rely on misleading advertisements that claim food is "lite" or "97%—free." As a result, misconceptions about fat and cholesterol are commonplace. This chapter, together with the shopping, cooking and fast food guides found in later chapters, will help you avoid these pitfalls and will make changing to a low-fat lifestyle simple and delicious.

Where do Calories Come From? Fat, carbohydrate and protein are the three nutrients that contribute calories to our diet. Different foods contain different amounts of each. For example, butter, margarine and all types of oil are almost exclusively fat. Sugars, starches and grains, on the other hand, are very high in carbohydrate. In fact, rice and potatoes have practically no fat at all (until they are covered with sour cream or margarine)! Foods high in protein include meats, poultry, fish and dairy products.

The Role of Fat in Weight Loss. There are several reasons why the most important factor in losing weight and keeping it off is the amount of fat you eat. First, ounce for ounce fat contains nearly two and one-half times the number of calories of carbohydrate or protein (see table). For example, an ounce of corn oil contains 252 calories, while an ounce of pure sugar (carbohydrate) contains only 112 calories. Furthermore, high-fat foods generally contain little or no fiber. In addition to the other well-publicized benefits of fiber, it contributes no calories to the diet but adds bulk which helps you feel full. An average sized potato, for instance, contains only 80 calories but fills your stomach much more than the 135 calories in the tablespoon of margarine you put on top. This is why it is so easy to lose control of the number of calories you eat when you choose high-fat foods.

CALORIES	Carbohydrate	Protein	Fat
Calories per gram	4	4	9
Calories per ounce	112	112	252

In addition, the way the body handles fat is different than the way it handles carbohydrate or protein. Fat in foods is very similar in composition to body fat. As a result, only 3 percent of its calories are used up in the conversion process. On the other hand, 23 percent of carbohydrate calories are burned up in its more complicated conversion to body fat. Several metabolic studies in humans have also shown that the production of body fat is closely related to the amount of fat consumed, *not to the number of calories*. Although it may seem strange, this means that calories from fat will make you gain weight more than calories from carbohydrate or protein. There is even recent evidence which suggests that our appetite is regulated in part by our carbohydrate intake. Researchers in Canada found that, at least in the short term, people eating a high-fat or a low-fat diet tended to eat until they met their daily carbohydrate requirements, regardless of the amount of fat they ate. Eating high fat foods tended to make subjects want to eat more. For these reasons, concentrating on eliminating fat from your diet is more important than counting calories.

What's the Big Fuss About Saturated Fats? Although all types of fat have the same number of calories and affect weight in the same manner, your cholesterol level is affected differently by each of the different types. There are two main categories of dietary fat: saturated and unsaturated. Advertisers often use these terms, but few consumers really understand the significance of each.

Saturated fats are "saturated" or fully loaded with hydrogen. These fats are readily converted by the liver into cholesterol. Unsaturated fats are not fully loaded with hydrogen. Some are almost fully loaded (monounsaturated), others less so (polyunsaturated). These fats are not as easily converted to cholesterol as saturated fats. Lowering your cholesterol level, therefore, requires not only avoiding cholesterol itself, but saturated fats as well.

What Foods Have Saturated and Unsaturated Fats? As a general rule, fats that come from animal products are saturated. For example, fats in red meat and poultry fall into this category. (Chicken breast is healthier simply because it is lower in fat than red meats.) Since milk and dairy products are animal products, their fat is also mainly saturated. In addition, a few plant oils contain saturated fats. These plants are simple to remember since they all come from tropical climates. They include palm and palm kernel oils, coconut oil and cocoa butter. All of the other vegetable oils such as corn, sunflower, safflower, soybean and cottonseed oils are mainly polyunsaturated, while olive, peanut and canola (rapeseed) oils are high in monounsaturated fat.

Saturated: Animal Fats, Coconut Oil, Cocoa Butter, Palm Oil, Palm Kernel Oil

Monounsaturated: Canola Oil, Olive Oil, Peanut Oil

Polyunsaturated: Corn Oil, Cottonseed Oil, Safflower Oil, Sunflower Oil, Soybean Oil

"The Catch": What Most Consumers Don't Know.

Although vegetable oils contain unsaturated fat, they can be made into saturated fat by a process called hydrogenation. This process is useful for manufacturers because it lengthens the shelf life of oils and gives less expensive vegetable oils important baking properties of more costly animal fats. Since unsaturated fats are liquid at room temperature, this process is also used to solidify vegetable oils to make products like margarine and shortening. The "catch" to consumers is that even though a product is advertised as containing 100% vegetable oil, due to hydrogenation it may be no healthier than animal fat. The key to avoiding this pitfall is reading the ingredient list on the package. The words "hydrogenated" or "partially hydrogenated" before *any* type of fat indicate that it is at least partially saturated.

So What Can I Eat? Now that you understand the importance of eliminating fat from your diet, the question remains, "what foods are 'low enough' in fat?" Authorities including the American Heart Association and the National Institutes of Health recommend a diet in which no more than 30% of total calories come from fat, with no more than 10% from saturated fat. These recommendations have recently been extended to include children over two years of age. New federal regulations which will take effect within the next few years require labels for most prepared foods indicating saturated fat content. For now, however, it is difficult to know just how much saturated fat is in a particular product. Two general rules to help meet the above recommendations are: **(1)** Choose products which are 30% fat or less; **(2)** Try to select products containing saturated fat (animal fat, tropical oils or hydrogenated vegetable oils), only if they are 20% fat or less. The shopping guide in Chapter 2 lists thousands of products which meet these requirements.

Watch Out, Weight Watchers! It cannot be overemphasized that while saturated and unsaturated fats do not contribute equally to your cholesterol level, all fats are concentrated sources of calories that contribute to weight gain. Products containing only "healthy" unsaturated fats can still be very fattening. Wesson canola oil, for instance, is "94% saturated fat-free." Although this is one of the best oils to use since it is low in saturated fat, it is still pure fat and should be used sparingly. Following a weight reduction, low cholesterol, or even a general healthy diet requires eating less *total* fat, not just less saturated fat.

FOODS WITH HIDDEN FAT

☞ Food Item	Serving Size	Calories	Grams of Fat	% Fat
Eggo Homestyle Waffles	1 waffle	120	5	38
Dunkin' Donuts Bran Muffin	1 muffin	3330	11	30
Dunkin' Donuts Plain Croissant	1 croissant	310	19	55
Ruffles Potato Chips	15 chips	148	10	61
French Fries	10 fries	158	8	47
Ritz Crackers	4 crackers	70	4	51
Wheatsworth Crackers	4 crackers	70	3	39
Charles Light Popcorn	0.5 oz.	50	2	36
Granola Breakfast Cereal	1 oz.	130	5	35
2% Low-Fat Milk	1 cup	121	5	35
American Cheese	1 slice	106	9	76
Wish Bone Light Classic Dressing, Ceasar	0.5 oz.	28	3	85
American Classic Cracked Wheat Crackers	4 crackers	70	4	51
Kraft Light Naturals Cheese	1 oz.	80	5	56
Natural Valley Peanut Butter Granola Bar	1 bar	120	6	45

Hidden Fat. Many people try to reduce the fat in their diet by avoiding some of the well-known high-fat items such as red meat, whole milk, butter, margarine, mayonnaise and bacon.

Cutting out such foods is a great start, but a lot of fat is hidden where you wouldn't necessarily suspect. Even foods which are thought of as "health foods" such as granola, oat bran muffins, wheat crackers and frozen yogurt can be very high in fat. Don't be taken in by a product that is "high fiber" or made with chicken or turkey. The table above gives several examples of foods with hidden fat.

Uncovering the Hidden Fat. With so much hidden fat, you need to be able to easily determine the amount of fat in foods to make appropriate choices. As mentioned above, authorities including the American Heart Association recommend that less than 30% of our calories come from fat. A simple way to put this into practice is by looking at nutritional information labels on food packages. Since a gram of fat has nine calories, an item which is 30% fat or less can have only one gram of fat for every 30 calories. (To get an idea of what a gram of fat is, remember that there are 5 grams of fat in a pat of butter or margarine). The nutrition label below indicates that Gorton's Natural Cut 90% Fat Free Breaded Fish Fillets contains 11 grams of fat and 230 calories in each serving. Although it is labeled "90% fat free," Gorton's Natural Cut Breaded Fish Fillets are actually 43% fat, far greater than the 30% guideline. Later in this chapter we will discuss how food manufacturers get away with such misleading labels.

Gorton's Natural Cut—Breaded Fish Fillets—90% Fat Free

Serving Size	2 fillets
Servings per package	3
Calories	230
Protein, grams	13
Carbohydrate, grams	19
Fat, grams	11
Polyunsaturated	5
Saturated	3
Monounsaturated and other	3
Cholesterol, mg	40
Sodium, mg	370

$$\% \text{ Calories From Fat} = \frac{\text{Grams of Fat per Serving x 9}}{\text{Total Calories per Serving}} \times 100$$

$$\text{Gorton's Natural Cut} = \frac{11 \text{ Grams x 9}}{230 \text{ Calories}} \times 100 = 43\% \text{ Fat}$$

What About Cholesterol? Cholesterol is a colorless, odorless substance which is contained only in animal products and does not contribute calories to the diet. It is an essential component of every cell in your body and a necessary building block for many hormones. The problem with cholesterol it that when too much is present in the wrong form in the blood, it increases your risk of heart attack, stroke and other serious medical conditions. As a result, authorities recommend that we consume no more than 300 milligrams of cholesterol per day.

With only a few easy-to-remember exceptions, foods high in cholesterol are also high in saturated fat. By avoiding foods high in saturated fat, you are automatically reducing your dietary cholesterol. The exceptions to this rule include organ meats (such as liver and kidney), eggs and shellfish including shrimp, lobster and crab. Although these foods are high in cholesterol, they are low in both saturated and unsaturated fat. Shellfish is so low in saturated fat that its total effect on your blood cholesterol level is small. As a result, many dietitians have recently begun allowing their patients on low cholesterol diets to eat shellfish.

In addition to avoiding saturated fat, a diet high in soluble fiber has been shown to have a cholesterol-lowering effect. This type of fiber is found in many fruits, vegetables, dried beans and oats. Although oat bran has been the focus of so much attention, beans are an even better source of this beneficial fiber. It is important to note that the overall effect of soluble fiber on reducing the risk of heart disease is relatively small and that watching your saturated fat intake and eliminating other risk factors are equally important.

Label Language. Remember when buying a product that its "label language" is intended to induce you to buy the product, not necessarily to convey clear, accurate information. Packaging terminology is very loosely regulated, so the wording of labels can be extremely misleading. Understanding the legal definition of the following terms will help you avoid high-fat products.

"Low-fat." The claim that a food is "low-fat" is often misleading. This can simply mean that the product is lower in fat than other similar products. For example, 2% "low-fat" milk is lower in fat than whole milk, but 36% of its calories come from fat and it is therefore not a low-fat food in the strict sense. Under the law there is no stipulation as to how much lower in fat a "low-fat" product must be. The difference is often trivial.

"Light" or "Lite." Products labelled "light" or "lite" are not necessarily low in fat. These words can mean anything from lighter in color, texture or taste, to lower in sodium, calories or fat. "Light" olive oil, for example, is lighter only in color and taste. It is certainly not lower in fat since all oils are 100% fat. There are many new brands of "light" potato chips. Ruffles Light potato chips contain one-third less fat than regular Ruffles, but at 45% fat should still be avoided. Extreme examples include "light" mayonnaise products which are simply regular mayonnaise diluted with water. The term "light" refers to the lower number of calories per tablespoon even though the product is still nearly 100% fat. Before buying a product labelled "light," check the nutritional information label to be sure it really is low-fat.

More specific guidelines exist for the use of these terms when relating to meat and poultry. The USDA requires that "lean," "light," or "low-fat" meats and poultry contain 25% less fat by weight than the maximum allowed for regular meat and poultry products.

"93% Fat-Free." Items that use this type of language can be particularly misleading. This claim always refers to a product's percentage of fat *by weight,* while what really matters is the percentage of fat *by calories.* To understand the difference, think of a glass of water (495 grams, no fat, no calories) and a pat of butter (5 grams, all fat, 45 calories). The pat of butter alone is 100% fat when measured by weight or by calories. Since the water is so much heavier than the butter, floating the butter in the water makes the water/butter combination (500 grams, 5 grams fat, 45 calories) "99% Fat-Free" when measured by weight. Since 100% of the calories still come from fat, this claim is obviously irrelevant. Eating the butter with the water is no healthier than eating the butter alone, but this type of advertising sure makes you think so.

Products advertised in this way include 2% "low-fat" milk and the new McDonald's McLean Deluxe sandwich. Two percent milk contains 2% milkfat by weight but 36% of its calories come from fat. The McLean Deluxe is billed as being "91% fat-free," but at 29% fat by calories, it barely qualifies as a low-fat item and is certainly not low in saturated fat.

"No Cholesterol." Beware of products that are promoted as "cholesterol-free" or as having "no cholesterol." Since cholesterol is found only in animal products, items containing only vegetable oils have no cholesterol but may still be high in total fat and saturated fat. A product that is "cholesterol-free" such as potato chips or french fries can be just as damaging to your heart (and waist!) as a cholesterol-containing product.

FOILING THE FRAUDS
CHAPTER 2

◆ A Look at the New Labelling Laws

To try to clear up some of the confusion caused by misleading label language, the Food and Drug Administration (FDA) has proposed an extensive set of regulations requiring more complete nutrition information, specifying how labels must be worded, and defining the vague words often used to make foods seem healthier. The proposed regulations are under review and may be modified before their scheduled effective date of May 8, 1993. (This date will likely be changed to 1994.) Although these regulations won't apply to foods overseen by the U.S. Department of Agriculture (USDA) such as meat and poultry, the USDA has announced its intention to create similar regulations for these products.

While the intent of these regulations is good and they will likely be helpful in reducing the problems talked about in Chapter 1, some understanding of the information that will (and won't) be required is necessary to avoid further confusion. Summarized below are the most pertinent proposed regulations. Understanding them will help you take advantage of this new information and choose the most nutritious products.

True Confessions: The New Nutrition Information Regulations. For now, nutrition information on food packages is completely optional. Under the new regulations, every product in package form must include a label which shows the serving size, number of servings per container, and the nutrition information per serving. Similar requirements are planned by the USDA for processed meats and poultry. The nutrition information must include the total calories, calories from fat, and the amount of fat, saturated fat, cholesterol, carbohydrate, protein, fiber, and sodium. The amount of carbohydrate has to be broken down into simple carbo-hydrate (sugars) and complex carbohydrate (starches). The percent of the government's recommended intake of vitamins and minerals must also be included. Further breakdown of fat content into monounsaturated and polyunsaturated will be optional. Nutrition labelling of items such as produce, raw meat and raw poultry will be voluntary.

Serving Size. Manufacturers have been and will continue to be allowed to decide on serving sizes for their products. Since the grams of fat, calories, etc. refer to the amount per serving, small serving sizes sometimes seem to be low-calorie or low-fat. To help prevent this misunderstanding, categories of foods will be assigned serving sizes defined by the FDA which will not be printed on labels, but will be used to determine whether claims such as "low-fat" and "low-calorie," can be made. (The meaning of these and other terms are given in the section on health and nutrient content claims below.) The reference serving sizes are supposed to be the amount eaten at a single sitting by someone four years of age or older.

Total Fat and Saturated Fat. Although the fat and saturated fat per serving will be on all labels, one very important piece of information, the percentage of calories from fat, will not be required. However, since the number of calories from fat will be included, the percentage of fat will be much easier to calculate than it is now. (Simply dividing the number of calories from fat by the total calories and multiplying by 100 gives this important value). It will also be possible to calculate the percentage of calories from saturated fat from the grams of saturated fat. As mentioned in Chapter 1, official guidelines say that no more than 30% of our calories should come from fat, and that no more than 10% should come from saturated fat.

$$\% \text{ Calories From Fat} = \frac{\text{Calories From Fat}}{\text{Total Calories}} \times 100$$

$$\% \text{ Calories From Saturated Fat} = \frac{\text{Grams of Saturated Fat} \times 9}{\text{Total Calories}} \times 100$$

Simple and Complex Carbohydrates. Under the new regulations carbohydrate content will have to be broken down into simple carbohydrates (sugar, both natural and added) and complex carbohydrates (starches). As you probably already know, a good nutritional principle is to cut down on sugars in favor of complex carbohydrates. Up until now it has been nearly impossible to know how much sugar is in foods. Using the new labels and remembering that one teaspoon of table sugar (sucrose) weighs about 4 grams will help us get an idea of how much sugar is in what we eat. This will be especially helpful for diabetics who have to watch their sugar intake carefully. Don't forget, however, that fruits, fruit juices and milk contain naturally occurring sugars which will be included under simple carbohydrates on the nutritional label.

Fiber. Several recent studies have suggested that a diet high in fiber reduces the risk of diseases including heart disease, diabetes, obesity, and certain types of cancer. Although these studies are not conclusive, the National Cancer Institute has recommended that we eat from 20 to 35 grams of fiber per day. The average American now eats only about 10 to 15 grams per day. The actual amount of fiber in different foods is almost never given on labels, leaving consumers to rely on manufacturers' claims which may or may not be accurate. The new regulations will provide this important information and eliminate the ambiguity.

Sodium. One of the guidelines for health improvement established by the USDA is to reduce sodium intake. There is evidence that some people who are "salt-sensitive" can lower their blood pressure by cutting down on salt. For those with high blood pressure, this can be an important way to reduce their risk of heart disease and stroke. (A benefit of lowering blood pressure in those who already have normal blood pressure has not yet been demonstrated). Although some people don't really need to lower their blood pressure and others won't respond to cutting back on sodium, the fact that a low-sodium diet has no health risks led the National Research Council to recommend a maximum daily sodium intake of 2,400 milligrams. (A typical American diet has over 4,000 milligrams of sodium per day). People with high blood pressure or certain other medical conditions may, on the advice of their physician, need to restrict their sodium intake even further. This will be a lot easier to do with the new labelling regulations since the amount of sodium per serving will be given on all packages.

The New Label Language: The Regulations on Health and Nutrient Content Claims. The current "Label Language" used on food packages is often vague and misleading, as discussed in Chapter 1. Some of the confusion arises from the absense of regulations stating the types of claims that manufacturers are allowed to make. One of the main purposes of the new labelling regulations is to clearly define the meaning of specific terms and the conditions under which health claims can be made. For example, manufacturers making nearly any type of health claim will be required to state the not-so-healthy aspects of their product *right next to the claim*, not hidden away in fine print. All claims implying a comparison with other products must specify the product being compared to and the specific differences. To illustrate this, the FDA wrote an example claim for "Lite Cheesecake" which reads, "1/3 fewer calories and 50% less fat than our regular cheesecake: lite cheesecake-200 calories, 4 grams fat; regular cheesecake-300 calories, 8 grams fat."

If a product satisfies a health claim because of the type of food it is made of and not because it was prepared differently, the claim must make it clear that all foods of that type are similar. For example, if a vegetable producer wished to advertise its broccoli as being "fat-free," it would have to call itself "broccoli, a fat-free food," so that consumers would clearly understand that all broccoli is inherently fat-free.

Listed below are the definitions for each of the specific terms allowed on package labels. Since each term has a very specific meaning, unless you really understand the definitions, the differences between "light," "less," "reduced," and "low" won't have much meaning. Because of this, reading and understanding nutrition information tables will still be as important as ever.

"Light" or "Lite." Products claiming to be "light" or "lite" must specify the attribute of the product which is referred to by the claim. For example, if the claim refers to the product being lighter in color or texture, this must be clearly stated. Products lower only in sodium cannot claim to be "light," but must use the words "reduced sodium" or "low sodium" instead. If the claim refers to the number of calories, it must be 1/3 lower than the regular product, and must have at least 40 calories less per serving, so that the difference is not trivial. Even if this requirement is met, if the product is over 50% fat by calories, it must have 50% less fat per serving than the regular product. As you see, foods will have to be significantly lower in fat than the regular product to be called "light," but this doesn't guarantee that it is actually low-fat. You will still need to figure it out from the nutrition information.

"Fat-Free." The terms "fat-free" and "nonfat" will only be allowed when a food contains less than 0.5 grams of fat per serving. In addition, the product must not contain *any* added fat or oil.

"Low-Fat." Foods can only be advertised as being low-fat if they have 3 grams of fat or less per serving *and* 3 grams or less per 100 grams of food. The second requirement is designed to eliminate products which are customarily consumed in small amounts but are still high in fat like butter or margarine. Since the key factor is the *percentage* of calories from fat and *not* the total grams of fat, items labelled "low-fat" may still be too high to qualify as a truly low-fat food.

"93% Fat-Free." Any product which calls itself any number of "% fat-free" must be low-fat as defined above. The number of grams of fat per serving must also be printed on the label near the claim. As discussed earlier, this claim still refers to the percentage of fat *by weight*, not *by calories*, and does not necessarily mean that a product is truly low-fat. Recall the example of the glass of water (495 grams, no fat, no calories) and pat of butter (5 grams, all fat, 45 calories). Floating the butter in the water makes the combination weigh 500 grams, with "only" 5 grams of fat, making it "99% fat-free," when measuring by weight (as products always do). Since water has no calories, all of the 45 calories in the water/butter combination still come from fat, making it 100% fat, as measured by calories. As a result of this type of confusion, it is generally best to ignore this type of claim—look at the label for the actual values and calculate the percentage of calories from fat.

"Lean" and "Extra Lean." The new regulations will define these terms for meat and poultry. "Lean" products must contain less than 10.5 grams of fat, less than 3.5 grams of saturated fat, and less than 94.5 milligrams of cholesterol per 100 grams. "Extra Lean" products must contain less than 4.9 grams of fat, less than 1.8 grams of saturated fat, and less than 94.5 milligrams of cholesterol per 100 grams.

"Saturated Fat-Free." The term "saturated fat-free" will only be allowed when a food contains less than 0.5 grams of saturated fat per serving. In addition, the product must not contain *any* added fat or oil.

"Low in Saturated Fat." Foods can only be advertised as being low in saturated fat if they contain 1 gram of saturated fat or less per serving *and* not more than 15% of its calories from saturated fat. (Recall that official guidelines recommend that no more than 10% of calories come from saturated fat). Any product making this or any other claim regarding saturated fat must state the level of total fat and cholesterol in the food in immediate proximity to the claim.

"Cholesterol Free." Foods labelled in this manner must contain no more than 2 milligrams of cholesterol per serving. In addition, products making any claim regarding cholesterol cannot contain more than 11.5 grams of fat per serving or per 100 grams of food, and no more than 2 grams of saturated fat per serving unless it is clearly indicated on the label adjacent to the claim. This will prevent extremely high fat foods such as french fries from promoting themselves as "cholesterol free."

"Low Cholesterol." Such products will be allowed to have no more than 20 milligrams of cholesterol per serving. Recall that the maximum recommended daily intake of cholesterol is 300 milligrams. The requirements for fat content are the same for all claims regarding cholesterol. (See "Cholesterol Free.")

"Calorie-Free." The term "calorie-free" will only be allowed when a food contains less than 5 calories per serving.

"Low-Calorie." Foods can only be advertised as being low-calorie if they contain 40 calories or less per serving *and* 40 calories or less per 100 grams of food.

"High in ..." The terms "high," "rich in," and "major source of" with respect to any nutrient can only be used if a product contains at least 20% of the recommended daily intake of that nutrient per serving. The words "source of," "good source of," or "important source of" can be used if it contains 10-19% of the recommended daily intake of the nutrient.

"Sodium Free." Products must contain no more than 5 milligrams of sodium per serving to be labelled as "sodium free" or "salt free." In addition, the product must contain no added sodium.

"Very Low Sodium." In order to be labelled "very low sodium," a product can contain no more than 35 milligrams of sodium per serving.

"Low Sodium." Products labelled in this manner must contain no more than 140 milligrams of sodium per serving.

"No Added Salt." This type of labelling can apply to foods which are not necessarily low in sodium. To prevent confusion, this statement can only be made on a label if no salt is added during processing, the regular product is normally processed with salt, and a statement that the product is not a sodium free food is placed adjacent to the claim.

"Reduced," "Less," and "Fewer." Under the new proposals, these terms are synonymous and can be used to describe any product which has been modified to reduce its content of a nutrient by at least the amount used to define the term "low" for that nutrient. For example, a product labelled as "reduced fat" must be reduced by at least 3 grams of fat per serving and per 100 grams of food, since this is the amount that defines an item as "low-fat." Since a product containing 20 mg of cholesterol or less is "low-cholesterol," a reduction of 20 mg of cholesterol per serving qualifies as "less cholesterol." No minimum percentage difference in the quantity of the nutrient is required to make this claim. However, details of the comparison item, as well as the actual and percentage reduction must also appear adjacent to the claim. As you can see, a product which remains very high in fat, cholesterol, sodium, etc. can make the claim of being "reduced" with only a minimal reduction. It will be important to carefully inspect the nutrition information to avoid being misled by this type of claim.

"A Good Source of Fiber." If a product claims to be a good source of fiber and is also high in fat, a statement of the total fat content per serving must be placed in immediate proximity to the claim. In addition, since some conflicting results have been found regarding the role of fiber in reducing the risk of cancer and heart disease, no claims that fiber reduces the risk of these diseases will be permitted on product packages.

Specific Health Claims. Health claims stating that a particular item reduces the risk of disease will be permitted only if specifically authorized by the FDA once clear scientific evidence exists to support a claim. In addition, the claim must describe the overall dietary changes which result in the reduced risk of disease. Listing of other risk factors for the disease is also recommended. A sample claim written by the FDA for a food low in saturated fat claiming to help reduce the risk of heart disease reads as follows: "High blood cholesterol is a major cause of coronary heart disease. Other important factors are a family history of heart disease, being overweight, high blood pressure, and cigarette smoking. A healthy diet low in saturated fat, total fat, and cholesterol will lower blood cholesterol levels and reduce the risk of heart disease in most people."

Summary: As you can see, the specific definitions for each of the terms allowed by the new regulations can be hard to remember. The words "low," "reduced," "less," etc. don't clearly distinguish the differences. The regulations will, at the very least, prohibit very unhealthy foods from making health claims by using vague terms as they do at present. Probably the most important difference will be the required nutrition information printed on the package. This will only be helpful, however, to those who learn to use it. An aisle by aisle nutritional tour of a supermarket given by a registered dietitian can be a valuable resource in helping you learn to use this information more effectively. Contact your local supermarket or a registered dietitian to find one in your area.

LOW-FAT
SHOPPING GUIDE
CHAPTER 3

Although leading a low-fat lifestyle may sound easy, finding out the amount of fat in foods at the grocery store can be difficult. Even once the new labelling requirements take effect and all products have a nutrition information label, calculating the percentage of calories from fat will still be tedious. Furthermore, as we have learned in the first two chapters, products promoted as "light" or "97% fat free" may nevertheless may be too high in fat, and actual calculation of the percentage of calories from fat is critical. This book includes an extensive listing of over 4,000 low-fat items to help you sort out high-fat from low-fat products. But before you take this list with you to the grocery store, review the helpful guidelines for selecting foods in the meat case, delicatessen, packaged meat, cheese, cereal, and bread sections.

The Meat Case. Contrary to popular belief, not all beef is high in fat and not all chicken or turkey is lean. Fat content varies considerably among the different parts of animals, and thus the fat content of the meat you buy is dependent upon the cut and grade.

Although most cuts of beef are high in fat, those derived from the round (rump) and shank portions tend to be the lowest. Even within these cuts a "select" or "good" grade should be chosen rather than the higher fat (though higher priced and better tasting) grades of "choice" and "prime." The cut, however, is more important in determining fat content than the grade.

Almost all types of ground beef are extremely high in fat. The terms "lean" and "extra-lean" mean only that these are lower in fat than regular ground beef. They are usually still *very* high in fat. The USDA regulations scheduled to take effect in 1993 will set maximum levels of fat for products labelled with these terms. "Lean" meats will contain less than 10.5 grams of fat per 100 grams of meat, while "extra lean" meats will contain less than 4.9 grams of fat per 100 grams. This still won't mean that these products derive less than 30% of their calories from fat.

Even though round and sirloin cuts of beef tend to be the leanest, be careful not to assume that pre-ground round or sirloin are low in fat. In fact, ground round is made from several different round cuts, both lean and fatty, and is not well trimmed. Consequently, ground round is equivalent to extra-lean ground beef at most supermarkets, and is about 58% fat. In most cases, pre-ground sirloin is a only a little lower in fat than ground round. And remember, 90% fat free means the meat is 10% fat *by weight*, which translates to 50-55% fat by calories in most beef cuts.

Your best bet is to choose a cut of top round or eye of round and have the meat department at your supermarket grind it for you. (Be sure they trim it first). Select grades of meat are not usually available in the supermarket, but the choice grade of both these meats are less than 30% of calories from fat (see table). Though more expensive, it shrinks less since it is lower in fat, and in the end may cost no more than the cheaper, fattier cuts. Since top round cuts are often on sale, having it ground can be even cheaper then pre-ground hamburger. Most supermarkets will gladly grind it for you free of charge. Stop by the meat section first and have your beef ground while you do your other shopping.

To make things even easier, new low-fat ground beef products are hitting the supermarkets. To make them lower in fat, fillers such as oat flour, oat bran and carrageenan seaweed are added. Similar products have been used by some fast food restaurants to make their hamburgers lower in fat. One such product using carrageenan as a filler is McDonald's McLean Deluxe. Most products using these types of fillers are still in the range of 42% fat by calories, compared with 52% fat or higher in the leanest types of ground beef commonly available. Healthy Choice Extra Lean Low Fat Ground Beef is, however, an exception. Using an oat flour based filler, Healthy Choice managed to decrease the fat drastically with only 28% of its calories coming from fat. Available in one and two pound packages, it is available in the fresh or frozen section of your supermarket. Since competition in this market is fierce, keep your eyes open for new contenders. For now, using Healthy Choice or having top round or eye of round ground for you by the butcher are your best bets.

◆ PROPORTION OF FAT IN SELECTED CUTS OF MEAT, POULTRY AND FISH
All meats are trimmed and skinless

Beef Cut	Percent Fat
Top Round (Choice)	25%
Eye of Round (Choice)	29%
Shank, Crosscut (Choice)	26%
Round Tip (Select)	28%
Top Sirloin (Select)	28%
Top Loin Steak (Select)	36%
Chuck Arm Pot Roast (Select)	29%
Tenderloin (Select)	42%
Porterhouse Steak (Choice)	45%
Rib Eye Steak (Choice)	47%
Ground Chuck	57%
Ground (Extra-Lean)	58%
Ground (Lean)	63%
Ground (Regular)	66%
Corned Beef Brisket	68%

Poultry Type	Percent Fat
Turkey Breast	19%
Chicken Breast	20%
Turkey Leg	35%
Chicken Leg	40%
Ground Turkey	45%
Chicken Thigh	50%
Chicken McNuggets	50%
Ground Chicken	55%
Turkey Sausage	69%
Turkey Bologna	72%

Seafood Type	Percent Fat
Lobster	5%
Scallops	7%
Cod	7%
Shrimp	10%
Clams	12%
Crab	16%
Tuna, White	16%
Halibut	19%
Swordfish	30%
Salmon, Chum	35%

Chicken, turkey, and fish are, generally speaking, good low-fat alternatives to beef. Certain poultry parts are high in fat, however, and should be avoided (see table). Ground chicken and turkey are often made by grinding the higher fat parts and can contain up to 55% fat. Ground skinless turkey breast, however, is an excellent choice.

As a note, when shopping or eating out remember that the way poultry and fish are prepared is extremely important in determining their fat content. Fried or breaded chicken or fish including Chicken McNuggets and many frozen dinner products are very high in fat and should be avoided. Furthermore, self-basting turkeys are often injected with oils which increase their fat content.

The Delicatessen. Choosing meats at the deli counter can pose other problems. To be certain that your choices are low-fat, have the clerk read you the specific nutrition information from the label. Don't assume that products made from chicken or turkey are low-fat. There is considerable variation from brand to brand since some products are basted or injected with fat during their preparation. For example, turkey breast is about 20% fat, but most prepared turkey breast sold at the deli is 28-32% fat. Products such as turkey ham can be as high as 50% fat, which is considerably higher than lower fat pork hams which are often as low as 32% fat. One of the lower fat turkey hams is Louis Rich which is also 32% fat. Healthy Choice's new line of deli meats are much lower in fat. Their hams are 25% fat while their turkey and chicken breast range between 4% to 17% fat. They even introduced a roast beef that contains only 22% fat by calories.

The Sandwich Meat Case. Prepackaged deli meats usually have nutrition information on the package, but in an effort to appear low-fat they may make the serving size small enough to have less than one gram of fat. For example, Butterball Fresh Deli Turkey Ham is "10 calories and less than one gram of fat per serving." It's impossible to tell how much less than one gram of fat is in each serving. Since one gram of fat has nine calories, this product could be as high as 80-90% fat.

Although unavailable to be included in the Shopping Guide, Healthy Choice offers a new line of low-fat luncheon meats which contain less than 30% calories from fat. These packaged meats along with some listed in the Shopping Guide would be good choices.

The Cheese Section. Most regular cheeses are up to 70-80% fat. Since it's difficult to conserve cheese flavor while reducing the fat below 30%, many of the good, lower fat cheeses don't qualify as truly low-fat. Several lower fat cheeses ranging from 40-60% fat have a very good flavor and, used in moderation, can be a good addition to your meals. A new product called Kaukauna Lite 50 is the first cheese available made with Simplesse, a fat substitute made from whey protein concentrate designed to cut the fat but provide the creamy, high-fat taste.

The Cereal Section. Most packaged cereals are low in fat and were included in our list. To make the healthiest choice you may want to follow a few more hints pertaining to cereals. Try to buy a cereal containing at least 2 grams of fiber and 6 grams or less of simple sugar per serving. For cereals containing fruit, 14 grams or less of simple sugar per serving is acceptable.

The Bread Section. While most breads are low-fat, some may not be exactly what you expect. If you have been buying wheat bread to get the whole grain goodness of whole wheat, you may be surprised to learn that the words "wheat flour" can mean any type of flour made from wheat. Be sure the ingredient list specifically says that the type of flour is "whole wheat," "100% whole wheat," "stone-ground wheat," or "cracked wheat." The words "wheat flour", "enriched flour" or "unbleached flour" generally mean "white flour." If possible, compare the actual fiber content between brands to make sure each slice has at least 2 grams of fiber.

The Shopping Guide. The following low-fat shopping list has been designed to help you find lower fat foods. Only those foods containing less than 30% fat by calories have been included. Nutrition information has also been included so comparison between brands can be made with ease. Over 4,000 name brand products and general items such as meats, pastas and dairy products are listed. Categories of food such as unprepared vegetables, fruits, fruit juices, and spices which are commonly known to be fat-free have been eliminated to make the list more manageable. Some related items such as vegetables packaged with sauces have been included since many contain fat. To make the list as easy to use as possible, it has been organized by section the way most grocery stores are laid out.

Your goal should be to have a diet with an overall average of 20 to 30% fat. (Remember that children younger than two should have no fat restriction.) Stick to the lower end of the range if you're interested in losing weight. These guidelines obviously don't totally restrict you from higher fat foods. You do, however, need to be sensible about the types and amounts of higher fat foods you eat or you'll never meet the 30% goal.

Despite the evidence pointing toward a high percentage of calories from fat as a major culprit, the total amount of fat is also important. In addition to eating sensible foods, you must limit yourself to sensible quantities. Avoid the temptation to dilute your fat with carbohydrate to keep the percentage of fat below 30%. For example, a serving of twenty french fries (16 grams of fat, 316 calories, 46% fat) is clearly high in fat. If, in addition to the fries you drink three 12 oz. glasses of Coca-Cola (0 grams of fat, 465 calories, 0% fat,) the total meal (16 grams of fat, 781 calories, 18.4% fat) becomes "low-fat." Obviously, drinking the Coke doesn't really make the fries any less fattening, so don't bother soothing your conscience with this ploy.

While we have made great efforts to contact all manufacturers of nationally distributed food products as well as many regional companies, this list is not exhaustive. New low-fat products are constantly being introduced, particularly with Americans' recent awareness of fat and cholesterol.

Many products list the quantity of fat as less than one (<1) gram of fat per serving. For those products with small serving sizes, this can prevent accurate calculation of the true percentage of fat. Such items which contain no ingredients with significant amounts of fat have been listed with a dash (-) in the %Fat column. All of the listed foods are 30% fat or less as prepared according to the manufacturer's directions. Modifying the preparation can make these foods even lower in fat. Details of how to do this are outlined in the Cooking Chapter.

As discussed in Chapter 2, restricting sodium intake to a sensible level is a good general principle for everyone to follow. To make this easier, we have included the sodium content of foods when possible. This information will be particularly useful to those with high blood pressure or others following a sodium restricted diet for other medical reasons.

Key to Product Tables

S. S.	Serving Size
CAL	Calories
FAT(g)	Fat (grams)
SOD(mg)	Sodium (milligrams)
CHL(mg)	Cholesterol (milligrams)
%FAT	percent of Fat

BAKERY

BAGELS

☞ International	S. S.	CAL	FAT(g)	SOD(mg)	CHL(mg)	%FAT
Bagel, Blueberry	1 bagel	230	1.0	230	0	3.9
Bagel, Cinnamon/Raisin	1/2 bagel	110	<1.0	110	0	<8.2
Bagel, Egg	1 bagel	228	1.0	270	0	3.9
Bagel, Oatbran	1 bagel	145	<1.0	180	0	<6.2
Bagel, Oatmeal/Raisin	1 bagel	220	1.0	220	0	4.1
Bagel, Onion	1 bagel	228	1.0	270	0	3.9
Bagel, Plain	1 bagel	228	1.0	270	0	3.9
Bagel, Sourdough	1 bagel	228	1.0	470	0	3.9
Bialys, Onion	1.5 oz.	110	<1.0	210	0	<8.2
Bialys, Plain	1.5 oz.	110	<1.0	210	0	<8.2
Junior Bagel, All Varieties	1 bagel	84	1.0	83	0	10.7

BREADS

☞ Arnold	S. S.	CAL	FAT(g)	SOD(mg)	CHL(mg)	%FAT
Bread, 1 1/2 Pound Country White	1 slice	100	2.0	200	0	18.0
Bread, 100% Stone Ground Whole Wheat	1 slice	50	<1.0	100	0	<18.0
Bread, Apple Walnut	1 slice	60	1.0	100	0	15.0
Bread, Bakery Light, Country Bran	1 slice	40	<1.0	80	0	<22.5
Bread, Bakery Light, Golden Wheat	1 slice	40	<1.0	90	0	<22.5
Bread, Bakery Light, Italian	1 slice	40	<1.0	90	0	<22.5
Bread, Bakery Light, Oatmeal	1 slice	40	<1.0	100	0	<22.5
Bread, Bakery Light, Rye, Soft	1 slice	40	<1.0	90	0	<22.5
Bread, Bakery Light, White, Premium	1 slice	40	<1.0	90	0	<22.5
Bread, Bakery Soft, Rye, Seeded	1 slice	70	1.0	160	0	12.9
Bread, Bakery Soft, Rye, Unseeded	1 slice	70	1.0	160	0	12.9
Bread, Bran'nola, Country Oat	1 slice	90	2.0	170	0	20.0
Bread, Bran'nola, Dark Wheat	1 slice	80	1.0	170	0	11.3
Bread, Bran'nola, Hearty Wheat	1 slice	90	2.0	200	0	20.0
Bread, Bran'nola, Nutty Grains	1 slice	90	2.0	140	0	20.0

BAKERY

☞ **Arnold**	S. S.	CAL	FAT(g)	SOD(mg)	CHL(mg)	%FAT
Bread, Bran'nola, Original	1 slice	80	1.0	135	0	11.3
Bread, Brick Oven, Wheat	1 slice	60	2.0	105	0	30.0
Bread, Brick Oven, Wheat, Light	1 slice	40	<1.0	80	0	<22.5
Bread, Brick Oven, White	1 slice	60	1.0	135	0	15.0
Bread, Brick Oven, White, Extra Fiber	1 slice	50	<1.0	90	0	<18.0
Bread, Brick Oven, White, Light	1 slice	40	<1.0	95	0	<22.5
Bread, Honey Wheat Berry	1 slice	80	1.0	140	0	11.3
Bread, Jewish Rye, Seeded	1 slice	70	<1.0	150	0	<12.9
Bread, Jewish Rye, Thin	1 slice	40	<1.0	95	0	<22.5
Bread, Jewish Rye, Unseeded	1 slice	70	<1.0	150	0	<12.9
Bread, Natural 12 Grain	1 slice	60	1.0	100	0	15.0
Bread, Natural Wheat	1 slice	80	1.0	180	0	11.3
Bread, Oatmeal	1 slice	60	1.0	95	0	15.0
Bread, Oatmeal Raisin	1 slice	60	<1.0	90	0	<15.0
Bread, Pumpernickel	1 slice	70	<1.0	160	0	<12.9
Bread, Raisin Cinnamon	1 slice	70	1.0	85	0	12.9
Bread, Rye, Dill	1 slice	70	1.0	160	0	12.9

☞ **Beefsteak**	S. S.	CAL	FAT(g)	SOD(mg)	CHL(mg)	%FAT
Bread, Rye, Hearty	1 slice	60	1.0	170	0	15.0
Bread, Rye, Mild	1 slice	70	1.0	180	0	12.9
Bread, Rye, Onion	1 slice	60	1.0	170	0	15.0
Bread, Rye, Soft	1 slice	60	1.0	170	0	15.0
Bread, Wheat, Hearty	1 slice	70	1.0	160	0	12.9
Bread, White, Robust	1 slice	70	1.0	140	0	12.9

☞ **Bread du Jour**	S. S.	CAL	FAT(g)	SOD(mg)	CHL(mg)	%FAT
Bread, Australian Wheat	1 slice	70	1.0	140	0	12.9
Bread, French	1 slice	70	1.0	150	0	12.9
Bread, French, Petite Loaves	1 loaf	230	2.0	540	0	7.8

☞ Colonial	S. S.	CAL	FAT(g)	SOD(mg)	CHL(mg)	%FAT
Bread, Oat Bran, Light	0.75 oz.	40	<1.0	100	0	<22.5
Bread, Wheat Berry, Light	0.75 oz.	40	<1.0	100	0	<22.5
Bread, Wheat, Light	0.75 oz.	40	<1.0	110	0	<22.5
Bread, White, Light	0.75 oz.	40	<1.0	110	0	<22.5

☞ Country Hearth	S. S.	CAL	FAT(g)	SOD(mg)	CHL(mg)	%FAT
Bread, 7 Whole Grain	1 slice	80	1.0	190	0	11.3
Bread, Bran 'N Honey	1 slice	70	1.0	160	0	12.9
Bread, Buttermilk, Old Fashioned	1 slice	70	1.0	190	0	12.9
Bread, D'Italia	1 slice	70	1.0	200	0	12.9
Bread, Deli Rye	1 slice	70	1.0	160	0	12.9
Bread, European Butter Sesame	1 slice	70	1.0	190	0	12.9
Bread, Grainola	1 slice	70	1.0	240	0	12.9
Bread, Honey & Oat	1 slice	70	1.0	180	0	12.9
Bread, Nature's Wheat	1 slice	70	1.0	160	0	12.9
Bread, Wheat Berry	1 slice	70	1.0	160	0	12.9
Bread, Wheat, Butter Split Top	1 slice	70	1.0	160	0	12.9
Bread, Wheat, Sandwich	1 slice	70	1.0	150	0	12.9
Bread, White, Butter Split Top	1 slice	70	1.0	160	0	12.9
Bread, White, Old Fashioned	1 slice	70	1.0	160	0	12.9
Bread, Whole Wheat, 100% Stone Ground	1 slice	70	1.0	160	0	12.9

☞ Dicarlo's	S. S.	CAL	FAT(g)	SOD(mg)	CHL(mg)	%FAT
Bread, French, Parisian	1 slice	70	1.0	170	0	12.9

BAKERY

☞ Earth Grains	S. S.	CAL	FAT(g)	SOD(mg)	CHL(mg)	%FAT
Bread, 100% Whole Wheat	1 oz.	70	1.0	<170	o	12.9
Bread, Cinnamon Swirl	1 oz.	80	2.0	150	0	22.5
Bread, Cracked Wheat	1 oz.	70	1.0	180	0	12.9
Bread, French	1 oz.	70	1.0	<200	0	12.9
Bread, French, International Hearth	1 oz.	70	1.0	180	0	12.9
Bread, French, Sourdough	1 oz.	70	1.0	<140	0	12.9
Bread, Gold'N Bran	1 oz.	70	1.0	150	0	12.9
Bread, Honey Oat and Nut	1 oz.	80	2.0	85	0	22.5
Bread, Honey Oat Berry	1 oz.	70	1.0	135	0	12.9
Bread, Honey Oat Bran	1 oz.	80	1.0	105	0	11.3
Bread, Honey Wheat Berry	1 oz.	70	1.0	160	0	12.9
Bread, Multi Grain	1 olz.	70	1.0	140	0	12.9
Bread, Onion & Garlic	1 oz.	70	1.0	140	0	12.9
Bread, Raisin Cinnamon	1 oz.	80	2.0	105	0	22.5
Bread, Rye, Dill	1 oz.	80	1.0	190	0	11.3
Bread, Rye, Extra Sour	1 oz.	70	1.0	200	0	12.9
Bread, Rye, Light	1 oz.	70	1.0	240	0	12.9
Bread, Rye, Light, Very Thin	1 oz.	70	1.0	230	0	12.9
Bread, Rye, Party	1 oz.	70	1.0	230	0	12.9
Bread, Rye, Pumpernickel	1 oz.	70	1.0	220	0	12.9
Bread, Sandwich, Salt Free	1 oz.	80	1.0	20	0	11.3
Bread, Sourdough, Light	0.75 oz.	40	1.0	115	0	22.5
Bread, Wheat Sandwich	1 oz.	70	1.0	150	0	12.9
Bread, Wheat, Lite 35	1.25 oz.	70	<1.0	170	0	<12.9
Bread, Wheat, Very Thin	1 oz.	70	1.0	150	0	12.9
Bread, White Sandwich	1 oz.	80	1.0	170	0	11.3
Bread, White, Lite 35	1.25 oz.	70	<1.0	190	0	<12.9
Bread, White, Very Thin	1 oz.	80	1.0	160	0	11.3
Mini Loaf, Country White	1 oz.	70	1.0	150	0	12.9
Mini Loaf, Cracked Wheat	1 oz.	70	1.0	170	0	12.9
Mini Loaf, Sourdough	1 oz.	80	1.0	210	0	11.3

☞ Freihofer's

	S.S.	CAL	FAT(g)	SOD(mg)	CHL(mg)	%FAT
Bread, 1886	1 slice	60	1.0	120	0	15.0
Bread, Cracked Wheat & Honey	1 slice	100	2.0	240	0	18.0
Bread, Italian	1 slice	70	1.0	135	0	12.9
Bread, Light Italian	1 slice	40	<1.0	115	0	<22.5
Bread, Light Oat	1 slice	40	<1.0	115	0	<22.5
Bread, Light Soft Rye	1 slice	40	<1.0	115	0	<22.5
Bread, Light Wheat	1 slice	40	<1.0	115	0	<22.5
Bread, Light White	1 slice	40	<1.0	115	0	<22.5
Bread, Low Sodium	1 slice	60	1.0	5	0	15.0
Bread, Oat Bran & Nut	1 slice	120	3.0	240	0	22.5
Bread, Old Fashion	1 slice	80	1.0	160	0	11.3
Bread, Pumpernickel	1 slice	60	0.0	200	0	0.0
Bread, Soft Rye (Seeded or Unseeded)	1 slice	70	1.0	170	0	12.9
Bread, Twelve Grain	1 slice	120	3.0	240	0	22.5
Bread, Wheat	1 slice	70	1.0	140	0	12.9
Bread, Wheat, 100% Whole	1 slice	100	2.0	240	0	18.0
Bread, Wheat, Hearty	1 slice	70	1.0	140	0	12.9
Bread, Wheat, Split Top	1 slice	70	1.0	150	0	12.9
Bread, White	1 slice	70	1.0	160	0	12.9
Bread, White, Buttercrust	1 slice	80	1.0	150	5	11.3
Bread, White, Country	1 slice	90	1.0	250	0	10.0
Bread, White, Hearty	1 slice	80	1.0	160	0	11.3
Bread, White, Sandwich	1 slice	70	1.0	140	0	12.9

☞ Fresh & Natural

	S.S.	CAL	FAT(g)	SOD(mg)	CHL(mg)	%FAT
Bread, Wheat	1 slice	70	1.0	130	0	12.9

☞ Grant's Farm

	S.S.	CAL	FAT(g)	SOD(mg)	CHL(mg)	%FAT
Bread, 100% Whole Wheat	1 oz.	70	1.0	160	0	12.9
Bread, 7-Grain, Light	0.75 oz.	40	<1.0	115	0	<22.5
Bread, Buttermilk	1 oz.	80	1.0	190	0	11.3

BAKERY

☞ Grant's Farm	S. S.	CAL	FAT(g)	SOD(mg)	CHL(mg)	%FAT
Bread, Honey Cracked Rye	1 oz.	70	1.0	190	0	12.9
Bread, Honey Grain	1 oz.	70	1.0	170	0	12.9
Bread, Honey Wheat Bran	1 oz.	70	1.0	120	0	12.9
Bread, Oat Bran	1 oz.	70	1.0	140	0	12.9
Bread, Oatmeal & Toasted Almond	1 oz.	80	2.0	135	0	22.5
Bread, Seven Grain	1 oz.	70	1.0	140	0	12.9
Bread, Wheat Berry	1 oz.	70	1.0	150	0	12.9
Bread, Wheat, Light	0.75 oz.	40	<1.0	115	0	<22.5
Bread, Wheat, Stone Ground	1 oz.	70	1.0	150	0	12.9
Bread, White, Light	0.75 oz.	40	<1.0	115	0	<22.5

☞ Home Pride	S. S.	CAL	FAT(g)	SOD(mg)	CHL(mg)	%FAT
Bread, Buttertop, Honey, Wheat	1 slice	100	2.0	210	<5	18.0
Bread, Buttertop, Seven Grain	1 slice	70	1.0	135	<5	12.9
Bread, Buttertop, Wheat	1 slice	70	1.0	170	<5	12.9
Bread, Buttertop, White	1 slice	70	1.0	170	<5	12.9
Bread, Light, Wheat	1 slice	40	<1.0	115	<5	<22.5
Bread, Light, White	1 slice	40	<1.0	115	<5	<22.5

☞ Kilpatrick's	S. S.	CAL	FAT(g)	SOD(mg)	CHL(mg)	%FAT
Bread, Oat Bran, Light	0.75 oz.	40	<1.0	100	0	<22.5
Bread, Wheat Berry, Light	0.75 oz.	40	<1.0	100	0	<22.5
Bread, Wheat, Light	0.75 oz.	40	<1.0	110	0	<22.5
Bread, White, Light	0.75 oz.	40	<1.0	110	0	<22.5

☞ Mrs. Baird's	S. S.	CAL	FAT(g)	SOD(mg)	CHL(mg)	%FAT
Bread, Buttered Split Top, Wheat	1 slice	80	1.0	140	0	11.3
Bread, Buttered Split Top, White	1 slice	70	2.0	140	0	25.7
Bread, Buttermilk	1 slice	75	1.0	140	0	12.0

☞ **Mrs. Baird's**	S. S.	CAL	FAT(g)	SOD(mg)	CHL(mg)	%FAT
Bread, Buttermilk, Wheat	1 slice	80	1.0	140	0	11.3
Bread, Enriched	1 slice	70	1.0	140	0	12.9
Bread, Enriched, Extra Thin	1 slice	70	1.0	140	0	12.9
Bread, Honey-n-Wheat	1 slice	60	1.0	120	0	15.0
Bread, Less Dark 'n Grainy	1 slice	40	<1.0	90	0	<22.5
Bread, Less Light, Wheat	1 slice	40	<1.0	90	0	<22.5
Bread, Light, Wheat	1 slice	40	<1.0	110	0	<22.5
Bread, Light, White	1 slice	40	<1.0	110	0	<22.5
Bread, Raisin Cinnamon Wheat	1 slice	70	1.0	90	0	12.9
Bread, Wheat, Extra Thin	1 slice	70	1.0	140	0	12.9
Bread, Wheat, Small	1 slice	70	1.0	140	0	12.9

☞ **Nissen**	S. S.	CAL	FAT(g)	SOD(mg)	CHL(mg)	%FAT
Bread, 'Taliano	1 slice	80	1.0	125	0	11.3
Bread, 100% Stone Grond Whole Wheat	1 slice	90	2.0	160	0	20.0
Bread, Canadian Brown Premium	1 slice	80	2.0	160	<5	22.5
Bread, Canadian White Premium	1 slice	90	2.0	190	0	22.5
Bread, Italian, Light	1 slice	40	<1.0	95	0	<22.5
Bread, Oatbran Premium with Hazelnuts	1 slice	70	<1.0	125	0	<12.9
Bread, Oatmeal Premium	1 slice	70	2.0	110	0	25.7
Bread, Oatmeal, Buttertop	1 slice	70	2.0	115	<5	25.7
Bread, Oatmeal, Light	1 slice	40	<1.0	75	0	<22.5
Bread, Raisin Premium	1 slice	60	1.0	70	0	15.0
Bread, Rye, Light	1 slice	70	1.0	160	<5	12.9
Bread, Rye, Pumpernickel	1 slice	70	1.0	170	<5	12.9
Bread, Rye, Russian Black	1 slice	70	1.0	180	<5	12.9
Bread, Rye, Soft	1 slice	70	1.0	170	<5	12.9
Bread, Sourdough Italian	1 slice	60	<1.0	210	0	<15.0
Bread, Vienna Premium	1 slice	60	<1.0	140	0	<15.0
Bread, Wheat, Buttertop	1 slice	60	1.0	95	<5	15.0
Bread, Wheat, Light	1 slice	40	<1.0	75	0	<22.5
Bread, White, Buttertop	1 slice	60	1.0	135	<5	15.0
Bread, White, Light	1 slice	40	<1.0	85	0	<22.5

BAKERY

☞ **Nissen**	S. S.	CAL	FAT(g)	SOD(mg)	CHL(mg)	%FAT
Bread, White, New England King	1 slice	70	<1.0	150	0	<12.9

☞ **Oatmeal Goodness**	S. S.	CAL	FAT(g)	SOD(mg)	CHL(mg)	%FAT
Bread, Light, Bran	1 slice	40	<1.0	95	0	<22.5
Bread, Light, Wheat	1 slice	40	<1.0	90	0	<22.5
Bread, Oatmeal/Bran	1 slice	80	1.0	150	0	11.3
Bread, Oatmeal/Sunflower Seeds	1 slice	80	1.0	150	0	11.3
Bread, Oatmeal/Wheat	1 slice	80	1.0	150	0	11.3

☞ **Oroweat**	S. S.	CAL	FAT(g)	SOD(mg)	CHL(mg)	%FAT
Bread, 100% Whole Wheat	1 slice	60	1.0	120	0	15.0
Bread, Black, Slim-Siced	1 slice	70	1.0	135	0	12.9
Bread, Bran'nola, Country Oat	2 slices	230	4.0	390	0	15.7
Bread, Bran'nola, Dark Wheat	1 slice	90	2.0	190	0	20.0
Bread, Original	1 slice	100	1.0	160	0	9.0
Bread, English Muffin Toasting	1slice	80	1.0	135	-	11.3
Bread, Grain	1 slice	110	2.0	210	0	16.4
Bread, Health Nut	1 slice	110	2.0	200	0	16.4
Bread, Honey Oat Berry	1 slice	100	1.0	125	0	9.0
Bread, Honey Wheat Berry	1 slice	90	1.0	180	0	10.0
Bread, Light, 9 Grain	1 slice	40	0.0	140	0	0.0
Bread, Light, 100% Whole Wheat	1 slice	40	0.0	140	0	0.0
Bread, Light, Country Oat	1 slice	40	0.0	140	0	0.0
Bread, Light, Hearty Rye	1 slice	40	0.0	140	0	0.0
Bread, Light, Old Fashioned White	1 slice	40	0.0	140	0	0.0
Bread, Oatmeal	1 slice	70	1.0	110	0	12.9
Bread, Oatnut	1 slice	100	2.0	200	0	18.0
Bread, Raisin and Cinnamon	1 slice	80	1.0	110	-	11.3
Bread, Raisin Walnut	1 slice	90	2.0	90	-	20.0
Bread, Royal Raisin Walnut	1 slice	90	2.0	90	-	20.0
Bread, Rye, Whole, Slim-Sliced	1 slice	70	1.0	135	0	12.9
Bread, Sourdough , Light	1 slice	40	0.0	115	0	0.0

☞ **Oroweat**	**S. S.**	**CAL**	**FAT(g)**	**SOD(mg)**	**CHL(mg)**	**%FAT**
Bread, Stone Ground 100% Whole Wheat	1 slice	60	1.0	125	0	15.0
Bread, Wheat, Thin Sliced	1 slice	50	1.0	90	0	18.0
Bread, White, Old Fashioned	1 slice	70	1.0	125	-	12.9
Bread, White, Thin Sliced	1 slice	50	1.0	90	0	18.0

☞ **Pepperidge Farm**	**S. S.**	**CAL**	**FAT(g)**	**SOD(mg)**	**CHL(mg)**	**%FAT**
Bread, Brown & Serve Italian	1 oz.	80	1.0	150	0	11.3
Bread, Cinnamon Swirl	1 slice	90	3.0	110	0	30.0
Bread, Cinnamon Swirl with Raisins	1 slice	90	2.0	100	0	20.0
Bread, Country White	2 slices	190	2.0	340	0	9.5
Bread, Cracked Wheat	1 slice	70	1.0	140	0	12.9
Bread, Crunchy Oat, 1 1/2 lb.	2 slices	190	4.0	290	0	18.9
Bread, Dijon Rye	1 slice	50	1.0	170	0	18.0
Bread, Family Pumpernickel	1 slice	80	1.0	230	0	11.3
Bread, Family Rye	1 slice	80	1.0	220	0	11.3
Bread, Family Rye, Seedless	1 slice	80	1.0	210	0	11.3
Bread, French Style	2 oz.	150	2.0	230	0	12.0
Bread, Hearty Sliced-7 Grain	2 slices	180	2.0	340	0	10.0
Bread, Honey Bran	1 slice	90	1.0	160	0	10.0
Bread, Italian	1 slice	70	1.0	125	0	12.9
Bread, Light Style Oatmeal	1 slice	45	0	95	0	0
Bread, Light Style Wheat	1 slice	45	0.0	90	0	0.0
Bread, Light Vienna	1 slice	45	0.0	100	0	0.0
Bread, Oatmeal	1 slice	70	1.0	160	0	12.9
Bread, Oatmeal, 1 1/2 lb.	1 slice	90	1.0	200	0	10.0
Bread, Oatmeal, Very Thin Sliced	1 slice	40	1.0	80	0	22.5
Bread, Sesame Wheat	2 slices	190	3.0	340	0	14.2
Bread, Soft Rye	1 slice	70	1.0	120	0	12.9
Bread, Sprouted Wheat	1 slice	70	2.0	100	0	25.7
Bread, Twin French	1 oz.	80	1.0	160	0	11.3
Bread, Vienna Thick Sliced	1 slice	70	1.0	125	0	12.9
Bread, Wheat, 1 1/2 lb.	1 slice	90	2.0	190	0	20.0
Bread, Wheat, Very Thin Sliced	1 slice	35	0.0	75	0	0.0

BAKERY

☞ Pepperidge Farm	S. S.	CAL	FAT(g)	SOD(mg)	CHL(mg)	%FAT
Bread, White, Sandwich	2 slices	130	2.0	260	0	13.8
Bread, White, Thin Sliced	1 slice	80	2.0	130	0	22.5
Bread, White, Toasting, White	1 slice	90	1.0	200	0	10.0
Bread, White, Very Thin Sliced	1 slice	40	0.0	80	0	0.0
Bread, Whole Wheat, Thin Sliced	1 slice	60	1.0	110	0	15.0
Party Pumpernickel Slices	4 slices	60	1.0	160	0	15.0
Party Rye Slices	4 slices	60	1.0	250	0	15.0

☞ Rainbo	S. S.	CAL	FAT(g)	SOD(mg)	CHL(mg)	%FAT
Bread, Country Meal	1 oz.	80	1.0	135	0	11.3
Bread, Honey Grain	1 oz.	70	1.0	170	0	12.9
Bread, Honey Grain, Family Recipe	1 oz.	70	1.0	180	0	12.9
Bread, IronKids	1 oz.	60	1.0	140	0	15.0
Bread, Oat Bran, Light	0.75 oz.	40	<1.0	100	0	<22.5
Bread, Oat, Family Recipe Split Top	1 oz.	70	1.0	140	0	12.9
Bread, Stone Ground, Family Recipe	1 oz.	70	1.0	110	0	12.9
Bread, Wheat	1 oz.	70	1.0	150	0	12.9
Bread, Wheat Berry, Light	0.75 oz.	40	<1.0	100	0	<22.5
Bread, Wheat, Family Recipe Honey Buttered Split Top	1 oz.	70	1.0	150	0	12.9
Bread, Wheat, Light	0.75 0z.	40	<1.0	110	0	<22.5
Bread, Wheat, Sandwich, Family Recipe	1 oz.	70	1.0	150	0	12.9
Bread, White, Enriched	1 oz.	70	1.0	140	0	12.9
Bread, White, Family Recipe Honey Buttered Split Top	1 oz.	80	1.0	150	0	11.3
Bread, White, Light	0.75 oz.	40	<1.0	110	0	<22.5
Bread, Whole Wheat	1 oz.	70	1.0	140	0	12.9

☞ Sunbeam	S. S.	CAL	FAT(g)	SOD(mg)	CHL(mg)	%FAT
Bread, Lite, Italian	1 slice	40	<1.0	100	0	<22.5
Bread, Lite, Wheat	1 slice	40	<1.0	100	0	<22.5
Bread, Lite, White	1 slice	40	<1.0	100	0	<22.5

☞Wonder	S. S.	CAL	FAT(g)	SOD(mg)	CHL(mg)	%FAT
Bread, 100% Whole Wheat	1 slice	60	1.0	130	0	15.0
Bread, 100% Whole Wheat, Soft	1 slice	60	1.0	130	0	15.0
Bread, 100% Whole Wheat, Stone Ground	1 slice	80	1.0	160	0	11.3
Bread, Cinnamon Raisin	1 slice	60	1.0	95	0	15.0
Bread, Cracked Wheat	1 slice	70	1.0	180	0	12.9
Bread, Family, Wheat	1 slice	70	1.0	150	0	12.9
Bread, French	1 slice	70	1.0	150	0	12.9
Bread, Golden/Country Style, Wheat	1 slice	70	1.0	160	0	12.9
Bread, Italian, Family	1 slice	70	1.0	170	0	12.9
Bread, Italian, Light	1 slice	40	0.0	115	0	0.0
Bread, Light, Wheat	1 slice	40	0.0	115	0	0.0
Bread, Light, White	1 slice	40	0.0	115	0	0.0
Bread, Sourdough, Light	1 slice	40	0.0	115	0	0.0
Bread, White	1 slice	70	1.0	150	0	12.9
Bread, with Buttermilk, White	1 slice	70	1.0	150	0	12.9

BREAD SHELLS

☞Boboli	S. S.	CAL	FAT(g)	SOD(mg)	CHL(mg)	%FAT
Italian Bread Shells	6" shell	300	7.0	620	5	21.0

BREADSTICKS

☞Angonoa's	S. S.	CAL	FAT(g)	SOD(mg)	CHL(mg)	%FAT
Breadsticks, Cheese	1 oz.	110	2.0	210	0	16.4
Breadsticks, Garlic	1 oz.	120	2.0	160	0	15.0
Breadsticks, Italian	1 oz.	120	2.0	240	0	15.0
Breadsticks, Low Sodium	1 oz.	120	4.0	15	0	30.0
Breadsticks, Onion	1 oz.	120	3.0	150	0	22.5
Breadsticks, Sesame Royale	1 oz.	120	4.0	200	0	30.0
Mini Breadsticks, Cheese	1 oz	110	2.0	160	0	16.4
Mini Breadsticks, Pizza	1 oz.	120	2.0	220	0	15.0
Mini Breadsticks, Sesame	1 oz.	120	4.0	200	0	30.0

BAKERY

☞Angonoa's	S. S.	CAL	FAT(g)	SOD(mg)	CHL(mg)	%FAT
Mini Breadsticks, Whole Wheat	1 oz.	120	4.0	170	0	30.0

☞Barbara's Bakery	S. S.	CAL	FAT(g)	SOD(mg)	CHL(mg)	%FAT
Bread Sticks, Italian Style	1 oz.	120	3.0	-	0	22.5
Bread Sticks, Regular	1 oz.	120	3.0	-	0	22.5
Sesame Sticks	1 oz.	130	4.0	-	-	27.7

☞Fattorie & Pandea	S. S.	CAL	FAT(g)	SOD(mg)	CHL(mg)	%FAT
Breadsticks, Sesame Seeds	3 sticks	65	2.0	100	-	27.7
Breadsticks, Traditional	3 sticks	60	1.0	100	-	15.0
Breadsticks, Whole Wheat	3 sticks	57	1.0	100	-	15.8

☞International	S. S.	CAL	FAT(g)	SOD(mg)	CHL(mg)	%FAT
Bialys Bread Sticks, All Varieties	1 stick	110	<1.0	210	0	<8.2

☞Oroweat	S. S.	CAL	FAT(g)	SOD(mg)	CHL(mg)	%FAT
Breadsticks, Plain	1 oz.	110	1.0	240	-	8.2
Breadsticks, Sesame	1 oz.	120	3.0	180	-	22.5

☞Stella D'Oro	S. S.	CAL	FAT(g)	SOD(mg)	CHL(mg)	%FAT
Breadsticks, Onion	1 stick	40	1.0	-	0	22.5
Breadsticks, Pizza	1 stick	45	1.0	-	0	20.0
Breadsticks, Regular	1 stick	40	1.0	55	0	22.5
Breadsticks, Sesame	1 stick	50	2.0	43	0	36.0
Breadsticks, Wheat	1 stick	40	1.0	-	0	22.5

BUNS/ROLLS

☞ **Arnold**	S. S.	CAL	FAT(g)	SOD(mg)	CHL(mg)	%FAT
Buns, Bran'nola Natural	1 bun	100	<1.0	160	0	<9.0
Buns, Hamburger	1 bun	120	2.0	220	0	15.0
Buns, Hot Dog	1 bun	110	2.0	180	0	16.4
Buns, Sandwich, Dutch Egg	1 bun	120	3.0	200	0	22.5
Rolls, Bakery Light	1 roll	80	<1.0	190	0	<11.3
Rolls, Dinner Party	1 roll	50	1.0	80	0	18.0
Rolls, Sandwich, Soft	1 roll	110	2.0	190	0	16.4

☞ **Bread du Jour**	S. S.	CAL	FAT(g)	SOD(mg)	CHL(mg)	%FAT
Rolls, Bavarian Wheat	1 roll	80	1.0	180	0	11.3
Rolls, Crusty Italian	1 roll	80	1.0	190	0	11.3

☞ **Dicarlo's**	S. S.	CAL	FAT(g)	SOD(mg)	CHL(mg)	%FAT
Rolls, French	1 roll	180	2.0	390	0	10.0
Rolls, Sourdough	1 roll	200	2.0	310	0	9.0

☞ **Earth Grains**	S. S.	CAL	FAT(g)	SOD(mg)	CHL(mg)	%FAT
Rolls, French	1 roll	100	1.0	270	0	9.0
Rolls, French, Sourdough	1 roll	100	1.0	160	0	9.0
Rolls, Kaiser	1 roll	190	2.0	520	0	9.5
Rolls, Onion	1 roll	490	2.0	53	0	3.7
Rolls, Submarine	1 roll	180	1.0	500	0	5.0
Rolls, Wheat	1 roll	110	1.0	260	0	8.2

☞ **Freihofer's**	S. S.	CAL	FAT(g)	SOD(mg)	CHL(mg)	%FAT
Buns, Hamburg	1 roll	110	2.0	280	0	16.4

BAKERY

☞ Freihofer's

	S. S.	CAL	FAT(g)	SOD(mg)	CHL(mg)	%FAT
Buns, Hot Dog	1 roll	90	1.0	200	0	10.0
Buns, New England Franks	1 roll	120	1.0	240	0	7.5
Rolls, Brown & Serve	1 roll	100	2.0	120	0	18.0
Rolls, Sandwich Mates	1 roll	110	1.0	210	0	8.2

☞ Home Pride

	S. S.	CAL	FAT(g)	SOD(mg)	CHL(mg)	%FAT
Rolls, Dinner, Wheat	1 roll	70	2.0	120	<5	25.7
Rolls, Dinner, White	1 roll	70	2.0	120	<5	25.7

☞ International

	S. S.	CAL	FAT(g)	SOD(mg)	CHL(mg)	%FAT
Bialys, Onion	1.5 oz.	110	<1.0	210	0	<8.2
Bialys, Plain	1.5 oz.	110	<1.0	210	0	<8.2
Rolls, Dinner, Hawaiian	1 roll	85	1.0	125	0	10.6

☞ Mrs. Baird's

	S. S.	CAL	FAT(g)	SOD(mg)	CHL(mg)	%FAT
Buns, Enriched	1 bun	160	4.0	280	0	22.5
Buns, Enriched, with Sesame Seeds	1 bun	160	4.0	280	0	22.5
Buns, Hot Dog, Enriched	1 bun	140	4.0	250	0	25.7
Buns, Wheat	1 bun	160	3.0	320	0	16.9
Rolls, Home Bake, Enriched	1 roll	90	3.0	140	0	30.0

☞ Nissen

	S. S.	CAL	FAT(g)	SOD(mg)	CHL(mg)	%FAT
Buns, Gourmet Sandwich	1 bun	180	4.0	320	0	20.0
Buns, Hamburger	1 bun	100	1.0	170	0	9.0
Buns, Hamburger, Light	1 bun	80	<1.0	190	0	<11.3
Buns, Sandwich	1 bun	140	2.0	240	0	12.9
Rolls, Brown 'N Serve White & Wheat	1 roll	70	1.0	135	0	12.9

☞ Nissen

	S. S.	CAL	FAT(g)	SOD(mg)	CHL(mg)	%FAT
Rolls, Dinner	1 roll	80	2.0	115	0	22.5
Rolls, Frankfurter	1 roll	100	1.0	170	0	9.0
Rolls, Hoagie	1 roll	180	3.0	370	0	15.0
Rolls, Hot Dog	1 roll	100	1.0	170	0	9.0
Rolls, Hot Dog, Light	1 roll	80	<1.0	190	0	<11.3
Rolls, Lanky Franks	1 roll	170	3.0	310	0	15.9
Rolls, New England Frankfurter, Light	1 roll	80	<1.0	190	0	<11.3
Rolls, New England Pan	1 roll	90	1.0	130	0	10.0
Rolls, Oatmeal Pan	1 roll	100	2.0	220	0	18.0

☞ Oroweat

	S. S.	CAL	FAT(g)	SOD(mg)	CHL(mg)	%FAT
Rolls, Health Nut	1 roll	160	3.0	200	0	16.9
Rolls, Honey Wheat Berry	1 roll	150	1.0	310	0	6.0

☞ Pepperidge Farm

	S. S.	CAL	FAT(g)	SOD(mg)	CHL(mg)	%FAT
Dinner Rolls, Country Style Classic	1 roll	50	1.0	90	0	18.0
Dinner Rolls, Enriched	1 roll	60	2.0	95	<5	30.0
Dinner Rolls, Finger Sesame Seeds	1 roll	60	2.0	85	<5	30.0
Dinner Rolls, Parker House	1 roll	60	1.0	80	5	15.0
Dinner Rolls, Party	1 roll	30	1.0	50	0	30.0
Dinner Rolls, Soft Family	1 roll	100	2.0	190	0	18.0
Frankfurter Rolls, Dijon	1 roll	160	5.0	230	0	28.1
Frankfurter Rolls, Top & Side Sliced	1 roll	140	3.0	270	0	19.3
Frankfurter Rolls, with Poppy Seeds	1 roll	130	2.0	280	0	13.8
Hamburger Buns	1 roll	130	2.0	240	0	13.8
Rolls, Brown 'n Serve Club	1 roll	100	1.0	190	0	9.0
Rolls, Brown 'n Serve French	1/2 roll	180	2.0	380	0	10.0
Rolls, Brown 'n Serve Hearth	1 roll	50	1.0	100	0	18.0
Rolls, French Style	1 rol	100	1.0	230	0	9.0
Rolls, Soft Hoagie	1 roll	210	5.0	320	0	21.4
Rolls, Sourdough Style French	1 roll	100	1.0	240	0	9.0

BAKERY

☞ **Pepperidge Farm**	S. S.	CAL	FAT(g)	SOD(mg)	CHL(mg)	%FAT
Sandwich Buns, Onion with Poppy Seeds	1 roll	150	3.0	260	0	18.0
Sandwich Buns, Potato	1 roll	160	4.0	260	0	22.5
Sandwich Buns, with Sesame Seeds	1 roll	140	3.0	230	0	19.3

☞ **Rainbo**	S. S.	CAL	FAT(g)	SOD(mg)	CHL(mg)	%FAT
Buns, Hamburger/Hot Dog	2 oz.	150	2.0	320	0	12.0

☞ **Wonder**	S. S.	CAL	FAT(g)	SOD(mg)	CHL(mg)	%FAT
Buns, Enriched	1 bun	70	1.0	160	0	12.9
Buns, Hamburger, Light	1 bun	80	1.0	210	0	11.3
Buns, Honey Wheat	1 bun	130	2.0	230	0	13.8
Buns, Hot Dog, Light	1 bun	80	1.0	210	0	11.3
Rolls, Bakery Style, Original	1 roll	140	2.0	280	0	12.9
Rolls, Bakery Style, Sourdough	1 roll	150	2.0	300	0	12.0
Rolls, Bakery Style, Wheat	1 roll	150	2.0	300	0	12.0
Rolls, Brown 'n Serve	1 roll	70	1.0	135	0	12.9
Rolls, Brown 'n Serve, with Buttermilk	1 roll	70	1.0	135	0	12.9
Rolls, Pan, Dinner or Biscuit	1 roll	80	1.0	140	0	11.3

CRUMPETS

☞ **Wolferman's**	S. S.	CAL	FAT(g)	SOD(mg)	CHL(mg)	%FAT
English Crumpets, Cinnamon	1.6 oz.	105	1.8	217	0	15.6
English Crumpets, Raspberry	1.6 oz.	95	0.6	263	0	6.1
Crumpets, Buttermilk	1	100	1.0	230	0	9.0
Crumpets, Cinnamon	1	90	1.0	259	0	10.0
Crumpets, Oat Bran	1	80	1.0	182	0	11.3
Crumpets, Original	1	90	0.0	216	0	0.0

MUFFINS

☞ **Arnold**	S. S.	CAL	FAT(g)	SOD(mg)	CHL(mg)	%FAT
Muffins, English, Bran'nola	1 muffin	140	1.0	220	0	6.4
Muffins, English, Extra Crisp	1 muffin	120	1.0	230	0	7.5
Muffins, English, Raisin	1 muffin	150	1.0	220	0	6.0
Muffins, English, Sourdough	1 muffin	120	1.0	250	0	7.5

☞ **Earth Grains**	S. S.	CAL	FAT(g)	SOD(mg)	CHL(mg)	%FAT
English Muffins, Oat Bran	2 oz.	120	1.0	410	0	7.5
English Muffins, Plain or Sourdough	2 oz.	120	1.0	390	0	7.5
English Muffins, Raisin	2.3 oz.	160	2.0	300	0	11.3
English Muffins, Sun Maid Raisin	2.5 oz.	160	1.0	180	0	5.6
English Muffins, Wheat Berry	2.3 oz.	140	1.0	470	0	6.4
English Muffins, Whole Wheat	2.3 oz.	130	1.0	420	0	6.9

☞ **Freihofer's**	S. S.	CAL	FAT(g)	SOD(mg)	CHL(mg)	%FAT
Muffins, English	1 muffin	130	1.0	320	0	6.9

☞ **Mrs. Baird's**	S. S.	CAL	FAT(g)	SOD(mg)	CHL(mg)	%FAT
Muffins, English	1 muffin	130	1.0	260	-	6.9

☞ **Nissen**	S. S.	CAL	FAT(g)	SOD(mg)	CHL(mg)	%FAT
Muffins, Corn	1 muffin	220	6.0	480	<5	24.5
Muffins, English	1 muffin	130	<1.0	220	0	<6.9
Muffins, English, Cinnamon Raisin	1 muffin	130	1.0	250	0	6.9
Muffins, English, Oatbran with Hazelnuts	1 muffin	130	2.0	190	0	13.8
Muffins, Raisin Bran	1 muffin	210	5.0	290	0	21.4

BAKERY

☞ Oatmeal Goodness

	S. S.	CAL	FAT(g)	SOD(mg)	CHL(mg)	%FAT
Muffins, English, Cinnamon Raisin	1 muffin	140	2.0	190	0	12.9
Muffins, English, Honey & Oatmeal	1 muffin	140	2.0	210	0	12.9

☞ Oroweat

	S. S.	CAL	FAT(g)	SOD(mg)	CHL(mg)	%FAT
Muffins, Blueberry	1 muffin	170	1.0	210	1	5.3
Muffins, Extra Crisp	1 muffin	130	1.0	260	-	6.9
Muffins, Health Nut	1 muffin	170	4.0	220	0	21.2
Muffins, Health Nut Raisin	1 muffin	200	4.0	220	0	18.0
Muffins, Oatnut Bran	1 muffin	160	2.0	230	0	11.3
Muffins, Sourdough	1 muffin	140	1.0	370	-	6.4

☞ Pepperidge Farm

	S. S.	CAL	FAT(g)	SOD(mg)	CHL(mg)	%FAT
English Muffins, Cinnamon Apple	1 muffin	140	1.0	210	0	6.4
English Muffins, Cinnamon Chip	1 muffin	160	3.0	180	0	16.9
English Muffins, Cinnamon Raisin	1 muffin	150	2.0	200	0	12.0
English Muffins, Regular	1 muffin	140	1.0	220	0	6.4
English Muffins, Sourdough	1 muffin	135	1.0	260	0	6.7

☞ Rainbo

	S. S.	CAL	FAT(g)	SOD(mg)	CHL(mg)	%FAT
Muffins, English	1 muffin	120	1.0	390	0	7.5

☞ Thomas'

	S. S.	CAL	FAT(g)	SOD(mg)	CHL(mg)	%FAT
Muffins, English, Bran Nut	1 muffin	140	3.0	200	0	19.3
Muffins, English, Honey Wheat	1 muffin	120	1.0	200	0	7.5
Muffins, English, Oat Bran	1 muffin	120	1.0	210	0	7.5
Muffins, English, Raisin	1 muffin	140	1.0	200	0	6.4
Muffins, English, Regular	1 muffin	120	1.0	210	0	7.5

☞Thomas'

	S. S.	CAL	FAT(g)	SOD(mg)	CHL(mg)	%FAT
Muffins, English, Sourdough	1 muffin	130	1.0	220	0	6.9
Toast-R-Cakes, Blueberry	1 cake	100	3.0	170	10	27.0
Toast-R-Cakes, Corn	1 cake	120	4.0	190	10	30.0
Toast-R-Cakes, Raisin	1 cake	100	3.0	180	10	27.0

☞Wolferman's

	S. S.	CAL	FAT(g)	SOD(mg)	CHL(mg)	%FAT
English Muffin, Apple Raisin Cinnamon	1/2 muffin	125	<1.0	223	<1	<7.2
English Muffin, Apple Strudel	1.7 oz.	113	2.1	218	0	16.6
English Muffin, Blueberry	1/2 muffin	110	1.0	208	0	8.2
English Muffin, Cheddar Cheese	1/2 muffin	120	2.0	324	<1	15.0
English Muffin, Cinnamon Raisin	1/2 muffin	110	1.0	229	0	8.2
English Muffin, Corn	1/2 muffin	120	1.0	209	1	7.5
English Muffin, Cranberry	1/2 muffin	120	1.0	219	0	7.5
English Muffin, Egg	1/2 muffin	112	1.0	237	<1	8.0
English Muffin, Garlic	1/2 muffin	110	1.0	240	0	8.2
English Muffin, Honey Bran	1/2 muffin	120	1.0	288	0	7.5
English Muffin, Low Sodium	1/2 muffin	110	1.0	119	0	8.2
English Muffin, Multi Grain	1/2 muffin	120	1.0	266	0	7.5
English Muffin, Oat Bran, Apple & Raisin	1/2 muffin	110	0.0	180	0	0.0
English Muffin, Original	1/2 muffin	110	1.0	249	0	8.2
English Muffin, Parmesan Cheese	1/2 muffin	120	1.0	220	<1	7.5
English Muffin, Raisin Rice	1/2 muffin	110	2.0	240	0	16.4
English Muffin, Sour Cream & Onion	1/2 muffin	120	2.0	234	<1	15.0
English Muffin, Sourdough	1/2 muffin	110	1.0	281	0	8.2
English Muffin, Wheat	1/2 muffin	100	1.0	211	0	9.0
Mini-English Muffin, Blueberry	1 muffin	70	0.0	140	0	0.0
Mini-English Muffin, Cheddar Cheese	1 muffin	80	1.0	223	<1	11.3
Mini-English Muffin, Cinnamon Raisin	1 muffin	80	0.0	154	0	0.0
Mini-English Muffin, Corn	1 muffin	80	1.0	135	<1	11.3
Mini-English Muffin, Oat Bran, Apple & Raisin	1 muffin	70	0.0	114	0	0.0
Mini-English Muffin, Original	1 muffin	75	0.0	170	0	0.0

BAKERY

BAKERY

☞ Wolferman's

	S. S.	CAL	FAT(g)	SOD(mg)	CHL(mg)	%FAT
Mini-English Muffin, Sourdough	1 muffin	75	1.0	203	<1	12.0
Mini-English Muffin, Wheat	1 muffin	75	0.0	142	0	0.0

☞ Wonder

	S. S.	CAL	FAT(g)	SOD(mg)	CHL(mg)	%FAT
Muffins, English	1 muffin	120	1.0	290	0	7.5
Muffins, English, Sourdough	1 muffin	120	1.0	240	0	7.5
Rounds, Raisin	1 round	140	2.0	220	0	12.9

PITAS AND PITA CHIPS

☞ International

	S. S.	CAL	FAT(g)	SOD(mg)	CHL(mg)	%FAT
Deli Farms Pita, Oat Bran	1 pocket	105	1.0	185	0	8.6
Deli Farms Pita, Onion	1 pocket	125	1.0	-	0	7.2
Deli Farms Pita, Plain	1 pocket	145	1.0	-	0	6.2
Deli Farms Pita, Plain, Junior	1 pocket	73	0.5	-	0	6.2
Deli Farms Pita, Plain, Large	1 pocket	232	1.0	-	0	3.9
Deli Farms Pita, Whole Wheat	1 pocket	125	1.0	-	0	7.2
Deli Farms Pita, Whole Wheat, Junior	1 pocket	63	0.5	-	0	7.1
Mr. Pita, Plain	1 pocket	79	<1.0	111	0	<11.4
Mr. Pita, Wheat	1 pocket	63	<1.0	111	0	<14.3

☞ New York Style

	S. S.	CAL	FAT(g)	SOD(mg)	CHL(mg)	%FAT
Pita Chips, Garlic	0.75 oz.	100	3.0	180	0	27.0
Pita Chips, Oat Bran	0.75 oz.	100	3.0	50	0	27.0
Pita Chips, Onion Poppy	0.75 oz.	100	3.0	180	0	27.0
Pita Chips, Plain Low Sodium	0.75 oz.	100	3.0	115	0	27.0
Pita Chips, Sesame	0.75 oz.	100	3.0	180	0	27.0

☞ **Sahara**	S. S.	CAL	FAT(g)	SOD(mg)	CHL(mg)	%FAT
Pita, 100% Whole Wheat	2 oz.	130	1.0	310	0	6.9
Pita, Oat Bran	1 oz.	80	<1.0	160	0	<11.3
Pita, Original Style	1 oz.	80	<1.0	150	0	<11.3

SWEET BAKERY

☞ **Aunt Fanny's**	S. S.	CAL	FAT(g)	SOD(mg)	CHL(mg)	%FAT
Cinnamon Duos	3.75 oz.	340	8.0	1135	-	21.2
Rolls, Caramel Nut	2 oz.	180	3.0	574	-	15.0
Rolls, Cinnamon	2 oz.	181	4.0	607	-	19.9
Rolls, Old Fashioned Apple Cinnamon	2 oz.	178	4.0	-	-	20.2

☞ **Dolly Madison**	S. S.	CAL	FAT(g)	SOD(mg)	CHL(mg)	%FAT
Carrot Cake	1 pkg.	400	10.0	740	-	22.5
Cupcake, Chocolate	1 cake	170	5.0	290	-	26.5
Cake, White Coconut Layer	1 slice	220	7.0	240	-	28.6
Creme Boats	1 cake	160	4.0	190	-	22.5
Creme Boats, Low Fat	1 cake	140	3.0	130	-	19.3
Dessert Cups	1 cake	100	2.0	110	-	18.0
Dessert Roll	1 cake	220	3.0	190	-	12.3
Frosty Angel	1 pkg.	310	9.0	460	-	26.1
Honey 'n Spice	1 pkg.	360	11.0	400	-	27.5
Zingers, Yellow	1 cake	140	4.0	100	-	25.7
Zingers, Creme	1 cake	110	3.0	90	-	24.5
Sweet Rolls, Apple	1 roll	210	5.0	210	-	21.4
Sweet Rolls, Cherry	1 roll	210	5.0	190	-	21.4
Sweet Rolls, Cinnamon	1 roll	210	5.0	210	-	21.4
Sweet Rolls, Cinnamon, Low Fat	1 roll	160	1.0	120	-	5.6
Low Fat Buttercrumb	1 cake	150	2.0	160	-	12.0
Low Fat Cake, Chocolate	1 cake	180	4.0	250	-	20.0
Low Fat Creme Boats	1 cake	140	3.0	130	-	19.3
Low Fat Creme Cakes	1 cake	90	2.0	90	-	20.0
Low Fat Cinnamon Rolls	1 roll	160	1.0	120	-	5.6

BAKERY

BAKERY

☞ **Drake's**	S. S.	CAL	FAT(g)	SOD(mg)	CHL(mg)	%FAT
Coffee Cake, Light & Fruity, Apple	1 cake	90	1.0	110	0	10.0
Coffee Cake, Light & Fruity, Raspberry	1 cake	90	1.0	105	0	10.0
Sunny Doodles	1 cake	100	3.0	100	0	27.0

☞ **Entenmann's Fat Free/Chol. Free**	S. S.	CAL	FAT(g)	SOD(mg)	CHL(mg)	%FAT
Buns, Apple	1 bun	150	0.0	140	0	0.0
Buns, Pineapple Cheese	1 bun	130	0.0	140	0	0.0
Buns, Raspberry Cheese	1 bun	150	0.0	120	0	0.0
Cake, Apple Spice	1 oz.	80	0.0	80	0	0.0
Cake, Banana Crunch	1 oz.	80	0.0	90	0	0.0
Cake, Blueberry Crunch	1 oz.	70	0.0	85	0	0.0
Cake, Chocolate Crunch	1 oz.	70	0.0	130	0	0.0
Cake, Chocolate Loaf	1 oz.	70	0.0	130	0	0.0
Cake, Chocolate, Fudge Iced	1.3 oz.	90	0.0	130	0	0.0
Cake, Cranberry Orange	1 oz.	70	0.0	95	0	0.0
Cake, Gold, Fudge Iced	1.3 oz.	90	0.0	100	0	0.0
Cake, Golden Chocolaty Chip Loaf	1 oz.	80	0.0	85	0	0.0
Cake, Golden French Crumb	1 oz.	70	0.0	80	0	0.0
Cake, Golden Loaf	1 oz.	70	0.0	100	0	0.0
Cake, Louisiana Crunch	1 oz.	80	0.0	100	0	0.0
Cake, Orange	1 oz.	70	0.0	95	0	0.0
Cake, Pineapple Crunch	1 oz.	70	0.0	85	0	0.0
Coffee Cake, Blueberry Cheese	1 oz.	90	0.0	100	0	0.0
Coffee Cake, Cinnamon Apple	1.3 oz.	90	0.0	90	0	0.0
Cookie, Fruit & Honey	2 cookies	80	0.0	110	0	0.0
Cookie, Home Style Apple	2 cookies	70	0.0	125	0	0.0
Cookie, Oatmeal Raisin	2 cookies	80	0.0	120	0	0.0
Cookie, Raisin	2 cookies	70	0.0	100	0	0.0
Loaf, Banana	1.3 oz.	90	0.0	125	0	0.0
Loaf, Marble	1 oz.	70	0.0	115	0	0.0
Loaf, Pineapple Crunch	1.3 oz.	90	0.0	135	0	0.0
Muffin, Blueberry	1 muffin	150	0.0	140	0	0.0
Muffin, Carrot Raisin	1 muffin	140	0.0	115	0	0.0

☞**Entenmann's Fat Free/Chol. Free**	S.S.	CAL	FAT(g)	SOD(mg)	CHL(mg)	%FAT
Muffin, Cinnamon Apple Raisin	1 muffin	160	0.0	140	0	0.0
Pastry Twist, Apple Cinnamon	1.1 oz.	90	0.0	75	0	0.0
Pastry Twist, Apricot	1.1 oz.	90	0.0	80	0	0.0
Pastry Twist, Lemon	1.1 oz.	90	0.0	80	0	0.0
Pastry Twist, Orange	1.1 oz.	90	0.0	70	0	0.0
Pastry Twist, Raspberry	1.1 oz.	90	0.0	75	0	0.0
Pastry, Cheese Filled Crumb	1.2 oz.	90	0.0	95	0	0.0
Pastry, Raspberry Cheese	1.3 oz.	100	0.0	90	0	0.0
Ring, Cinnamon	1 oz.	80	0.0	75	0	0.0
Ring, Holiday	1 oz.	80	0.0	55	0	0.0

☞**Freihofer's**	S.S.	CAL	FAT(g)	SOD(mg)	CHL(mg)	%FAT
Buns, Cinnamon	1 bun	98	0.0	120	0	0.0
Cake, Angel Food	1.25 oz.	90	0.0	290	0	0.0
Cake, Raisin Pound	1 oz.	80	1.0	70	0	11.3
Coffee Ring, Cheese	1.3 oz.	90	1.0	90	0	10.0
Coffee Ring, Cinnamon	1.2 oz.	100	1.0	110	0	9.0
Cookie, Oatmeal Raisin Nut	2 cookies	100	3.0	55	0	30.0
Ring, Cinnamon Apple	1.3 oz.	90	1.0	100	0	10.0
Ring, Raspberry Cheese	1.3 oz.	90	1.0	115	0	10.0
Strip, Apple Raisin	1.3 oz.	90	1.0	80	0	10.0
Strip, Cheese	1.3 oz.	90	1.0	90	0	10.0
Strip, Cherry Cheese	1.3 oz.	90	1.0	80	0	10.0
Strip, Strawberry Cheese	1.3 oz.	90	1.0	80	0	10.0
Twist, Lemon	1.1 oz.	90	1.0	95	0	10.0
Twist, Raspberry	1.1 oz.	100	1.0	80	0	9.0

☞**Hostess**	S.S.	CAL	FAT(g)	SOD(mg)	CHL(mg)	%FAT
Coffee Cake, Cinnamon Crumb, 97% Fat Free	1 cake	80	1.0	95	0	11.3
Cup Cakes Lights, Chocolate Cake with Chocolate Frosting	1 cake	110	1.0	160	0	8.2

BAKERY

☞ Hostess

☞ Hostess	S. S.	CAL	FAT(g)	SOD(mg)	CHL(mg)	%FAT
Cup Cakes Lights, Chocolate Cake with Creamy Filling	1 cake	130	2.0	190	0	13.8
Cup Cakes Lights, Raspberry Filled	1 cake	130	1.0	170	0	6.9
Cup Cakes, Chocolate	1 cake	180	6.0	290	5	30.0
Cup Cakes, Orange	1 cake	160	5.0	150	10	28.1
Dessert Cups	1 cup	90	2.0	170	15	20.0
Lights, Apple Spice	1 cake	130	1.0	150	0	6.9
Lights, Vanilla Pudding Filled	1 cake	130	1.0	180	0	6.9
Lil Angels	1 cake	90	2.0	95	2	20.0
Muffins, Apple Streusel, 97% Fat Free	1 muffin	100	1.0	160	0	9.0
Muffins, Blueberry, 97% Fat Free	1 muffin	100	1.0	160	0	9.0
Sno Balls	1 cake	150	4.0	160	2	24.0
Sweet Roll, Cinnamon	1 roll	140	4.0	170	20	25.7
Twinkies	1 cake	150	5.0	200	20	30.0
Twinkies Lights	1 cake	110	2.0	160	0	16.4
Twinkies, Banana	1 cake	150	5.0	200	20	30.0
Twinkies, Fruit' n Creme-Strawberry	1 cake	140	3.0	180	20	19.3

☞ Little Debbie

☞ Little Debbie	S. S.	CAL	FAT(g)	SOD(mg)	CHL(mg)	%FAT
Coffee Cake	2.1 oz.	230	6.0	220	<2	23.5
Easter Puffs	1.3 oz.	150	4.0	60	<2	24.0
Figaroos	1.5 oz.	160	4.0	105	<2	22.5
Fudge Round	1.2 oz.	150	5.0	75	<2	30.0
Golden Cremes	2.5 oz.	270	9.0	260	<2	30.0
Marshmallow Supremes	1.1 oz.	130	4.0	55	<2	27.7
Pie, Apple	3.0 oz.	310	9.0	200	<2	26.1
Pie, Pecan	3.0 oz.	330	11.0	300	<2	30.0

☞ Manor

☞ Manor	S. S.	CAL	FAT(g)	SOD(mg)	CHL(mg)	%FAT
Deluxe Fruitcake	2 oz.	210	6.0	75	-	25.7

☞ **Nissen**	S. S.	CAL	FAT(g)	SOD(mg)	CHL(mg)	%FAT
Angel Ring	1 oz.	70	<1.0	190	0	<12.9
Buns, Apple Cinnamon	1 bun	150	4.0	200	0	24.0
Buns, Cinnamon	1 bun	140	4.0	180	<5	25.7
Buns, Hot Cross	1 bun	100	1.0	180	0	9.0
Buns, Raspberry	1 bun	150	4.0	190	0	24.0
Cake, Angel, Orange Chiffon	1 oz.	70	<1.0	190	0	<12.9
Dessert Shells	1 shell	80	2.0	160	0	22.5
Sponge Layers	1 layer	370	8.0	710	<5	19.5

☞ **Pet**	S. S.	CAL	FAT(g)	SOD(mg)	CHL(mg)	%FAT
Cake, Applesauce	2.5 oz.	234	7.0	230	-	26.9
Cake, Fudge	2.5 oz.	222	6.0	402	-	24.3
Fingers, Devil's Food	3 oz.	288	9.0	438	-	28.1
Fingers, Raspberry	3 oz.	303	9.0	337	-	26.7
Fingers, Spice	3 oz.	290	9.0	433	-	27.9
Fingers, Vanilla	3 oz.	301	9.0	388	-	26.9
Rolls, Caramel Nut	2 oz.	180	3.0	574	-	15.0
Rolls, Cinnamon	2 oz.	181	4.0	607	-	19.9
Rolls, Cinnamon Raisin	2 oz.	181	3.0	562	-	14.9
Rolls, Pecan	2 oz.	184	4.0	537	-	19.6
Rolls, Strawberry	2 oz.	165	3.0	127	5	16.4

☞ **Rainbo Break Cake**	S. S.	CAL	FAT(g)	SOD(mg)	CHL(mg)	%FAT
Angelfood Cake	1 oz.	70	0.0	100	-	0.0
Carrot Cakes	2 cakes	370	12.0	380	20	29.2
Dessert Sets	1 cup	100	1.0	115	-	9.0
Filled Twins	2 twins	310	10.0	260	15	29.0
Rolls, Apple Sweet	1 roll	120	2.0	150	0	15.0
Rolls, Cherry Sweet	1 roll	130	2.0	125	0	13.8
Rolls, Cinnamon Nut	2 rolls	330	11.0	220	-	30.0
Rolls, Cinnamon Raisin Sweet	1 roll	120	3.0	110	0	22.5
Rolls, Cinnamon Sweet	1 roll	120	3.0	125	0	22.5

BAKERY

☞Rainbo Break Cake	S.S.	CAL	FAT(g)	SOD(mg)	CHL(mg)	%FAT
Rolls, Pecan Sweet	1 roll	120	3.0	120	0	22.5

☞Tastykake	S.S.	CAL	FAT(g)	SOD(mg)	CHL(mg)	%FAT
Cupcake, Tastylight, Chocolate	1 cake	100	1.3	116	0	11.7
Cupcake, Tastylight, Vanilla	1 cake	100	1.2	121	0	13.5
Cupcakes, Chocolate	1 cake	100	2.6	122	4	23.4
Fudge Bar	1 bar	205	6.8	155	6	29.9
Junior, Coconut	1 cake	296	6.0	304	49	18.2
Junior, Koffee Kake	1 cake	261	8.5	212	40	29.3
Junior, Lemon	1 cake	306	4.0	255	-	11.8
Junior, Orange	1 cake	337	9.2	236	51	24.6
Kreme Kup	1 cake	86	2.8	13	4	29.3
Krimpet, Butterscotch	1 cake	103	2.6	83	22	22.7
Krimpet, Jelly	1 cake	85	1.0	82	21	10.6
Krimpet, Strawberry	1 cake	101	2.0	84	20	17.8
Mini Donuts, Honey Wheat	1 donut	40	1.2	48	3	27.0
Mini Donuts, Powdered Sugar	1 donut	42	1.3	71	4	27.9
Pie, Blueberry	1 pie	308	9.4	410	0	27.5
Pie, Cherry	1 pie	298	9.7	306	0	29.3
Pie, French Apple	1 pie	353	10.7	225	0	27.3
Pie, Strawberry	1 pie	342	11.4	303	0	30.0
Tasty Twist	1 twist	18	0.6	-	-	30.0

BAKING MIXES

ALL PURPOSE BAKING MIXES

☞ Bisquick

	S. S.	CAL	FAT(g)	SOD(mg)	CHL(mg)	%FAT
Baking Mix	1/2 cup	240	8.0	700	0	30.0

☞ Hain

	S. S.	CAL	FAT(g)	SOD(mg)	CHL(mg)	%FAT
Baking Mix, Whole Wheat	1 1/2 oz.	150	1.0	680	-	6.0

☞ Hodgson Mill

	S. S.	CAL	FAT(g)	SOD(mg)	CHL(mg)	%FAT
Insta-Bake Baking Mix, Whole Wheat	2 oz.	216	6.5	345	-	27.1

☞ Jiffy

	S. S.	CAL	FAT(g)	SOD(mg)	CHL(mg)	%FAT
Biscuit Mix, Baking	1.1 oz.	102	2.9	215	<1	25.6
Biscuit Mix, Buttermilk	1 oz.	120	3.4	300	1	25.5

☞ Martha White

	S. S.	CAL	FAT(g)	SOD(mg)	CHL(mg)	%FAT
BixMix Biscuit Mix	1 biscuit	90	2.0	240	<2	20.0

☞ Robin Hood/ Gold Medal

	S. S.	CAL	FAT(g)	SOD(mg)	CHL(mg)	%FAT
Biscuit Mix	1/8 mix	90	3.0	270	0	30.0

BAKING MIXES

BROWNIE MIXES

☞ Betty Crocker	S. S.	CAL	FAT(g)	SOD(mg)	CHL(mg)	%FAT
Brownie Mix, Carmel Swirl	1 brownie	120	4.0	115	10	30.0
Brownie Mix, Light Fudge	1 brownie	100	1.0	90	0	9.0

☞ Jiffy	S. S.	CAL	FAT(g)	SOD(mg)	CHL(mg)	%FAT
Brownie Mix, Fudge	0.66 oz.	80	2.0	85	15	22.5

☞ Pillsbury	S. S.	CAL	FAT(g)	SOD(mg)	CHL(mg)	%FAT
Brownie Mix, Lovin' Lite	1 brownie	100	2.0	80	10	18.0
Brownie Mix, Lovin' Lite*	1 brownie	100	2.0	85	0	18.0
*No Cholesterol Recipe						

CAKE MIXES

☞ Betty Crocker	S. S.	CAL	FAT(g)	SOD(mg)	CHL(mg)	%FAT
Angelfood Cake Mix, Confetti	1/12 cake	150	0.0	30	0	0.0
Angelfood Cake Mix, Lemon Custard	1/12 cake	150	0.0	300	0	0.0
Angelfood Cake Mix, Traditional	1/12 cake	130	0.0	170	0	0.0
Angelfood Cake Mix, White	1/12 cake	150	0.0	300	0	0.0
Classic Dessert Mix, Chocolate Pudding	1/6 cake	230	5.0	250	-	19.6
Classic Dessert Mix, Lemon Chiffon	1/12 cake	200	5.0	200	-	22.5
Classic Dessert Mix, Lemon Pudding	1/6 cake	230	5.0	270	0	19.6
Supermoist Cake Mix, Butter Pecan*	1/12 cake	220	7.0	320	0	28.6
Supermoist Cake Mix, Carrot*	1/12 cake	220	6.0	300	0	24.6
Supermoist Cake Mix, Cherry Chip	1/2 cake	190	3.0	370	0	14.2
Supermoist Cake Mix, Devil's Food*	1/12 cake	220	7.0	430	0	28.6
Supermoist Cake Mix, Golden Vanilla*	1/12 cake	220	7.0	270	0	28.6
Supermoist Cake Mix, Lemon*	1/12 cake	220	7.0	280	0	28.6
Supermoist Cake Mix, Marble*	1/12 cake	210	7.0	290	0	30.0
Supermoist Cake Mix, Milk Chocolate*	1/12 cake	210	7.0	340	0	30.0

☞ **Betty Crocker**	S. S.	CAL	FAT(g)	SOD(mg)	CHL(mg)	%FAT
Supermoist Cake Mix, Sour Cream White*	1/12 cake	180	3.0	290	0	15.0
Supermoist Cake Mix, Spice*	1/12 cake	220	7.0	320	0	28.6
Supermoist Cake Mix, White*	1/12 cake	220	7.0	270	0	28.6
Supermoist Cake Mix, Yellow*	1/12 cake	220	7.0	300	0	28.6
Supermoist Light Cake Mix, Devil's Food	1/12 cake	200	4.0	340	55	18.0
Supermoist Light Cake Mix, Devil's Food*	1/12 cake	180	3.0	370	0	15.0
Supermoist Light Cake Mix, White	1/12 cake	180	3.0	330	0	15.0
Supermoist Light Cake Mix, Yellow	1/12 cake	200	4.0	310	55	18.0
Supermoist Light Cake Mix, Yellow*	1/12 cake	190	3.0	330	0	14.2
*No Cholesterol Recipe						

☞ **Duncan Hines**	S. S.	CAL	FAT(g)	SOD(mg)	CHL(mg)	%FAT
Layer Cake Mix, Angelfood	1/12 cake	140	0.0	130	0	0.0
Layer Cake Mix, Banana*	1/12 cake	200	5.0	290	0	22.5
Layer Cake Mix, Dark Dutch Fudge*	1/12 cask	200	6.0	370	0	27.0
Layer Cake Mix, Devil's Food*	1/12 cake	200	6.0	370	0	27.0
Layer Cake Mix, French Vanilla*	1/12 cake	200	5.0	290	0	22.5
Layer Cake Mix, Fudge Marble*	1/12 cake	200	5.0	290	0	22.5
Layer Cake Mix, Lemon Supreme*	1/12 cake	200	5.0	290	0	22.5
Layer Cake Mix, Orange Supreme*	1/12 cake	200	5.0	290	0	22.5
Layer Cake Mix, Pineapple Supreme*	1/12 cake	200	5.0	290	0	22.5
Layer Cake Mix, Spice*	1/12 cake	200	5.0	290	0	22.5
Layer Cake Mix, Strawberry Supreme*	1/12 cake	200	5.0	290	0	22.5
Layer Cake Mix, Swiss Chocolate*	1/12 cake	200	6.0	370	0	27.0
Layer Cake Mix, Yellow*	1/12 cake	200	5.0	290	0	22.5
DeLights, Devil's Food	1/12 cake	180	5.0	345	35	25.0
DeLights, Fudge Marble	1/12 cake	180	4.0	250	35	20.0
DeLights, Yellow	1/12 cake	180	4.0	275	35	20.0
DeLights, Lemon	1/12 cake	180	4.0	275	35	20.0
*Must use "Lite"Recipe						

BAKING MIXES

☞ Jiffy	S. S.	CAL	FAT(g)	SOD(mg)	CHL(mg)	%FAT
Cake Mix, Dark Fudge	0.9 oz.	80	2.0	180	10	22.5
Cake Mix, Devil's Food	0.9 oz.	80	2.0	170	15	22.5
Cake Mix, Golden Yellow	0.9 oz.	80	2.0	120	15	22.5
Cake Mix, Spice	0.9 oz.	80	2.0	125	15	22.5
Cake Mix, White	0.9 oz.	80	2.0	110	0	22.5

☞ Krusteaz	S. S.	CAL	FAT(g)	SOD(mg)	CHL(mg)	%FAT
Cake Mix, White	1/12 pkg.	183	4.0	350	0	19.7

☞ Martha White	S. S.	CAL	FAT(g)	SOD(mg)	CHL(mg)	%FAT
Pound Cake Mix	1/10 cake	120	4.0	110	20	30.0

☞ Pillsbury	S. S.	CAL	FAT(g)	SOD(mg)	CHL(mg)	%FAT
Cake Mix, Bundt Tunnel of Lemon	1/16 cake	270	9.0	280	40	30.0
Cake Mix, Bundt Tunnel of Lemon*	1/16 cake	260	8.0	280	0	27.7
Lovin' Lites Cake Mix, Angelfood	1/8 loaf	90	0.0	210	0	0.0
Lovin' Lites Cake Mix, Devil's Food	1/12 cake	170	3.0	380	35	15.9
Lovin' Lites Cake Mix, Devil's Food*	1/12 cake	160	2.0	380	0	11.3
Lovin' Lites Cake Mix, White	1/12 cake	180	3.0	310	35	15.0
Lovin' Lites Cake Mix, White*	1/12 cake	170	2.0	310	0	10.6
Lovin' Lites Cake Mix, Yellow	1/12 cake	180	3.0	300	35	15.0
Lovin' Lites Cake Mix, Yellow*	1/12 cake	170	2.0	310	0	10.6
Pillsbury Plus Cake Mix, Banana*	1/12 cake	190	4.0	280	0	18.9
Pillsbury Plus Cake Mix, Carrot*	1/12 cake	190	5.0	300	0	23.7
Pillsbury Plus Cake Mix, Chocolate Chip*	1/12 cake	190	5.0	280	0	23.7
Pillsbury Plus Cake Mix, Dark Chocolate*	1/12 cake	180	5.0	340	0	25.0
Pillsbury Plus Cake Mix, Funfetti*	1/12 cake	230	2.0	290	0	7.8
Pillsbury Plus Cake Mix, German Chocolate*	1/12 cake	180	4.0	280	0	20.0

☞ Pillsbury	S. S.	CAL	FAT(g)	SOD(mg)	CHL(mg)	%FAT
Pillsbury Plus Cake Mix, Lemon*	1/12 cake	180	3.0	280	0	15.0
Pillsbury Plus Cake Mix, Strawberry*	1/12 cake	190	4.0	310	0	18.9
Pillsbury Plus Cake Mix, White*	1/12 cake	190	4.0	290	0	18.9
Pillsbury Plus Cake Mix, Yellow*	1/12 cake	190	5.0	300	0	23.7
*No Cholesterol Recipe						

☞ Sweet 'n Low	S. S.	CAL	FAT(g)	SOD(mg)	CHL(mg)	%FAT
Cake Mix, Banana	1/10 cake	90	2.0	40	<5	20.0
Cake Mix, Chocolate	1/10 cake	90	2.0	40	<5	20.0
Cake Mix, Lemon	1/10 cake	90	2.0	40	<5	20.0
Cake Mix, Lite Gingerbread	1/10 cake	90	2.0	20	<5	20.0
Cake Mix, White	1/10 cake	90	2.0	40	<5	20.0
Cake Mix, Yellow	1/10 cake	90	2.0	40	<5	20.0

CORN BREAD MIXES

☞ Aunt Jemima	S. S.	CAL	FAT(g)	SOD(mg)	CHL(mg)	%FAT
Easy Mix, Corn Bread	1/8 brd.	196	6.3	679	13	28.9
Flako Corn Muffin Mix	1 muffin	116	3.3	351	-	25.6

☞ Krusteaz	S. S.	CAL	FAT(g)	SOD(mg)	CHL(mg)	%FAT
Honey Cornbread Mix	1/16 pkg.	120	3.0	230	0	22.5

☞ Martha White	S. S.	CAL	FAT(g)	SOD(mg)	CHL(mg)	%FAT
Cotton Pickin' Corn Bread Mix	1/6 pkg.	110	2.0	360	0	16.4

BAKING MIXES

BAKING MIXES

☞ Pillsbury	S. S.	CAL	FAT(g)	SOD(mg)	CHL(mg)	%FAT
Ballard Corn Bread Mix	1/8 recipe	150	3.0	580	30	18.0

☞ Robin Hood/ Gold Medal	S. S.	CAL	FAT(g)	SOD(mg)	CHL(mg)	%FAT
Corn Bread Mix, White	1/6 mix	140	4.0	490	-	25.7
Corn Bread Mix, Yellow	1/6 mix	150	5.0	500	-	30.0
Corn Muffin Mix	1/6 mix	130	2.0	250	-	13.8

FROSTINGS

☞ Betty Crocker	S. S.	CAL	FAT(g)	SOD(mg)	CHL(mg)	%FAT
Frosting Mix, Creamy Deluxe Light, Chocolate	1/12 tub	130	2.0	60	0	13.9
Frosting Mix, Creamy Deluxe Light, Milk Chocolate	1/12 tub	140	2.0	50	0	12.9
Frosting Mix, Creamy Deluxe Light, Vanilla	1/12 tub	140	2.0	30	0	12.9
Frosting Mix, Creamy, Milk Chocolate	1/12 mix	170	5.0	40	0	26.5
Frosting Mix, Creamy, Vanilla	1/12 mix	170	5.0	50	0	26.5
Frosting Mix, Fluffy	1/12 mix	70	0.0	40	0	0.0

☞ Jiffy	S. S.	CAL	FAT(g)	SOD(mg)	CHL(mg)	%FAT
Frosting Mix, Carmel	0.75 oz.	100	3.0	100	0	27.0
Frosting Mix, Fudge	0.75 oz.	90	3.0	160	0	30.0
Frosting Mix, White	0.75 oz.	100	3.0	100	0	27.0

☞ Krusteaz	S. S.	CAL	FAT(g)	SOD(mg)	CHL(mg)	%FAT
Frosting Mix, Fudge	1/12 pkg.	130	2.0	50	0	13.8
Frosting Mix, White	1/12 pkg.	130	2.0	50	0	13.8

🖙 Pillsbury	S. S.	CAL	FAT(g)	SOD(mg)	CHL(mg)	%FAT
Lovin' Lites Frosting, Chocolate Fudge	1/12 can	120	2.0	90	0	15.0
Lovin' Lites Frosting, Milk Chocolate	1/12 can	130	2.0	95	0	13.8
Lovin' Lites Frosting, Vanilla	1/12 can	130	2.0	70	0	13.8

MUFFIN MIXES

🖙 Betty Crocker	S. S.	CAL	FAT(g)	SOD(mg)	CHL(mg)	%FAT
Muffin Mix, Apple Cinnamon	1 muffin	120	4.0	140	25	30.0
Muffin Mix, Apple Cinnamon*	1 muffin	110	3.0	140	0	24.5
Muffin Mix, Light Muffins, Mild Blueberry	1 muffin	70	<1.0	140	20	<12.9
Muffin Mix, Light Muffins, Wild Blueberry*	1 muffin	70	<1.0	140	0	<12.9
Muffin Mix, Twice the Blueberries	1 muffin	120	4.0	140	0	30.0
Muffin Mix, Twice the Blueberries*	1 muffin	110	3.0	140	0	24.5
Muffin Mix, Wild Blueberry	1 muffin	120	4.0	150	25	30.0
Muffin Mix, Wild Blueberry*	1 muffin	110	3.0	150	0	24.5
*No Cholerterol Recipe						

🖙 Duncan Hines	S. S.	CAL	FAT(g)	SOD(mg)	CHL(mg)	%FAT
Muffin Mix, Blueberry, Bakery Style	1 muffin	190	6.0	250	-	28.4
Muffin Mix, Blueberry, Regular Style	1 muffin	120	3.0	185	-	22.5

🖙 Hodgson Mill	S. S.	CAL	FAT(g)	SOD(mg)	CHL(mg)	%FAT
Muffin Mix, Whole Wheat	1 muffin	140	3.0	330	-	19.3

🖙 Jiffy	S. S.	CAL	FAT(g)	SOD(mg)	CHL(mg)	%FAT
Muffin Mix, Honey Date	1.2 oz.	120	4.0	190	20	30.0

☞ Krusteaz	S. S.	CAL	FAT(g)	SOD(mg)	CHL(mg)	%FAT
Muffin Mix, Blueberry, Imitation	2 oz.	170	4.0	300	5	21.2
Muffin Mix, Blueberry, Real	2 oz.	124	2.0	218	27	14.5

☞ Pillsbury	S. S.	CAL	FAT(g)	SOD(mg)	CHL(mg)	%FAT
Lovin' Lites, Blueberry Muffin Mix	1 muffin	100	1.0	160	20	9.0
Lovin' Lites, Blueberry Muffin Mix*	1 muffin	100	1.0	160	0	9.0
*No Cholesterol Recipe						

☞ Martha White	S. S.	CAL	FAT(g)	SOD(mg)	CHL(mg)	%FAT
Muffin Mix, Apple-Cinnamon	1 muffin	140	3.0	250	<2	19.3
Muffin Mix, Blackberry	1 muffin	140	3.0	250	<2	19.3
Muffin Mix, Blueberry	1 muffin	140	3.0	260	<2	19.3
Muffin Mix, Bran	1 muffin	150	5.0	330	35	30.0
Muffin Mix, Orangeberry	1 muffin	140	3.0	220	<2	19.3
Muffin Mix, Raspberry	1 muffin	140	3.0	180	<2	19.3
Muffin Mix, Strawberry	1 muffin	140	3.0	270	<2	19.3

☞ Robin Hood/ Gold Medal	S. S.	CAL	FAT(g)	SOD(mg)	CHL(mg)	%FAT
Muffin Pouch Mix, Applesauce	1 muffin	160	5.0	240	-	28.1
Muffin Pouch Mix, Banana	1 muffin	150	5.0	240	-	30.0
Muffin Pouch Mix, Caramel	1 muffin	150	5.0	230	-	30.0
Muffin Pouch Mix, Honey Bran	1 muffin	170	5.0	240	-	26.5
Muffin Pouch Mix, Oat	1 muffin	150	5.0	220	45	30.0
Muffin Mix, Honey Bran	1/12 pkg.	140	4.0	290	0	25.7
Muffin Mix, Oat Bran	2.25 oz.	210	6.0	340	0	25.7

BAKING MIXES

PANCAKE MIXES

☞ Aunt Jemima	S. S.	CAL	FAT(g)	SOD(mg)	CHL(mg)	%FAT
Pancake Batter, Blueberry	3.6 oz.	204	4.0	688	27	17.6
Pancake Batter, Buttermilk	3.6 oz.	180	2.3	778	27	11.5
Pancake Batter, Original	3.6 oz.	183	2.4	763	19	11.8
Pancake Mix, Buttermilk Complete	three 4"	230	2.0	610	10	7.8
Pancake Mix, Light Buttermilk Complete	three 4"	130	2.0	570	-	13.8
Pancake Mix, Original*	three 4"	170	3.0	600	0	15.9
Pancake Mix, Original Complete	three 4"	250	3.0	910	15	10.8
Pancake Mix, Whole Wheat*	three 4"	190	5.0	550	0	23.7
*No Cholesterol Recipe						

☞ Betty Crocker	S. S.	CAL	FAT(g)	SOD(mg)	CHL(mg)	%FAT
Pancake Mix, Complete Buttermilk	three 4"	210	3.0	500	-	12.9

☞ Bisquick	S. S.	CAL	FAT(g)	SOD(mg)	CHL(mg)	%FAT
Shake 'N Pour Pancake & Waffle Mix, Apple Cinnamon	three 4"	270	3.0	880	0	10.0
Shake 'N Pour Pancake & Waffle Mix, Blueberry	three 4"	280	3.0	840	0	9.6
Shake 'N Pour Pancake & Waffle Mix, Buttermilk	three 4"	250	3.0	880	0	10.8
Shake 'N Pour Pancake & Waffle Mix, Original	three 4"	250	3.0	880	0	10.8

☞ Hungry Jack	S. S.	CAL	FAT(g)	SOD(mg)	CHL(mg)	%FAT
Pancake Mix, Complete Packets	three 4"	180	3.0	650	0	15.0
Pancake Mix, Extra Lights	three 4"	190	6.0	490	55	28.4
Pancake Mix, Extra Lights*	three 4"	170	4.0	500	0	21.2
Pancake Mix, Extra Lights Complete	three 4"	180	3.0	730	0	15.0
*No Cholesterol Recipe						

BAKING MIXES

☞Krusteaz	S.S.	CAL	FAT(g)	SOD(mg)	CHL(mg)	%FAT
Tempura Batter Mix	1 oz.	102	0.0	480	0	0.0

☞Martha White	S.S.	CAL	FAT(g)	SOD(mg)	CHL(mg)	%FAT
FlapStax Pancake Mix	1 pancake	80	1.0	320	<1	11.3

☞Robin Hood/ Gold Medal	S.S.	CAL	FAT(g)	SOD(mg)	CHL(mg)	%FAT
Pouch Pancake Mix, Buttermilk	1/8 mix	110	3.0	280	-	24.5

PIZZA CRUST MIXES

☞Jiffy	S.S.	CAL	FAT(g)	SOD(mg)	CHL(mg)	%FAT
Pizza Crust Mix	0.81 oz.	90	2.0	160	0	20.0

☞Martha White	S.S.	CAL	FAT(g)	SOD(mg)	CHL(mg)	%FAT
Pizza Crust Mix, Deep Dish	1/8 pkg.	110	<1.0	110	0	<8.2
Pizza Crust Mix, Regular	1/8 pkg.	100	2.0	125	0	18.0

☞Robin Hood/ Gold Medal	S.S.	CAL	FAT(g)	SOD(mg)	CHL(mg)	%FAT
Pizza Crust Mix	1/6 mix	110	1.0	220	-	8.2

QUICKBREAD AND MISCELLANEOUS BAKING MIXES

☞Aunt Jemima	S.S.	CAL	FAT(g)	SOD(mg)	CHL(mg)	%FAT
Easy Mix, Coffee Cake	1/8 cake	156	4.4	279	1	25.4

☞ Betty Crocker	S. S.	CAL	FAT(g)	SOD(mg)	CHL(mg)	%FAT
Classic Dessert Mix, Gingerbread	1/9 cake	220	7.0	330	30	28.6
Classic Dessert Mix, Date Bar	1 bar	60	2.0	35	0	30.0

☞ Pillsbury	S. S.	CAL	FAT(g)	SOD(mg)	CHL(mg)	%FAT
Gingerbread Mix	1/ 9 cake	180	5.0	300	0	25.0
Quickbread Mix, Apple Cinnamon	1/12 cake	180	6.0	170	20	30.0
Quickbread Mix, Apple Cinnamon*	1/12 cake	190	6.0	170	0	28.4
Quickbread Mix, Banana	1/12 cake	170	5.0	200	35	26.5
Quickbread Mix, Blueberry	1/12 cake	180	6.0	170	0	30.0
Quickbread Mix, Cranberry	1/12 cake	170	4.0	160	0	21.2
Quickbread Mix, Date	1/12 cake	160	3.0	150	0	16.9
Hot Roll Mix*	2 rolls	240	4.0	370	25	15.0
*No Cholesterol Recipe						

BAKING SECTION

BARLEY

☞ **Generic**	S. S.	CAL	FAT(g)	SOD(mg)	CHL(mg)	%FAT
Barley, Medium Pearled	1/4 cup	172	.05	0	-	2.6
Barley, Pearled, Quick	1/3 cup	172	.05	0	-	2.6

COCOA

☞ **Hershey's**	S. S.	CAL	FAT(g)	SOD(mg)	CHL(mg)	%FAT
Cocoa	1/3 cup	120	4.0	10	0	30.0
European Cocoa	1/3 cup	90	3.0	15	0	30.0

☞ **Nestle**	S. S.	CAL	FAT(g)	SOD(mg)	CHL(mg)	%FAT
Cocoa	1/2 cup	180	6.0	6	-	30.0

CORN MEAL

☞ **Generic**	S. S.	CAL	FAT(g)	SOD(mg)	CHL(mg)	%FAT
Corn Meal, Enriched White	3 Tbsp.	102	.05	1	-	4.4
Corn Meal, Enriched Yellow	3 Tbsp.	102	0.5	1	-	4.4
Corn Meal, White, Bolted	3 Tbsp.	99	0.7	337	-	6.4
Corn Meal, White, Buttermilk, Self-Rising	3 Tbsp.	101	1.1	439	-	9.8
Corn Meal, White, Enriched, Bolted, Self-Rising	3 Tbsp.	99	0.9	382	-	8.2
Corn Meal, White, Self-Rising	3 Tbsp.	98	0.5	381	-	4.6
Corn Meal, Yellow, Self-Rising	3 Tbsp.	100	1.0	490	-	9.0

EVAPORATED AND SWEETENED CONDENSED MILK

BAKING SECTION

☞ Carnation

	S. S.	CAL	FAT(g)	SOD(mg)	CHL(mg)	%FAT
Evaporated Low-Fat Milk	1/2 cup	110	3.0	130	-	24.5
Evaporated Skim Milk	1/2 cup	100	0.3	147	-	2.7
Sweetened Condensed Milk	1/8 cup	123	3.1	43	-	22.7

☞ Dairymate

	S. S.	CAL	FAT(g)	SOD(mg)	CHL(mg)	%FAT
Evaporated Light Skimmed Milk	1/2 cup	100	<1.0	150	10	<9.0

☞ Pet

	S. S.	CAL	FAT(g)	SOD(mg)	CHL(mg)	%FAT
Evaporated Light Skimmed Milk	1/2 cup	100	<1.0	150	10	<9.0

FLOUR

☞ Generic

	S. S.	CAL	FAT(g)	SOD(mg)	CHL(mg)	%FAT
Flour, All-Purpose	1 cup	400	1.0	0	0	2.3
Flour, Bread	1 cup	400	2.0	0	0	4.5
Flour, Cracked Wheat	1 cup	320	2.0	3	0	5.6
Flour, Graham	1 cup	320	2.0	3	0	5.6
Flour, Oat Flour	1 cup	390	3.0	0	0	6.9
Flour, Rye	1 cup	450	2.0	0	0	4.0
Flour, Self-Rising	1 cup	380	1.0	1500	0	2.4
Flour, Unbleached	1 cup	400	1.0	0	0	2.3
Flour, Whole Wheat	1 cup	350	2.0	0	0	5.1

MISCELLANEOUS

☞ Kellogg's

	S. S.	CAL	FAT(g)	SOD(mg)	CHL(mg)	%FAT
Corn Flake Crumbs	1 oz.	100	0.0	290	0	0.0
Croutettes	0.7 oz.	70	0.0	260	-	0.0

☞ **Krusteaz**	S. S.	CAL	FAT(g)	SOD(mg)	CHL(mg)	%FAT
Wheat Germ	1 oz.	103	2.0	1	0	17.5

☞ **Nabisco**	S. S.	CAL	FAT(g)	SOD(mg)	CHL(mg)	%FAT
Cracker Meal	1/4 cup	110	0.0	10	0	0.0

NONFAT DRY MILK

☞ **Generic**	S. S.	CAL	FAT(g)	SOD(mg)	CHL(mg)	%FAT
Nonfat Dry Milk	5 Tbsp.	80	0.0	125	5	0.0

TORTILLA MIX

☞ **Quaker**	S. S.	CAL	FAT(g)	SOD(mg)	CHL(mg)	%FAT
Masa Harina de Maiz	2 tortillas	137	1.5	5	-	9.9
Masa Trigo	2 tortillas	149	4.0	794	0	24.2

BREAKFAST SECTION

BREAKFAST BARS

☞Kellogg's	S. S.	CAL	FAT(g)	SOD(mg)	CHL(mg)	%FAT
Nutri Grain Cereal Bars, All Flavors	1 bar	150	5.0	65	0	30.0

☞Quaker	S. S.	CAL	FAT(g)	SOD(mg)	CHL(mg)	%FAT
Chewy Granola Bars, S'Mores	1 bar	130	4.0	85	0	27.7
Chewy Granola Bars, Honey Graham Cinnamon	1 bar	120	4.0	105	0	30.0

BREAKFAST BEVERAGE MIXES

☞Carnation	S. S.	CAL	FAT(g)	SOD(mg)	CHL(mg)	%FAT
Hot Cocoa Mix, 70-Calorie	1 cup	70	<1.0	135	1	<12.9
Hot Cocoa Mix, Chocolate Fudge	1 cup	110	1.0	135	1	8.2
Hot Cocoa Mix, Chocolate Mint	1 cup	110	1.0	120	1	8.2
Hot Cocoa Mix, Milk Chocolate	1 cup	110	1.0	130	1	8.2
Hot Cocoa Mix, Rich Chocolate	1 cup	110	1.0	120	0.5	8.2
Hot Cocoa Mix, Sugar Free Diet	1 cup	25	<1.0	140	1	-
Hot Cocoa Mix, Sugar Free Mocha	1 cup	50	<1.0	140	2	<18.0
Hot Cocoa Mix, Sugar Free Rich Chocolate	1 cup	50	<1.0	160	3	<18.0
Hot Cocoa Mix, with Chocolate Marshmallows	1 cup	110	1.0	120	2	8.2
Hot Cocoa Mix, with Marshmallows	1 cup	110	1.0	120	0.5	8.2
Instant Breakfast*, Chocolate	1 cup	216	1.4	261	6	5.8
Instant Breakfast*, Chocolate Malt	1 cup	216	2.4	286	7	10.0
Instant Breakfast*, Coffee	1 cup	216	0.4	276	7	1.7
Instant Breakfast*, No Sugar Added, Chocolate	1 cup	156	1.4	241	6	8.1
Instant Breakfast*, No Sugar Added, Chocolate Malt	1 cup	156	2.4	261	6	13.8
Instant Breakfast*, No Sugar Added, Strawberry	1 cup	156	0.4	246	7	2.3

☞ Carnation

	S. S.	CAL	FAT(g)	SOD(mg)	CHL(mg)	%FAT
Instant Breakfast*, No Sugar Added, Vanilla	1 cup	156	0.4	246	7	2.3
Instant Breakfast*, Strawberry	1 cup	216	0.4	336	7	1.7
Instant Breakfast*, Vanilla	1 cup	216	0.4	261	7	1.7
Instant Breakfast**, Chocolate	1 cup	251	5.7	257	20	20.4
Instant Breakfast**, Chocolate Malt	1 cup	251	6.7	282	21	24.0
Instant Breakfast**, Coffee	1 cup	251	4.7	272	21	16.9
Instant Breakfast**, No Sugar Added, Chocolate	1 cup	191	5.7	237	20	26.9
Instant Breakfast**, No Sugar Added, Strawberry	1 cup	191	4.7	242	21	22.1
Instant Breakfast**, No Sugar Added, Vanilla	1 cup	191	4.7	242	21	22.1
Instant Breakfast**, Strawberry	1 cup	251	4.7	332	21	16.9
Instant Breakfast**, Vanilla	1 cup	251	4.7	257	21	16.9
*with skim milk, **with 2% milk						

☞ Pillsbury

	S. S.	CAL	FAT(g)	SOD(mg)	CHL(mg)	%FAT
Instant Breakfast*, Chocolate	1 cup	216	<1.4	226	4	<5.8
Instant Breakfast*, Chocolate Malt	1 cup	216	0.4	261	4	1.7
Instant Breakfast*, Strawberry	1 cup	216	0.4	226	4	1.7
Instant Breakfast*, Vanilla	1 cup	226	0.4	226	4	1.6
Instant Breakfast**, Chocolate	1 cup	250	5.0	220	20	18.0
Instant Breakfast**, Chocolate Malt	1 cup	250	5.0	250	20	18.0
Instant Breakfast**, Strawberry	1 cup	250	5.0	220	20	18.0
Instant Breakfast**, Vanilla	1 cup	260	5.0	220	20	17.3
*with skim milk, **with 2% milk						

☞ Swiss Miss

	S. S.	CAL	FAT(g)	SOD(mg)	CHL(mg)	%FAT
Cocoa, Bavarian Chocolate	6 oz.	110	3.0	170	2	24.5
Cocoa, Diet	6 oz.	20	<1.0	180	2	-
Cocoa, Double Rich	6 oz.	110	3.0	180	2	24.5
Cocoa, Lite	6 oz.	70	<1.0	180	1	<12.9

☞ **Swiss Miss**	S. S.	CAL	FAT(g)	SOD(mg)	CHL(mg)	%FAT
Cocoa, Milk Chocolate	6 oz.	110	3.0	170	2	24.5
Cocoa, Rich	6 oz.	120	2.0	105	0	15.0
Cocoa, Sugar Free	6 oz.	50	<1.0	190	2	<18.0
Cocoa, Sugar Free with Sugar Free Marshmallows	6 oz.	50	<1.0	180	2	<18.0
Cocoa, White Chocolate	6 oz.	120	2.0	40	0	15.0
Cocoa, with Mini Marshmallows	6 oz.	110	3.0	170	2	24.5

DRY CEREALS

☞ **General Mills**	S. S.	CAL	FAT(g)	SOD(mg)	CHL(mg)	%FAT
Basic 4	3/4 cup	170	2.0	290	0	10.6
Body Buddies, Natural Fruit	1 cup	110	1.0	280	0	8.2
Booberry	1 cup	110	1.0	210	0	8.2
Cheerios	1.25 cup	110	2.0	290	0	16.4
Cheerios, Apple Cinnamon	3/4 cup	110	2.0	180	0	16.4
Cheerios, Honey Nut	3/4 cup	110	1.0	250	0	8.2
Cinnamon Toast Crunch	3/4 cup	120	3.0	210	0	22.5
Clusters	1/2 cup	110	2.0	140	0	16.4
Cocoa Puffs	1 cup	110	1.0	170	0	8.2
Count Chocula	1 cup	110	1.0	210	0	8.2
Country Corn Flakes	1 cup	110	1.0	260	0	8.2
Crispy Wheats 'N Raisins	3/4 cup	100	1.0	140	0	9.0
Fiber One	1/2 cup	60	1.0	140	0	15.0
Frankenberry	1 cup	110	1.0	210	0	8.2
Fruity Yummy Mummy	1 cup	110	1.0	160	0	8.2
Golden Grahams	3/4 cup	110	1.0	280	0	8.2
Kaboom	1 cup	110	1.0	270	0	8.2
Kix	1.5 cup	110	1.0	260	0	8.2
Lucky Charms	1 cup	110	1.0	180	0	8.2
Natural Valley, Cinnamon & Raisin	1/3 cup	120	4.0	90	0	30.0
Oatmeal Crisp	1 cup	110	2.0	180	0	16.4
Oatmeal Raisin Crisp	1/2 cup	110	2.0	170	0	16.4
Raisin Nut Bran	1/2 cup	110	3.0	140	0	24.5
S'Mores Grahams	3/4 cup	160	2.0	310	0	11.3

☞ General Mills	S. S.	CAL	FAT(g)	SOD(mg)	CHL(mg)	%FAT
Total	1 cup	100	1.0	200	0	9.0
Total Corn Flakes	1 cup	110	<1.0	200	0	<8.2
Total Raisin Bran	1 cup	140	1.0	190	0	6.4
Triples	3/4 cup	150	1.0	310	0	6.0
Trix	1 cup	110	1.0	140	0	8.2
Wheaties	1 cup	100	1.0	200	0	9.0

☞ Kellogg's	S. S.	CAL	FAT(g)	SOD(mg)	CHL(mg)	%FAT
All-Bran	1/3 cup	70	1.0	260	0	12.9
All-Bran with Extra Fiber	1/2 cup	50	0.0	140	0	0.0
Apple Jacks	1 cup	110	0.0	125	0	0.0
Apple Raisin Crisp	2/3 cup	130	0.0	230	0	0.0
Bran Buds	1/3 cup	70	1.0	200	0	12.9
Bran Flakes	2/3 cup	90	0.0	220	0	0.0
Cocoa Krispies	3/4 cup	110	0.0	190	0	0.0
Common Sense Oat Bran	1/2 cup	100	1.0	250	0	9.0
Common Sense Oat Bran with Raisins	1/2 cup	130	1.0	250	0	7.5
Corn Flakes	1 cup	100	0.0	290	0	0.0
Corn Pops	1 cup	110	0.0	90	0	0.0
Crispix	1 cup	110	0.0	220	0	0.0
Double Dip Crunch	2/3 cup	120	2.0	160	0	15.0
Fiberwise	2/3 cup	90	1.0	140	0	10.0
Froot Loops	1 cup	110	1.0	125	0	8.2
Frosted Flakes	3/4 cup	110	0.0	200	0	0.0
Frosted Krispies	3/4 cup	110	0.0	220	0	0.0
Frosted Mini-Wheats	4 biscuits	100	0.0	0	0	0.0
Frosted Mini-Wheats, Bite Size	1/2 cup	100	0.0	0	0	0.0
Fruitful Bran	2/3 cup	120	0.0	220	0	0.0
Fruity Marshmallow Krispies	1.25 cup	140	0.0	210	0	0.0
Granola, Low-Fat	1/3 cup	120	2.0	60	0	15.0
Just Right with Fiber Nuggets	2/3 cup	100	1.0	200	0	9.0
Just Right with Fruit & Nuts	3/4 cup	140	1.0	190	0	6.4
Kenmei Rice Bran	3/4 cup	110	1.0	230	0	8.2
Müeslix Crispy Blend	2/3 cup	150	2.0	150	0	11.3

BREAKFAST SECTION

☞ Kellogg's

	S. S.	CAL	FAT(g)	SOD(mg)	CHL(mg)	%FAT
Müeslix Golden Crunch	1/2 cup	120	2.0	170	0	15.0
Nut & Honey Crunch	2/3 cup	110	1.0	200	0	8.2
Nut & Honey Crunch O's	2/3 cup	110	2.0	190	0	16.4
Nutri-Grain Almond Raisin	2/3 cup	140	2.0	220	0	12.9
Nutri-Grain Raisin Bran	1 cup	130	1.0	200	0	6.9
Nutri-Grain Wheat	2/3 cup	90	0.0	170	0	0.0
Oatbake Honey Bran	1/3 cup	110	3.0	190	0	24.5
Oatbake Raisin Nut	1/3 cup	110	3.0	200	0	24.5
Product 19	1 cup	100	0.0	320	0	0.0
Raisin Bran	3/4 cup	120	1.0	210	0	7.5
Rice Krispies	1 cup	110	0.0	290	0	0.0
Shredded Wheat, Whole Grain	1/2 cup	90	0.0	0.0	0	0.0
Squares, Apple Cinnamon	1/2 cup	90	0.0	5	0	0.0
Squares, Blueberry	1/2 cup	90	0.0	5	0	0.0
Squares, Raisin	1/2 cup	90	0.0	0	0	0.0
Squares, Strawberry	1/2 cup	90	0.0	5	0	0.0
Special K	1 cup	110	0.0	230	0	0.0

☞ Nabisco

	S. S.	CAL	FAT(g)	SOD(mg)	CHL(mg)	%FAT
100% Bran Cereal	1/2 cup	70	1.0	180	0	12.9
Fruit Wheats, Apple	1/2 cup	90	0.0	15	0	0.0
Shredded Wheat	1 biscuit	80	1.0	0	0	11.3
Shredded Wheat 'n Bran	2/3 cup	90	0.0	0	0	0.0
Shredded Wheat with Oat Bran	2/3 cup	100	1.0	130	0	9.0
Shredded Wheat, Spoon Size	2/3 cup	90	1.0	0	0	10.0
Team Flakes	1 cup	110	1.0	180	0	8.2

☞ Post

	S. S.	CAL	FAT(g)	SOD(mg)	CHL(mg)	%FAT
Alpha-Bits	1 oz.	110	1.0	190	0	8.2
C.W. Post Hearty Granola	1 oz.	130	4.0	80	0	27.7
Cocoa Pebbles	1 oz.	110	1.0	160	0	8.2

BREAKFAST SECTION

☞ Post	S. S.	CAL	FAT(g)	SOD(mg)	CHL(mg)	%FAT
Fruit & Fibre, Dates, Raisins, Walnuts with Oat Clusters	1.25 oz.	120	2.0	170	0	15.0
Fruit & Fibre, Peaches, Raisins & Almonds with Oat Clusters	1.25 oz.	120	2.0	170	0	15.0
Fruit & Fibre, Tropical Fruit with Oat Clusters	1.25 oz.	120	3.0	170	0	22.5
Fruity Pebbles	1 oz.	110	1.0	160	0	8.2
Grape-Nuts	1 oz.	110	0.0	170	0	0.0
Grape-Nuts Flakes	1 oz.	100	1.0	160	0	9.0
Honey Bunches of Oats with Almonds	1 oz.	120	3.0	160	0	22.5
Honey Bunches of Oats, Honey Roasted	1 oz.	110	2.0	180	0	16.4
Honeycomb	1 oz.	110	0.0	170	0	0.0
Natural Bran Flakes	1 oz.	90	0.0	240	0	0.0
Natural Raisin Bran	1.4 oz.	120	1.0	200	0	7.5
Oat Flakes	1 oz.	110	1.0	130	0	8.2
Post Toasties	1 oz.	110	0.0	310	0	0.0
Raisin Grape-Nuts	1 oz.	100	0.0	140	0	0.0
Smurf-Magic Berries	1 oz.	120	1.0	60	0	7.5
Super Golden Crisp	1 oz.	110	0.0	45	0	0.0

☞ Quaker	S. S.	CAL	FAT(g)	SOD(mg)	CHL(mg)	%FAT
Cap'n Crunch	3/4 cup	113	1.7	241	-	13.5
Cap'n Crunch's Crunchberries	3/4 cup	113	1.7	247	-	13.5
Cap'n Crunch's Peanut Butter Crunch	3/4 cup	119	3.0	281	-	22.7
Crunchy Bran	2/3 cup	89	1.3	316	-	13.1
King Vitamin	1 1/2 cup	110	1.0	280	-	8.2
Kretschmer Honey Crunch Wheat Germ	1/4 cup	105	2.8	2	-	24.0
Kretschmer Wheat Germ	1/4 cup	103	3.4	2	0	29.7
Life	2/3 cup	101	1.7	186	-	15.1
Life, Cinnamon	2/3 cup	101	1.7	182	-	15.1
Oat Squares	1/2 cup	105	1.6	159	-	13.7
Oh!s, Crunchy Nut	1 cup	127	4.2	164	-	29.8
Oh!s, Honey Graham	1 cup	122	3.2	217	-	23.6
Popeye Sweet Crunch	1 cup	113	1.8	254	-	14.3

☞ Quaker	S. S.	CAL	FAT(g)	SOD(mg)	CHL(mg)	%FAT
Puffed Rice	1 cup	54	0.1	1	0	1.7
Puffed Wheat	1 cup	50	0.2	1	0	3.6
Shredded Wheat	2 biscuits	132	0.6	1	-	4.1
Unprocessed Bran	2 Tbsp.	8	0.2	0	-	22.5

☞ Ralston Purina	S. S.	CAL	FAT(g)	SOD(mg)	CHL(mg)	%FAT
Almond Delight	3/4 cup	110	2.0	200	0	16.4
Bill & Ted's Excellent Cereal	1 cup	110	0.0	160	0	8.2
Bran News, Cinnamon	3/4 cup	100	0.0	160	0	0.0
Chex, Corn	1 cup	110	0.0	310	0	0.0
Chex, Double	2/3 cup	100	0.0	190	0	0.0
Chex, Honey Graham	2/3 cup	110	1.0	180	0	8.2
Chex, Honey Nut Oat	1/2 cup	100	1.0	220	0	9.0
Chex, Multi-Bran	2/3 cup	90	0.0	200	0	0.0
Chex, Rice	1.13 cup	110	0.0	280	0	0.0
Chex, Rice, Frosted Juniors	3/4 cup	110	0.0	200	0	0.0
Chex, Wheat, Whole Grain	2/3 cup	100	1.0	230	0	9.0
Cookie-Crisp, Chocolate Chip	1 cup	110	1.0	190	0	8.2
Muesli, Apple Almond	1/2 cup	150	2.0	140	0	12.0
Muesli, Cranberry Walnut	1/2 cup	150	3.0	95	0	18.0
Muesli, Date Almond	1/2 cup	140	2.0	95	0	12.9
Muesli, Peach Pecan	1/2 cup	150	3.0	95	0	18.0
Muesli, Raspberry Almond	1/2 cup	150	3.0	95	0	18.0
Prince of Thieves	1 cup	110	1.0	70	0	8.2
Slimer! and the Real Ghostbusters	1 cup	110	1.0	115	0	8.2
Sunflakes	1 cup	100	1.0	240	0	9.0
Teenage Mutant Ninja Turtles	1 cup	110	0.0	190	0	0.0
The Addam's Family	1 cup	110	1.0	65	0	8.2
The Jetsons	3/4 cup	110	1.0	160	0	8.2

☞ Wonder	S. S.	CAL	FAT(g)	SOD(mg)	CHL(mg)	%FAT
Corn Flakes, Apple Cinnamon	1 cup	110	0.0	65	0	8.2

BREAKFAST SECTION

☞Wonder	S.S.	CAL	FAT(g)	SOD(mg)	CHL(mg)	%FAT
Honey Nut Crispy Rice	1 cup	110	1.0	205	0	0.0
Crunchy Graham Oat Rings	3/4 cup	110	1.0	125	0	8.2

GRANOLAS

☞Post	S.S.	CAL	FAT(g)	SOD(mg)	CHL(mg)	%FAT
C.W. Post Hearty Granola	1 oz.	130	4.0	80	0	27.7

☞Kellog's	S.S.	CAL	FAT(g)	SOD(mg)	CHL(mg)	%FAT
Naural Valley, Cinnamon & Raisin	1/3 cup	120	4.0	90	0	30.0
Granola, Low-Fat	1/3 cup	120	2.0	60	0	15.0

☞Quaker	S.S.	CAL	FAT(g)	SOD(mg)	CHL(mg)	%FAT
100% Natural, Low-Fat	1/4 cup	110	2.0	15	0	16.0

HOT CEREALS

☞Aunt Jemima	S.S.	CAL	FAT(g)	SOD(mg)	CHL(mg)	%FAT
Hominy Grits, Regular, Enriched White Quick	3 Tbsp.	101	0.2	1	-	1.8

☞Highspire	S.S.	CAL	FAT(g)	SOD(mg)	CHL(mg)	%FAT
Maltex	1 oz.	105	1.0	0	0	8.6
Maypo, 30 Second	1 oz.	100	1.0	0	0	9.0
Maypo, Vermont Style	1 oz.	105	1.0	0	0	8.6
Maypo, with Oat Bran	1.25 oz.	130	2.0	1	0	13.8
Wheatena	1 oz.	100	1.0	0	0	9.0

☞Nabisco

	S. S.	CAL	FAT(g)	SOD(mg)	CHL(mg)	%FAT
Cream of Rice	1 oz.	100	0.0	0	0	0.0
Cream of Wheat, Instant	1 oz.	100	<1.0	0	<5	<9.0
Cream of Wheat, Mix 'n Eat, Apple and Cinnamon	1.25 oz.	130	0.0	250	0	0.0
Cream of Wheat, Mix 'n Eat, Maple Brown Sugar	1.25 oz.	130	0.0	180	0	0.0
Cream of Wheat, Mix 'n Eat, Brown Sugar Cinnamon	1.25 oz.	130	0.0	230	0	0.0
Cream of Wheat, Mix 'n Eat, Original	1 oz.	100	0.0	170	0	0.0
Cream of Wheat, Quick	1 oz.	100	<1.0	80	<5	<9.0
Cream of Wheat, Regular	1 oz.	100	0.0	0	0	0.0

☞Pillsbury

	S. S.	CAL	FAT(g)	SOD(mg)	CHL(mg)	%FAT
Farina	2.3 cup	80	<1.0	270	0	<11.3

☞Quaker

	S. S.	CAL	FAT(g)	SOD(mg)	CHL(mg)	%FAT
Hominy Grits, Regular, Enriched White Quick	3 Tbsp.	101	0.2	1	-	1.8
Hominy Grits, White, Instant	1 pkg.	79	0.1	440	-	1.1
Hominy Grits, With Cheddar Cheese Flavor, Instant	1 pkg.	104	1.0	497	0	8.7
Hominy Grits, With Imitation Bacon Bits, Instant	1 pkg.	101	0.4	590	-	3.6
Hominy Grits, With Imitation Ham Bits, Instant	1 pkg..	99	0.3	800	0	2.7
Hominy Grits, Yellow, Enriched, Quick	3 Tbsp.	101	0.2	1	-	1.8
Instant Quaker Oatmeal with Apples & Cinnamon	1 pkg.	120	1.0	130	0	7.5
Instant Quaker Oatmeal with Cinnamon & Spice	1 pkg.	160	2.0	320	0	11.3
Instant Quaker Oatmeal with Maple & Brown Sugar	1 pkg.	150	2.0	320	0	12.0
Instant Quaker Oatmeal with Raisin, Date & Walnut	1 pkg.	140	4.0	220	0	25.7
Instant Quaker Oatmeal with Raisins & Spice	1 pkg.	150	2.0	270	0	12.0

BREAKFAST SECTION

☞ Quaker	S. S.	CAL	FAT(g)	SOD(mg)	CHL(mg)	%FAT
Instant Quaker Oatmeal, Peaches & Cream Flavors	1 pkg.	130	2.0	180	0	13.8
Instant Quaker Oatmeal, Regular Flavor	1 pkg.	90	2.0	270	0	20.0
Instant Quaker Oatmeal, Strawberries & Cream Flavors	1 pkg.	130	2.0	200	0	13.8
Quaker and Mother's Oat Bran	2/3 cup, cooked	90	2.0	0	0	20.0
Quaker and Mother's Whole Wheat Hot Natural Cereal	2/3 cup, cooked	90	1.0	0	0	10.0
Quaker Extra Instant Oatmeal, Apple & Spices	1 pkg.	130	2.0	190	0	13.8
Quaker Extra Instant Oatmeal, Raisin & Spices	1 pkg.	130	2.0	120	0	13.8
Quaker Extra Instant Oatmeal, Regular Flavor	1 pkg.	100	2.0	220	0	18.0
Quaker Oats, Quick and Old Fashioned	2/3 cup, cooked	100	2.0	0	0	18.0

☞ Ralston Purina	S. S.	CAL	FAT(g)	SOD(mg)	CHL(mg)	%FAT
Hot Cereal, High Fiber	1/3 cup, uncooked	90	1.0	0	0	10.0

TOASTER PASTRIES

☞ Kellogg's	S. S.	CAL	FAT(g)	SOD(mg)	CHL(mg)	%FAT
Frosted Pop Tarts Toaster Pastries, Blueberry	1 pastry	210	6.0	210	0	25.7
Frosted Pop Tarts Toaster Pastries, Brown Sugar Cinnamon	1 pastry	210	7.0	190	0	30.0
Frosted Pop Tarts Toaster Pastries, Cherry	1 pastry	200	5.0	220	0	22.5
Frosted Pop Tarts Toaster Pastries, Chocolate Fudge	1 pastry	200	5.0	220	0	22.5
Frosted Pop Tarts Toaster Pastries, Chocolate Vanilla Creme	1 pastry	200	5.0	230	0	22.5
Frosted Pop Tarts Toaster Pastries, Dutch Apple	1 pastry	210	6.0	200	0	25.7
Frosted Pop Tarts Toaster Pastries, Grape	1 pastry	200	5.0	200	0	22.5

☞ Kellogg's	S. S.	CAL	FAT(g)	SOD(mg)	CHL(mg)	%FAT
Frosted Pop Tarts Toaster Pastries, Raspberry	1 pastry	200	5.0	210	0	22.5
Frosted Pop Tarts Toaster Pastries, Strawberry	1 pastry	200	5.0	190	0	22.5
Pop Tarts Toaster Pastries, Blueberry	1 pastry	210	6.0	210	0	25.7
Pop Tarts Toaster Pastries, Cherry	1 pastry	210	6.0	220	0	25.7
Pop Tarts Toaster Pastries, Strawberry	1 pastry	210	6.0	200	0	25.7

☞ Merico	S. S.	CAL	FAT(g)	SOD(mg)	CHL(mg)	%FAT
Toaster Pastry, Apple, Frosted	1 pastry	210	6.0	150	0	25.7
Toaster Pastry, Blueberry	1 pastry	210	6.0	150	0	25.7
Toaster Pastry, Blueberry, Frosted	1 pastry	210	7.0	140	0	30.0
Toaster Pastry, Cherry	1 pastry	210	6.0	260	0	25.7
Toaster Pastry, Cherry, Frosted	1 pastry	210	7.0	150	0	30.0
Toaster Pastry, Cinnamon, Frosted	1 pastry	220	7.0	150	0	28.6
Toaster Pastry, Grape, Frosted	1 pastry	210	7.0	140	0	30.0
Toaster Pastry, Strawberry	1 pastry	210	6.0	125	0	25.7
Toaster Pastry, Strawberry, Frosted	1 pastry	210	7.0	140	0	30.0

☞ Nabisco	S. S.	CAL	FAT(g)	SOD(mg)	CHL(mg)	%FAT
Toastettes, Apple	1 tart	190	5.0	170	0	23.7
Toastettes, Blueberry	1 tart	190	5.0	200	0	23.7
Toastettes, Cherry	1 tart	190	5.0	200	0	23.7
Toastettes, Strawberry	1 tart	190	5.0	200	0	23.7
Toastettes, Frosted, Apple	1 tart	190	5.0	170	0	23.7
Toastettes, Frosted, Blueberry	1 tart	190	5.0	200	0	23.7
Toastettes, Frosted, Brown Sugar Cinnamon	1 tart	190	5.0	180	0	23.7
Toastettes, Frosted, Cherry	1 tart	190	5.0	200	0	23.7
Toastettes, Frosted, Fruit Punch	1 tart	190	5.0	200	0	23.7
Toastettes, Frosted, Fudge	1 tart	200	5.0	280	0	22.5
Toastettes, Frosted, Strawberry	1 tart	190	5.0	200	0	23.7

CANNED GOODS

◆ Canned Vegetables With No Other Added Ingredients Are All Acceptable But May Be High In SODIUM

CANNED BEANS AND TOMATO PRODUCTS

☞ B&M	S. S.	CAL	FAT(g)	SOD(mg)	CHL(mg)	%FAT
Baked Beans, Barbecue	8 oz.	280	4.0	850	5	12.9
Baked Beans, Hot N Spicy	8 oz.	240	3.0	990	<5	11.3
Baked Beans, Maple	8 oz.	240	2.0	890	<5	7.5
Baked Beans, Pea Beans	8 oz.	270	6.0	750	5	20.0
Baked Beans, Red Kidney Beans	8 oz.	240	4.0	680	5	15.0
Baked Beans, Tomato	8 oz.	230	3.0	1010	-	11.7
Baked Beans, Vegetarian, 50 % Less Sodium	8 oz.	230	3.0	370	0	11.7
Baked Beans, with Honey	8 oz.	240	3.0	890	0	11.3
Baked Beans, Yellow Eye Beans	8 oz.	250	5.0	810	5	18.0

☞ Campbell's	S. S.	CAL	FAT(g)	SOD(mg)	CHL(mg)	%FAT
Beans, Barbecue	7 7/8 oz.	210	4.0	900	-	17.1
Beans, Home Style	8 oz.	220	4.0	820	-	16.4
Beans, Hot Chili	7.75 oz.	180	4.0	870	-	20.0
Beans, Old Fashioned in Molasses & Brown Sugar Sauce	8 oz.	230	3.0	730	-	11.7
Beans, Pork & Beans in Tomato Sauce	8 oz.	200	3.0	770	-	13.5
Beans, Vegetarian	7.75 oz.	170	1.0	780	-	5.3

☞ Contadina	S. S.	CAL	FAT(g)	SOD(mg)	CHL(mg)	%FAT
Italian Paste	1/4 cup	65	1.0	520	0	13.8
Pizza Sauce, Original	1/4 cup	30	<1.0	330	0	<30.0

CANNED GOODS

☞ Contadina

	S. S.	CAL	FAT(g)	SOD(mg)	CHL(mg)	%FAT
Pizza Sauce, Pizza Squeeze	1/4 cup	30	<1.0	330	0	<30.0
Pizza Sauce, with Italian Cheese	1/4 cup	30	<1.0	380	0	<30.0

☞ Del Montel

	S. S.	CAL	FAT(g)	SOD(mg)	CHL(mg)	%FAT
Vegetable Classics, Corn and Carrots	1/2 cup	70	2.0	330	-	25.7
Vegetable Classics, Peas and Mushrooms	1/2 cup	70	2.0	430	-	25.7
Vegetable Classics, Santa Fe Style Corn	1/2 cup	90	3.0	370	-	30.0

☞ Friends

	S. S.	CAL	FAT(g)	SOD(mg)	CHL(mg)	%FAT
Baked Beans, Maple	8 oz.	240	2.0	890	<5	7.5
Beans, Red Kidney, with Pork	8 oz.	270	4.0	990	4	13.3
Beans, Pea, Small, with Pork	8 oz.	260	5.0	890	<5	17.3

☞ Hunt

	S. S.	CAL	FAT(g)	SOD(mg)	CHL(mg)	%FAT
Beans, Red Kidney	4 oz.	100	<1.0	400	0	<9.0
Beans, Small Red	4 oz.	90	<1.0	560	0	<10.0
Pork and Beans	4 oz.	135	1.0	430	1	6.7

☞ Progresso

	S. S.	CAL	FAT(g)	SOD(mg)	CHL(mg)	%FAT
Beans, Black	1/2 cup	90	1.0	350	0	10.0
Beans, Cannellini	1/2 cup	80	<1.0	220	0	<11.3
Beans, Chick	1/2 cup	110	1.0	200	0	7.5
Beans, Fava	1/2 cup	90	<1.0	420	-	<10.0
Beans, Pinto	1/2 cup	110	<1.0	410	0	<8.2
Beans, Red Kidney	1/2 cup	100	<1.0	210	0	<9.0
Beans, Roman	1/2 cup	110	<1.0	420	-	<8.2

☞ Ranch Style

	S. S.	CAL	FAT(g)	SOD(mg)	CHL(mg)	%FAT
Beans	7.5 oz.	200	4.0	960	-	18.0
Beans, Dark Red Kidneys	7.5 oz.	170	1.0	900	-	5.3
Beans, Ole Fashioned Navies	7.5 oz.	160	2.0	890	-	11.3
Beans, Pinto with Jalapeño	7.5 oz.	180	2.0	1420	-	10.0
Beans, Premium Pintos	7.5 oz.	160	1.0	890	-	5.6
Blackeye Peas	7.5 oz.	170	2.0	920	-	10.6
Blackeyes with Jalapeño	7.5 oz.	180	2.0	1290	-	10.0

☞ S&W

	S. S.	CAL	FAT(g)	SOD(mg)	CHL(mg)	%FAT
Beans, Barbecue, Texas Style	1/2 cup	135	1.0	550	-	6.7
Beans, Brick Oven Baked	1/2 cup	160	2.0	560	-	11.3
Beans, Butter	1/2 cup	100	1.0	440	-	9.0
Beans, Chili	1/2 cup	130	1.0	520	-	6.9
Beans, Dark Red Kidney	1/2 cup	120	1.0	569	-	7.5
Beans, Dark Red Kidney, Lite, 50% Less Salt	1/2 cup	120	1.0	355	-	7.5
Beans, Garbanzo	1/2 cup	110	1.0	470	-	8.2
Beans, Garbanzo, Lite, 50% Less Salt	1/2 cup	110	1.0	295	-	8.2
Beans, Maple Sugar	1/2 cup	150	1.0	586	-	6.0
Beans, Pork 'N	1/2 cup	130	2.0	135	-	13.8
Beans, Smoky Ranch	1/2 cup	130	2.0	569	-	13.8
Chili Makin's	1/2 cup	100	1.0	782	-	9.0

☞ Van Camp's

	S. S.	CAL	FAT(g)	SOD(mg)	CHL(mg)	%FAT
Beans, Baked	1 cup	260	2.0	1020	-	6.9
Beans, Baked, Deluxe	1 cup	320	4.0	970	-	11.3
Beans, Brown Sugar	1 cup	290	5.1	640	-	15.8
Beans, Butter	1 cup	162	0.5	710	-	2.8
Beans, Kidney, Dark Red	1 cup	182	0.5	830	-	2.5
Beans, Kidney, Light Red	1 cup	184	0.5	650	-	2.4

☞**Van Camp's**	S.S.	CAL	FAT(g)	SOD(mg)	CHL(mg)	%FAT
Beans, Kidney, Red, New Orleans Style	1 cup	178	.6	940	-	3.0
Beans, Mexican Style Chili	1 cup	210	2.4	730	-	10.3
Beans, Red	1 cup	194	0.6	928	-	2.8
Beans, Vegetarian Style	1 cup	206	0.6	950	-	2.6
Pork and Beans	1 cup	216	1.9	1000	0	7.9

CANNED BEAN SALADS

☞**S&W**	S.S.	CAL	FAT(g)	SOD(mg)	CHL(mg)	%FAT
Marinated Garden Salad	1/2 cup	60	0.0	670	-	0.0
Marinated Mixed Bean Salad	1/2 cup	90	1.0	730	-	10.0

CANNED CHILI

☞**Dennison's**	S.S.	CAL	FAT(g)	SOD(mg)	CHL(mg)	%FAT
Lite Chicken Chili	7.5 oz.	190	2.0	870	35	9.5
Lite Chili with Beans	7.5 oz.	180	2.0	890	40	10.0

☞**Hain**	S.S.	CAL	FAT(g)	SOD(mg)	CHL(mg)	%FAT
Chili, Spicy Tempeh	7.5 oz.	160	4.0	1350	0	22.5
Chili, Spicy Vegetarian	7.5 oz.	160	1.0	1060	0	5.6
Chili, Spicy Vegetarian, Reduced Sodium	7.5 oz.	170	1.0	200	0	5.3
Chili, Spicy with Chicken	7.5 oz.	130	2.0	1030	40	13.8

☞**Hunt**	S.S.	CAL	FAT(g)	SOD(mg)	CHL(mg)	%FAT
Manwich Chili Fixins	5.3 oz.	110	<1.0	900	0	<8.2
Manwich Extra Thick and Chunky Sauce	2.5 oz.	60	<1.0	640	0	<15.0
Manwich Mexican	2.5 oz.	60	1.0	460	0	25.7

☞ **Hunt**	S. S.	CAL	FAT(g)	SOD(mg)	CHL(mg)	%FAT
Manwich Sloppy Joe Sauce	2.5 oz.	35	<1.0	390	0	<22.5

CANNED ENTREES

☞ **Chef Boyardee**	S. S.	CAL	FAT(g)	SOD(mg)	CHL(mg)	%FAT
ABC's & 123's in Cheese Flavored Sauce	8.6 oz.	200	1.0	1020	2	4.5
ABC's & 123's in Sauce	7.5 oz.	160	1.0	830	2	5.6
Dinosaurs in Cheese Flavored Sauce	7.5 oz.	160	1.0	790	1	5.6
Lasagna	7.5 oz.	240	8.0	1090	22	30.0
Macaroni Shells	7.5 oz.	150	1.0	930	-	6.0
Mini Cannelloni	7.5 oz.	230	7.0	1050	14	27.4
Mini Ravioli, Beef	7.5 oz.	210	5.0	1140	12	21.4
Pac Man in Tomato Sauce	7.5 oz.	150	1.0	830	2	6.0
Ravioli, Beef, in Tomato and Meat Sauce	7.5 oz.	220	5.0	1120	15	20.5
Ravioli, Cheese, in Beef and Tomato Sauce	7.5 oz.	200	3.0	1205	11	13.5
Ravioli, Cheese, in Tomato Sauce	7.5 oz.	200	5.0	990	5	22.5
Sharks in Cheese Flavored Sauce	7.5 oz.	170	1.0	780	2	5.3
Sharks with Meatballs	7.5 oz.	230	7.0	890	15	27.4
Smurf Beef Ravioli and Pasta with Meat Sauce	7.5 oz.	230	5.0	1160	11	19.6
Smurf in Cheese Flavored Sauce	7.5 oz.	150	1.0	830	2	6.0
Tic Tac Toes in Cheese Flavored Sauce	7.5 oz.	160	1.0	870	-	5.6
Zooroni with Meatballs in Sauce	7.5 oz.	240	8.0	970	17	30.0

☞ **Franco-American**	S. S.	CAL	FAT(g)	SOD(mg)	CHL(mg)	%FAT
Beef Raviolio's in Meat Sauce	7.5 oz.	250	8.0	920	-	28.8
CircusO's Pasta in Tomato and Cheese Sauce	7.63 oz.	170	2.0	860	-	10.6
Spaghetti in Tomato Sauce with Cheese	7.63 oz.	180	2.0	840	-	10.0
SpaghettiO's in Tomato & Cheese Sauce	7.5 oz.	170	2.0	860	-	10.6

CANNED GOODS

☞ Franco-American

	S.S.	CAL	FAT(g)	SOD(mg)	CHL(mg)	%FAT
Sporty0's in Tomato & Cheese Sauce	7.5 oz.	170	2.0	860	-	10.6
Teddy0's in Tomato & Cheese Sauce	7.5 oz.	170	2.0	900	-	10.6

☞ Healthy Choice

	S.S.	CAL	FAT(g)	SOD(mg)	CHL(mg)	%FAT
Beef Stew	7.5 oz.	140	2.0	540	35	12.9
Chili, Spicy with Beans and Ground Turkey	7.5 oz.	210	5.0	530	40	21.4
Chili, Turkey, with Beans	7.5 oz.	200	5.0	560	45	22.5
Lasagna with Meat Sauce	7.5 oz.	220	5.0	530	25	20.5
Soup, Chunky Beef Vegetable	7.5 oz.	110	1.0	490	20	8.2
Soup, Chunky Chicken Noodle & Vegetable	7.5 oz.	160	4.0	500	45	22.5
Spaghetti Rings	7.5 oz.	140	0.0	460	0	0.0
Spaghetti with Meat Sauce	7.5 oz.	150	3.0	390	20	18.0

☞ Hunt's

	S.S.	CAL	FAT(g)	SOD(mg)	CHL(mg)	%FAT
Homestyle, Oriental Style Chicken and Noodles	1 cup	170	4.0	1610	-	21.2
Homestyle, Noodles and Chicken	1 cup	160	4.0	1510	-	22.5
Homestyle, Tomato Sauce with Macaroni and Beef	1 cup	160	4.0	1150	-	22.5
Homestyle, Noodles and Sauce with Beef	1 cup	160	5.0	1280	-	28.1

☞ Sweet Sue

	S.S.	CAL	FAT(g)	SOD(mg)	CHL(mg)	%FAT
Chicken & Dumplings	1 oz.	25	0.8	105	3	29.9
Chicken and Egg Noodles	1 oz.	27	0.4	108	4	14.3
Dumplings with Gravy	1 oz.	20	0.3	45	<1	15.2

☞ **Van Camp's**	S. S.	CAL	FAT(g)	SOD(mg)	CHL(mg)	%FAT
Noodlee Weenee	1 cup	245	8.5	1245	-	31.2
Spaghettee Weenee	1 cup	243	7.4	1128	-	27.4

CANNED FISH AND POULTRY

☞ **Bumble Bee**	S. S.	CAL	FAT(g)	SOD(mg)	CHL(mg)	%FAT
Tuna, Chunk Light In Water	2 oz.	60	1.0	310	30	15.0
Tuna, Chunk White In Water	2 oz.	70	2.0	310	30	25.7
Tuna, Solid White In Water	2 oz.	70	2.0	310	30	25.7

☞ **Chicken of the Sea**	S. S.	CAL	FAT(g)	SOD(mg)	CHL(mg)	%FAT
50% Less Salt Chunk Light	2 oz.	60	1.0	135	-	15.0
Chunk Light Tuna in Spring Water	2 oz.	60	1.0	310	-	15.0
Dietetic Chunk White Tuna	2 oz.	60	1.0	30	-	15.0
Lite-Chunk	2 oz.	70	2.0	310	-	25.7
Pink Salmon	2 oz.	60	2.0	280	-	30.0
Sockeye Red Salmon	2 oz.	60	2.0	280	-	30.0
Solid White Albacore Tuna in Spring Water	2 oz.	60	1.0	310	-	15.0

☞ **Doxsee**	S. S.	CAL	FAT(g)	SOD(mg)	CHL(mg)	%FAT
Chopped Clams, Liquid & Solids	6.5 oz.	90	<1.0	1020	-	<10.0
Clam Juice	3 fl. oz.	4	0.0	110	-	0.0

☞ **Honey Boy**	S. S.	CAL	FAT(g)	SOD(mg)	CHL(mg)	%FAT
Chum Salmon	3.5 oz.	124	4.0	-	65	29.0

☞ Hormel	S.S.	CAL	FAT(g)	SOD(mg)	CHL(mg)	%FAT
Chunk White & Dark Chicken	2.5 oz.	90	3.0	210	45	30.0
Chunk White Turkey	2.5 oz.	70	1.0	390	30	12.9

☞ Progresso	S.S.	CAL	FAT(g)	SOD(mg)	CHL(mg)	%FAT
Minced Clams	1/2 cup	70	<1.0	140	26	<12.9

☞ S & W	S.S.	CAL	FAT(g)	SOD(mg)	CHL(mg)	%FAT
Clams, Fancy Chopped	2 oz.	28	0.0	280	-	0.0
Clams, Fancy Minced	2 oz.	28	0.0	280	-	0.0
Clams, Whole Baby Chowder	2 oz.	33	0.0	-	-	0.0
Crab, Dungeness	3.25 oz.	81	2.0	920	-	22.2
Oysters, Fancy Whole	2 oz.	95	3.0	-	-	28.4
Shrimp, Deveined Medium Whole	2 oz.	65	0.0	-	-	0.0
Tuna, Chunk Light Fancy	2 oz.	60	1.0	500	-	15.0

☞ Snow's	S.S.	CAL	FAT(g)	SOD(mg)	CHL(mg)	%FAT
Minced Clams, Liquid & Solids	6.5 oz.	90	<1.0	1020	-	<10.0

☞ StarKist	S.S.	CAL	FAT(g)	SOD(mg)	CHL(mg)	%FAT
Tuna, Chunk Light in Pure Distilled Water, Diet	6.13 oz.	35	<1.0	35	25	<25.7
Tuna, Chunk Light in Spring Water	6.13 oz.	60	<1.0	250	25	<15.0
Tuna, Chunk Light in Spring Water, 60% Less Salt	6.13 oz.	65	1.0	120	25	13.8
Tuna, Chunk Light in Spring Water, Hickory Smoke Flavor	6.13 oz.	50	<1.0	250	25	<18.0
Tuna, Chunk Light in Spring Water, Weight Watchers, No Salt Added	6.13 oz.	60	<1.0	210	25	<15.0

☞ **StarKist**	S. S.	CAL	FAT(g)	SOD(mg)	CHL(mg)	%FAT
Tuna, Chunk White in Pure Distilled Water, Diet	6.13 oz.	70	1.0	35	25	12.9
Tuna, Chunk White in Spring Water, 60% Less Salt	6.13 oz.	70	<1.0	120	25	<12.9
Tuna, Solid Light in Spring Water	6.13 oz.	60	<1.0	250	25	<15.0
Tuna, Solid Light in Spring Water, Prime Catch	6.13 oz.	60	<1.0	250	25	<15.0
Tuna, Solid White in Spring Water	6.13 oz.	70	1.0	250	25	12.9
Tuna, Solid White in Spring Water, Weight Watchers, No Salt Added	6.13 oz.	70	1.0	210	25	12.9

☞ **Swanson**	S. S.	CAL	FAT(g)	SOD(mg)	CHL(mg)	%FAT
Premium Chunk White and Dark Turkey	2.5 oz.	90	3.0	280	-	30.0
Premium Chunk White Turkey	2.5 oz.	80	1.0	260	-	11.3

CANNED AND PACKAGED SOUPS

☞ **Campbell's**	S. S.	CAL	FAT(g)	SOD(mg)	CHL(mg)	%FAT
Chunky, Bean with Ham Old Fashioned	9 5/8 oz.	250	8.0	960	-	28.8
Chunky, Beef	9.5 oz.	170	4.0	970	-	21.2
Chunky, Beef	10.75 oz.	200	5.0	1100	-	22.5
Chunky, Chicken Nuggets with Vegetables & Noodles	10.75 oz.	190	6.0	1060	-	28.4
Chunky, Chicken with Rice	9.5 oz.	140	4.0	1060	-	25.7
Chunky, Chicken, Old Fashioned	9.5 oz.	150	4.0	1070	-	24.0
Chunky, Chicken, Old Fashioned	10.75 oz.	180	5.0	1220	-	25.0
Chunky, Chili Beef	9.5 oz.	260	6.0	990	-	20.8
Chunky, Chili Beef	11 oz.	290	7.0	1120	-	21.7
Chunky, Clam Chowder, Manhattan Style	9.5 oz.	150	4.0	980	-	24.0
Chunky, Clam Chowder, Manhattan Style	10.75 oz.	160	4.0	1110	-	22.5
Chunky, Creole Style	9.5 oz.	220	7.0	800	-	28.6
Chunky, Creole Style	10.75 oz.	240	8.0	910	-	30.0
Chunky, Minestrone	9.5 oz.	160	4.0	870	-	22.5

CANNED GOODS

☞ **Campbell's**	S. S.	CAL	FAT(g)	SOD(mg)	CHL(mg)	%FAT
Chunky, Peppersteak	9.5 oz.	160	3.0	920	-	16.9
Chunky, Peppersteak	10.75 oz.	180	3.0	1050	-	15.0
Chunky, Split Pea with Ham	9.5 oz.	210	5.0	950	-	21.4
Chunky, Split Pea with Ham	10.75 oz.	230	6.0	1080	-	23.5
Chunky, Steak and Potato	9.5 oz.	170	4.0	1000	-	21.2
Chunky, Steak and Potato	10.75 oz.	200	5.0	1140	-	22.5
Chunky, Vegetable	9.5 oz.	150	4.0	970	-	24.0
Chunky, Vegetable	10.75 oz.	160	4.0	1100	-	22.5
Chunky, Vegetable Beef, Old Fashioned	9.5 oz.	160	5.0	970	-	28.1
Chunky, Vegetable Beef, Old Fashioned	10.75 oz.	190	6.0	1100	-	28.4
Condensed Soup, Bean with Bacon	8 oz.	140	4.0	840	-	25.7
Condensed Soup, Bean, Homestyle	8 oz.	130	1.0	700	-	6.9
Condensed Soup, Beef	8 oz.	80	2.0	830	-	22.5
Condensed Soup, Beef Broth (Bouillon)	8 oz.	16	0.0	820	-	0.0
Condensed Soup, Chicken & Stars	8 oz.	60	2.0	870	-	30.0
Condensed Soup, Chicken Barley	8 oz.	70	2.0	850	-	25.7
Condensed Soup, Chicken Broth & Noodles	8 oz.	45	1.0	860	-	20.0
Condensed Soup, Chicken Gumbo	8 oz.	60	2.0	900	-	30.0
Condensed Soup, Chicken Noodle	8 oz.	60	2.0	900	-	30.0
Condensed Soup, Chicken Noodle-O's	8 oz.	70	2.0	820	-	25.7
Condensed Soup, Clam Chowder, Manhattan Style	8 oz.	70	2.0	820	-	25.7
Condensed Soup, Consommé	8 oz.	25	0.0	750	-	0.0
Condensed Soup, Cream of Tomato, Homestyle	8 oz.	110	3.0	810	-	24.5
Condensed Soup, French Onion	8 oz.	60	2.0	900	-	30.0
Condensed Soup, Green Pea	8 oz.	160	3.0	820	-	16.9
Condensed Soup, Minestrone	8 oz.	80	2.0	900	-	22.5
Condensed Soup, Potato (half milk, half water)	8 oz.	120	4.0	900	-	30.0
Condensed Soup, Special Request, Bean with Bacon	8 oz.	140	4..0	470	-	25.7
Condensed Soup, Special Request, Chicken Noodle	8 oz.	60	2.0	440	-	30.0
Condensed Soup, Special Request, Tomato	8 oz.	90	2.0	430	-	20.0

☞ **Campbell's**	S. S.	CAL	FAT(g)	SOD(mg)	CHL(mg)	%FAT
Condensed Soup, Special Request, Tomato (2% milk)	8 oz.	150	4.0	490	-	24.0
Condensed Soup, Special Request, Vegetable	8 oz.	90	2.0	500	-	20.0
Condensed Soup, Special Request, Vegetable Beef	8 oz.	70	2.0	470	-	25.7
Condensed Soup, Split Pea with Ham & Bacon	8 oz.	160	4.0	780	-	22.5
Condensed Soup, Teddy Bear	8 oz.	70	2.0	790	-	25.7
Condensed Soup, Tomato	8 oz.	90	2.0	680	-	20.0
Condensed Soup, Tomato (2% milk)	8 oz.	150	4.0	740	-	24.0
Condensed Soup, Tomato Bisque	8 oz.	120	3.0	820	-	22.5
Condensed Soup, Tomato, Old Fashioned	8 oz.	110	2.0	730	-	16.4
Condensed Soup, Turkey Noodle	8 oz.	70	2.0	880	-	25.7
Condensed Soup, Vegetable	8 oz.	90	2.0	830	-	20.0
Condensed Soup, Vegetable Beef	8 oz.	70	2.0	780	-	25.7
Condensed Soup, Vegetable, Homestyle	8 oz.	60	2.0	880	-	30.0
Condensed Soup, Vegetable, Old Fashioned	8 oz.	60	2.0	880	-	30.0
Condensed Soup, Vegetable, Vegetarian	8 oz.	80	2.0	790	-	22.5
Condensed Soup, Won Ton	8 oz.	40	1.0	850	-	22.5
Condensed Soup, Zesty Tomato	8 oz.	100	2.0	760	-	18.0
Cup 2 Minute Soup Mix, Chicken Noodle with White Meat	6 oz.	90	2.0	770	-	20.0
Cup 2 Minute Soup Mix, Noodle with Chicken Broth	6 oz.	90	2.0	910	-	20.0
Healthy Request, Bean with Bacon	8 oz.	140	4.0	470	5	25.7
Healthy Request, Chicken Noodle	8 oz.	60	2.0	460	15	30.0
Healthy Request, Chicken with Rice	8 oz.	60	2.0	480	10	30.0
Healthy Request, Cream of Mushroom	8 oz.	60	2.0	460	<5	30.0
Healthy Request, Hearty Chicken Noodle	8 oz.	80	2.0	470	25	22.5
Healthy Request, Hearty Minestrone	8 oz.	90	3.0	430	<2	30.0
Healthy Request, Hearty Vegetable	8 oz.	110	3.0	480	0	24.5
Healthy Request, Hearty Vegetable Beef	8 oz.	120	3.0	490	15	22.5

CANNED GOODS

☞ Campbell's	S. S.	CAL	FAT(g)	SOD(mg)	CHL(mg)	%FAT
Healthy Request, Tomato (made with skim milk)	8 oz.	130	2.0	490	<5	13.8
Healthy Request, Tomato (made with water)	8 oz.	90	2.0	220	430	20.0
Healthy Request, Vegetable	8 oz.	90	2.0	500	<5	20.0
Healthy Request, Vegetable Beef	8 oz.	70	2.0	490	5	25.7
Home Cookin', Bean with Bacon	10.75 oz.	210	4.0	1000	-	17.1
Home Cookin', Beef with Vegetables and Pasta	10.75 oz.	140	2.0	1060	-	12.9
Home Cookin', Chicken Gumbo with Sausage	10.75 oz.	140	4.0	1090	-	25.7
Home Cookin', Chicken Minestrone	10.75 oz.	180	6.0	950	-	30.0
Home Cookin', Chicken with Noodles	10.75 oz.	140	4.0	1150	-	25.7
Home Cookin', Country Vegetable	10.75 oz.	120	2.0	1070	-	15.0
Home Cookin', Hearty Lentil	10.75 oz.	170	2.0	930	-	10.6
Home Cookin', Minestrone	10.75 oz.	140	3.0	1220	-	19.3
Home Cookin', Split Pea with Ham	10.75 oz.	230	1.0	1310	-	3.9
Home Cookin', Tomato Garden	10.75 oz.	150	3.0	930	-	18.0
Home Cookin', Vegetable Beef	10.75 oz.	140	3.0	1160	-	19.3
Low Fat Block Ramen Noodle Soup, Beef flavor	8 oz.	160	1.0	890	-	5.6
Low Fat Block Ramen Noodle Soup, Chicken flavor	8 oz.	160	1.0	940	-	5.6
Low Fat Block Ramen Noodle Soup, Oriental flavor	8 oz.	150	1.0	940	-	6.0
Low Fat Block Ramen Noodle Soup, Pork flavor	8 oz.	150	1.0	1140	-	6.0
Low Fat Cup-A-Ramen, Beef flavor with Vegetables	8 oz.	220	2.0	1600	-	8.2
Low Fat Cup-A-Ramen, Chicken flavor with Vegetables	8 oz.	220	2.0	1500	-	8.2
Low Fat Cup-A-Ramen, Oriental flavor with Vegetables	8 oz.	220	2.0	1400	-	8.2
Low Fat Cup-A-Ramen, Shrimp flavor with Vegetables	8 oz.	230	2.0	1290	-	7.8
Low Sodium, Chicken Broth	10.5 oz.	30	1.0	85	-	30.0
Low Sodium, Chicken with Noodles	10.75 oz.	170	5.0	90	-	26.5
Low Sodium, Chunky Vegetable Beef	10.75 oz.	180	5.0	90	-	25.0
Low Sodium, Split Pea	10.75 oz.	230	4.0	30	-	15.7

☞ Campbell's	S. S.	CAL	FAT(g)	SOD(mg)	CHL(mg)	%FAT
Low Sodium, Tomato with Tomato Pieces	10.5 oz.	190	3.0	45	-	14.2
Microwavable Cup Soup, Beef flavor Noodle	1.35 oz.	130	2.0	1270	-	13.8
Microwavable Cup Soup, Chicken flavor Noodle	1.35 oz.	140	3.0	1340	-	19.3
Microwavable Cup Soup, Hearty Noodle with Vegetables	1.7 oz.	180	2.0	1320	-	10.0
Microwavable Cup Soup, Noodle Soup with Broth	1.35 oz.	130	2.0	1360	-	13.8
Quality Soup and Recipe Mix, Chicken Noodle	8 oz.	100	2.0	710	-	18.0
Quality Soup and Recipe Mix, Hearty Noodle	8 oz.	90	1.0	840	-	10.0
Quality Soup and Recipe Mix, Noodle	8 oz.	110	2.0	700	-	16.4
Quality Soup and Recipe Mix, Onion	8 oz.	30	0.0	700	-	0.0
Quality Soup and Recipe Mix, Vegetable	8 oz.	40	0.0	710	-	0.0

☞ College Inn	S. S.	CAL	FAT(g)	SOD(mg)	CHL(mg)	%FAT
Broth, Beef	1/2 can	16	0	960	0	0.0

☞ Hain	S. S.	CAL	FAT(g)	SOD(mg)	CHL(mg)	%FAT
Chicken Vegetable	8 oz.	110	3.0	790	10	24.5
Chicken Vegetable, No Salt Added	8 oz.	100	3.0	85	10	27.0
Creamy Mushroom	9.5 oz.	120	4.0	900	5	30.0
Italian Vege-Pasta	9.5 oz.	160	5.0	910	20	28.1
Italian Vege-Pasta, Low Sodium	9.5 oz.	150	5.0	90	20	30.0
Minestrone	9.5 oz.	170	3.0	930	0	15.9
Minestrone, No Salt Added	9.5 oz.	160	4.0	75	0	22.5
Mushroom Barley	9.5 oz.	80	2.0	780	5	22.5
New England Clam Chowder	9.25 oz.	150	4.0	780	15	24.0
Soup Mix, Lentil Savory	3/4 cup	130	2.0	810	8	13.8
Soup Mix, Minestrone Savory	3/4 cup	110	1.0	870	6	8.2

☞ Hain

	S. S.	CAL	FAT(g)	SOD(mg)	CHL(mg)	%FAT
Soup Mix, Onion Savory	3/4 cup	50	2.0	900	2	36.0
Soup Mix, Onion Savory, No Added Salt	3/4 cup	50	1.0	470	2	18.0
Soup Mix, Vegetable Savory	3/4 cup	80	1.0	730	-	11.3
Soup Mix, Vegetable Savory, No Added Salt	3/4 cup	80	1.0	330	-	11.3
Vegetable Broth	9.5 oz.	45	0.0	600	0	0.0
Vegetable Broth, Low Sodium	9.5 oz.	40	0.0	85	0	0.0
Vegetable Split Pea	9.5 oz.	170	1.0	970	0	5.3
Vegetable Split Pea, No Salt Added	9.5 oz.	170	1.0	70	0	5.3
Vegetarian Lentil	9.5 oz.	160	3.0	690	0	16.9
Vegetarian Lentil, No Salt Added	9.5 oz.	160	3.0	65	0	16.9
Vegetarian Vegetable	9.5 oz.	150	4.0	790	0	24.0
Vegetarian Vegetable, No Salt Added	9.5 oz.	150	5.0	80	0	30.0

☞ Healthy Choice

	S. S.	CAL	FAT(g)	SOD(mg)	CHL(mg)	%FAT
Bean and Ham	7.5 oz.	220	4.0	480	5	16.5
Chicken Noodle, Old Fashioned	7.5 oz.	160	2.0	520	0	11.3
Chicken with Rice	7.5 oz.	140	4.0	510	15	25.7
Chunky Beef Vegetable	7.5 oz.	110	1.0	490	20	8.2
Chunky Chicken Noodle & Vegetable	7.5 oz.	160	4.0	500	45	22.5
Country Vegetable	7.5 oz.	120	1.0	540	0	7.5
Hearty Beef	7.5 oz.	120	1.0	580	20	7.5
Hearty Chicken	7.5 oz.	150	5.0	530	35	30.0
Minestrone	7.5 oz.	160	2.0	520	0	11.3
Split Pea and Ham	7.5 oz.	170	3.0	460	10	15.9
Tomato Garden	7.5 oz.	130	3.0	510	5	20.8
Vegetable Beef	7.5 oz.	130	1.0	530	15	6.9

☞ Knorr

	S. S.	CAL	FAT(g)	SOD(mg)	CHL(mg)	%FAT
Soup Mix, Cauliflower	1 cup	100	3.0	750	-	27.0

☞Knorr	S. S.	CAL	FAT(g)	SOD(mg)	CHL(mg)	%FAT
Soup Mix, Chick 'n Pasta	1 cup	90	2.0	850	-	20.0
Soup Mix, Chicken Flavored Noodle	1 cup	100	2.0	720	-	18.0
Soup Mix, Country Barley	1 cup	120	2.0	940	-	15.0
Soup Mix, French Onion	1 cup	50	1.0	970	-	18.0
Soup Mix, Hearty Minestrone	1 cup	130	2.0	940	-	13.8
Soup Mix, Oxtail Hearty Beef	1 cup	70	2.0	1120	-	25.7
Soup Mix, Tomato Basil	1 cup	90	3.0	940	-	30.0
Soup Mix, Vegetable	1 cup	35	1.0	840	-	25.7

☞Lipton	S. S.	CAL	FAT(g)	SOD(mg)	CHL(mg)	%FAT
Cup-A-Soup, Chicken 'N Rice	3/4 cup	47	0.8	667	-	15.4
Cup-A-Soup, Chicken Flavored Broth	3/4 cup	20	0.6	605	1	27.7
Cup-A-Soup, Chicken Noodle	3/4 cup	48	1.1	671	-	20.6
Cup-A-Soup, Chicken Noodle with Chicken Meat	3/4 cup	46	1.0	660	-	19.5
Cup-A-Soup, Chicken Vegetable	3/4 cup	47	0.6	566	8	11.5
Cup-A-Soup, Country Style Harvest Vegetable	3/4 cup	91	1.2	459	-	11.9
Cup-A-Soup, Country Style Hearty Chicken	3/4 cup	69	1.1	688	-	14.4
Cup-A-Soup, Hearty Chicken Flavor and Noodles	3/4 cup	110	1.6	587	-	13.1
Cup-A-Soup, Lite Chicken Florentine	3/4 cup	42	0.5	481	6	10.6
Cup-A-Soup, Lite Creamy Tomato and Herb	3/4 cup	66	0.3	305	2	4.1
Cup-A-Soup, Lite Golden Broccoli	3/4 cup	42	1.2	427	1	26.0
Cup-A-Soup, Lite Lemon Chicken	3/4 cup	48	0.4	419	4	7.6
Cup-A-Soup, Lots-A-Noodles, Garden Vegetable	7/8 cup	123	1.5	720	-	10.9
Cup-A-Soup, Onion	3/4 cup	27	0.5	665	0	16.6
Cup-A-Soup, Ring Noodle	3/4 cup	47	0.7	650	-	13.4
Cup-A-Soup, Spring Vegetable	3/4 cup	33	0.8	746	6	21.9
Cup-A-Soup, Tomato	3/4 cup	103	0.9	524	-	7.9
Soup Mix, Beef Flavor Mushroom	8 oz.	38	0.5	763	-	11.9
Soup Mix, Beefy Onion	8 oz.	24	0.7	639	0	25.8

CANNED GOODS

☞ Lipton	S. S.	CAL	FAT(g)	SOD(mg)	CHL(mg)	%FAT
Soup Mix, Chicken Noodle	8 oz.	82	1.8	702	-	19.8
Soup Mix, Chicken Noodle with Diced White Chicken	8 oz.	81	1.8	795	-	20.1
Soup Mix, Country Vegetable	8 oz.	80	0.7	803	0	7.9
Soup Mix, Giggle Noodle Soup with Real Chicken Broth	8 oz.	72	1.6	708	-	20.0
Soup Mix, Golden Onion with Real Chicken Broth	8 oz.	62	1.5	716	-	21.8
Soup Mix, Hearty Chicken Noodle	8 oz.	83	1.3	753	-	14.2
Soup Mix, Hearty Noodle with Vegetables	8 oz.	75	1.6	687	-	19.1
Soup Mix, Instant, Beef Oriental	1 cup	177	0.8	912	-	4.1
Soup Mix, Instant, Chicken Oriental Noodle	1 cup	180	1.7	785	-	8.5
Soup Mix, Instant, Garden Vegetable Oriental	1 cup	199	1.0	915	-	4.5
Soup Mix, Instant, Oriental Noodle	1 cup	198	1.3	781	-	5.9
Soup Mix, Noodle with Real Chicken Broth	8 oz.	62	1.5	708	-	21.6
Soup Mix, Onion	8 oz.	20	0.2	632	-	9.0
Soup Mix, Onion Mushroom	8 oz.	41	0.9	683	0	19.9
Soup Mix, Ring-O-Noodle with Real Chicken Broth	8 oz.	67	1.5	708	-	20.3
Soup Mix, Vegetable	8 oz.	39	0.5	640	-	11.7

☞ Pritikin	S. S.	CAL	FAT(g)	SOD(mg)	CHL(mg)	%FAT
Chicken	7.25 oz.	80	1.0	170	5	11.3
Chicken Broth	6.85 oz.	12	0.0	135	0	0.0
Chicken Gumbo	7.38 oz.	60	1.0	180	5	15.0
Chicken Vegetable	7.25 oz.	60	1.0	150	5	15.0
Lentil	7.38 oz.	80	0	160	0	0.0
Minestrone	7.38 oz.	70	0.0	120	0	0.0
Navy Bean	7.38 oz.	90	<1.0	160	0	<10.0
Split Pea	7.4 oz.	120	<1.0	160	0	<7.5
Tomato	7.25 oz.	70	0.0	135	0	0.0
Turkey Vegetable	7.38 oz.	50	<1.0	160	5	<18.0
Vegetable	7.38 oz.	60	0.0	120	0	0..0

☞ Progresso	S. S.	CAL	FAT(g)	SOD(mg)	CHL(mg)	%FAT
Beef Barley	9.5 oz.	140	4.0	780	30	25.7
Beef Minestrone	9.5 oz.	170	5.0	910	-	26.5
Beef Noodle	9.5 oz.	170	4.0	1030	40	21.2
Beef Vegetable	9.5 oz.	150	3.0	790	-	18.0
Chicken Barley	9.25 oz.	100	2.0	710	20	18.0
Chicken Broth	4 oz.	8	0.0	360	<5	0.0
Chicken Minestrone	9.5 oz.	130	3.0	870	20	20.8
Chicken Noodle	9.5 oz.	120	4.0	920	35	30.0
Chicken Rice	9.5 oz.	130	3.0	750	20	20.8
Chicken Vegetable	9.5 oz.	140	4.0	710	25	25.7
Escarole in Chicken Broth	9.5 oz.	30	1.0	1100	<5	30.0
Green Split Pea	9.5 oz.	160	3.0	1050	<5	16.9
Ham and Bean	9.5 oz.	140	2.0	950	10	12.9
Hearty Beef	9.5 oz.	160	4.0	820	35	22.5
Hearty Chicken	9.5 oz.	130	4.0	960	30	27.7
Hearty Minestrone	9.25 oz.	110	2.0	740	<5	16.4
Home Style Chicken	9.5 oz.	110	3.0	740	20	24.5
Lentil	9.5 oz.	140	4.0	840	0	25.7
Manhattan Clam Chowder	9.5 oz.	120	2.0	1050	-	15.0
Minestrone	9.5 oz.	130	4.0	1010	0	27.7
Split Pea with Ham	9.5 oz.	150	5.0	880	15	30.0
Tomato	9.5 oz.	110	3.0	1140	0	24.5
Tortellini	9.5 oz.	90	3.0	840	10	30.0
Vegetable	9.5 oz.	90	2.0	1190	<5	20.0

COOKIES

COOKIES

☞ Archway	S. S.	CAL	FAT(g)	SOD(mg)	CHL(mg)	%FAT
Apricot Filled	1	100	3.0	80	5	27.0
Blueberry Filled	1	100	3.0	90	5	27.0
Cherry Filled	1	100	3.0	90	0	27.0
Cinnamon Apple	1	100	3.0	140	5	24.0
Date Filled Oatmeal	1	100	3.0	100	5	27.0
Dutch Cocoa	1	100	3.0	95	5	27.0
Fruit 'N Honey	1	100	3.0	120	5	27.0
Gingersnaps	1	35	1.0	30	0	25.7
Lemon Drop	1	85	2.0	110	5	21.2
Molasses	1	110	3.0	160	10	24.5
Molasses, Old Fashioned	1	120	3.0	140	5	22.5
Oatmeal	1	110	3.0	100	5	24.5
Oatmeal Bran, Apple	1	105	3.0	115	5	25.7
Oatmeal Bran, Apricot	1	105	2.0	115	5	17.1
Oatmeal Bran, Bluberry	1	105	3.0	110	5	25.7
Oatmeal Bran, Rasberry	1	105	3.0	110	5	25.7
Oatmeal, Apple Filled	1	100	3.0	110	5	27.0
Oatmeal, Raisin Bran	1	110	3.0	85	0	24.5
Raspberry Filled	1	100	3.0	80	5	27.0
Soft Sugar Drop	1	90	3.0	90	5	30.0
Strawberry Filled	1	100	3.0	90	5	27.0
Sugar	1	100	3.0	130	0	27.0
Vanilla Wafer	1	30	1.0	30	0	30.0
Windmill	1	140	3.0	135	0	19.3

☞ Barbara's Bakery	S. S.	CAL	FAT(g)	SOD(mg)	CHL(mg)	%FAT
California Lemon & Orange	2	39	1.0	-	-	23.1
Chocolate & Vanilla Crisps	0.5 oz.	70	2.0	-	0	25.7
Fruit & Nut	2	125	2.0	-	0	14.4

COOKIES

COOKIES

☞ Barbara's Bakery

	S. S.	CAL	FAT(g)	SOD(mg)	CHL(mg)	%FAT
Ginger Snaps	2	39	1.0	-	-	23.1
Oatmeal Raisin	2	102	2.0	-	0	17.6
Tropical Coconut	2	64	2.0	-	0	28.1

☞ Break Cake

	S. S.	CAL	FAT(g)	SOD(mg)	CHL(mg)	%FAT
Apple Sandwich Cakes	1	90	3.0	70	5	30.0
Hermit Cookie	1	230	7.0	280	10	27.4
Marshmallow Pie, Banana	1	150	5.0	80	0	30.0
Marshmallow Pie, Chocolate	1	150	5.0	70	0	30.0
Marshmallow Pie, Devil's Food	1	140	4.0	85	-	25.7
Marshmallow Pie, Double Decker Chocolate	1	360	11.0	170	-	27.5

☞ FFV

	S. S.	CAL	FAT(g)	SOD(mg)	CHL(mg)	%FAT
Animal Crackers	9	130	4.0	120	0	27.7
Bars, Fig	1	110	3.0	95	0	24.5
Bars, Fig, Whole Wheat	1	130	3.0	100	0	20.8
Bars, Oatmeal Apple	1	70	2.0	55	0	25.7
Bars, Peach Apricot	1	70	1.0	50	0	12.9
Bars, Peach Apricot, Whole Wheat	1	130	3.0	100	0	20.8
Bars, Raspberry, Oat Bran	1	150	5.0	100	0	30.0
Cookies, Oatmeal	5	130	4.0	150	3	27.7
Devilsfood Trolley Cakes	2	120	2.0	80	-	15.0
Ginger Boys	7	120	4.0	170	0	30.0
Ginger Snaps	5	130	4.0	140	0	27.7
Jelly Tarts	1	60	2.0	55	0	30.0
Royal Kreem Pilot Bread	1	60	2.0	60	-	30.0
Tango	2	160	5.0	50	-	28.1

☞ Grandma's	S. S.	CAL	FAT(g)	SOD(mg)	CHL(mg)	%FAT
Old Time Molasses	2	320	9.0	520	5	25.3
Soft Raisin	2	320	10.0	280	10	28.1

☞ Keebler	S. S.	CAL	FAT(g)	SOD(mg)	CHL(mg)	%FAT
Alpha Graham Cookies	6	70	2.0	55	0	25.7
Baby Bear Cookies	3	70	2.0	55	0	25.7
Danish Wedding Cookies	2	60	2.0	40	0	30.0
Fig Bars	1	60	2.0	70	0	30.0
Grahams, Cinnamon Crisp	4	70	2.0	85	0	25.7
Iced Animal Cookies	3	70	2.0	65	0	25.7

☞ LU	S. S.	CAL	FAT(g)	SOD(mg)	CHL(mg)	%FAT
Crokine	2	37	0.0	70	-	0.0
Maria LU Whole Wheat & Cinnamon	1	45	1.0	55	-	20.0
Petit Beurre	1	40	1.0	45	-	22.5
Pims	2	97	2.4	25	-	22.3

☞ Mother's	S. S.	CAL	FAT(g)	SOD(mg)	CHL(mg)	%FAT
Bakery Wagon, Apple Cinnamon	1	100	3.0	100	2	27.0
Bakery Wagon, Apple Walnut Raisin	1	100	3.0	110	2	27.0
Bakery Wagon, Date Filled Oatmeal	1	90	3.0	100	2	30.0
Bakery Wagon, Honey Fruit Bar	1	100	3.0	70	2	27.0
Bakery Wagon, Oatmeal Chocolate Chunk	1	100	3.0	80	2	27.0
Bakery Wagon, Raspberry Filled	1	90	3.0	125	2	30.0
Dinosaur Grrrahams, Original	1	72	2.0	52	-	25.0
Fig Bars	2	112	2.0	86	-	16.1
Fig Bars, Whole Wheat	2	122	2.0	103	-	14.8
Mini Dinosaur, Chocolate	7	70	2.0	45	-	25.7

COOKIES

☞ **Mother's**	S.S.	CAL	FAT(g)	SOD(mg)	CHL(mg)	%FAT
Mini Dinosaur, Cinnamon	7	70	2.0	40	-	25
Mini Dinosaur, Original	7	60	1.0	40	-	15.0

☞ **Nabisco**	S.S.	CAL	FAT(g)	SOD(mg)	CHL(mg)	%FAT
Barnum's Animal Crackers	5	60	2.0	70	0	30.0
Bugs Bunny Graham Cookies	5	60	2.0	70	0	30.0
Chocolate Chip Snaps	3	70	2.0	50	0	25.7
Chocolate Snaps	4	70	2.0	75	<2	25.7
Devils Food Cakes	1	70	1.0	40	0	12.9
Famous Chocolate Wafers	2 1/2	70	2.0	110	<2	25.7
Ginger Snaps, Old Fashioned	2	60	1.0	80	0	15.0
Honey Maid Cinnamon Grahams	2	60	1.0	85	0	15.0
Honey Maid Honey Grahams	2	60	1.0	90	0	15.0
Newtons, Apple	1	70	2.0	70	0	25.7
Newtons, Fig	1	60	1.0	60	0	15.0
Newtons, Raspberry	1	70	2.0	70	0	25.7
Newtons, Strawberry	1	70	2.0	70	0	25.7
Newtons, Variety Pack	1	120	3.0	110	0	22.5
Nilla Wafers	3 1/2	60	2.0	45	<5	30.0
SnackWell's Cinnamon Graham Snacks	4	50	0.0	50	0	0.0
Snack Well's Chocolate Chip Cookies (bite size)	6	60	1.0	85	0	15.0
SnackWell's Devil's Food Cookie Cake	1	60	0.0	30	0	0.0
Snack Well's Oatmeal Raisin Cookies	1	60	1.0	65	0	15.0
Social Tea Biscuits	3	70	2.0	60	<5	25.7
Teddy Grahams, Chocolate Graham Snacks	11	60	2.0	90	0	30.0
Teddy Grahams, Cinnamon Graham Snacks	11	60	2.0	90	0	30.0
Teddy Grahams, Honey Graham Snacks	11	60	2.0	90	0	30.0
Teddy Grahams, Vanilla Graham Snacks	11	60	2.0	75	0	30.0

COOKIES

☞ **Peak Freans**	S. S.	CAL	FAT(g)	SOD(mg)	CHL(mg)	%FAT
Arrowroot	1	38	0.0	0	-	0.0
Ginger Crisp	1	39	0.0	0	-	0.0
Golden Sugar Biscuits with Currants	1	79	0.0	0	-	0.0

☞ **Pepperidge Farm**	S. S.	CAL	FAT(g)	SOD(mg)	CHL(mg)	%FAT
Distinctive Cookies, Chantilly	1	80	2.0	35	<5	22.5
Distinctive Cookies, Linzer	1	120	4.0	55	<5	30.0
Distinctive Cookies, Zurich	1	60	2.0	30	0	30.0
Wholesome Choice, Apple Oatmeal Tart	1	70	2.0	45	0	22.0
Wholesome Choice, Carrot Walnut	1	60	1.0	45	0	18.0
Wholesome Choice, Cranberry Honey	1	60	2.0	50	0	25.0
Wholesome Choice, Date Walnut	1	60	2.0	45	0	28.0
Wholesome Choice, Oatmeal Raisin	1	60	1.0	50	0	17.0
Wholesome Choice, Raspberry Tart	1	70	2.0	35	0	21.0

☞ **R.W. Frookie**	S. S.	CAL	FAT(g)	SOD(mg)	CHL(mg)	%FAT
Animal Frackers	6	60	2.0	25	0	30.0
Animal Frackers, Chocolate	6	60	2.0	25	0	30.0
Apple Spice, Fat Free	1	50	0.0	80	0	0.0
Oatmeal Raisin, Fat Free	1	50	0.0	75	0	0.0

☞ **Salerno**	S. S.	CAL	FAT(g)	SOD(mg)	CHL(mg)	%FAT
Dinosaur Grrrahams	1	70	2.0	50	0	25.7

☞ **Stella D'oro**	S. S.	CAL	FAT(g)	SOD(mg)	CHL(mg)	%FAT
Almond Toast (Mendel)	1	60	1.0	-	0	15.0

COOKIES

☞ Stella D'oro	S. S.	CAL	FAT(g)	SOD(mg)	CHL(mg)	%FAT
Anginetti	1	30	1.0	-	0	30.0
Anisette Sponge	1	50	1.0	-	0	18.0
Anisette Toast	1	50	1.0	-	0	18.0
Anisette Toast, Jumbo	1	110	1.0	-	0	8.2
Breadsticks, Onion	1	40	1.0	-	0	22.5
Breadsticks, Pizza	1	45	1.0	-	0	20.0
Breadsticks, Regular	1	40	1.0	55	0	22.5
Breadsticks, Sesame	1	50	2.0	43	0	36.0
Breadsticks, Wheat	1	40	1.0	-	0	22.5
Dutch Apple Bars	1	110	3.0	-	1	24.5
Egg Biscuits, Sugared	1	80	1.0	-	1	11.3
Egg Jumbo	1	50	1.0	-	0	18.0
Fruit Slices	1	60	2.0	-	0	30.0

☞ Sunshine	S. S.	CAL	FAT(g)	SOD(mg)	CHL(mg)	%FAT
Animal Crackers	13	130	4.0	160	0	27.7
Fig Bars	1	50	1.0	35	<2	18.0
Ginger Snaps	5	100	3.0	120	0	27.0
Golden Fruit Raisin Biscuits	1	70	1.0	40	<2	12.9
Graham, Honey	1	60	2.0	90	0	30.0
Grahamy Bears	4	60	2.0	55	0	30.0
Oatmeal Cookies, Country Style	1	60	2.0	55	0	30.0

CRACKERS

CRACKERS

☞**Bremner**	S. S.	CAL	FAT(g)	SOD(mg)	CHL(mg)	%FAT
Wafers, Plain	14	119	3.3	165	0	25.0

☞**Carr's**	S. S.	CAL	FAT(g)	SOD(mg)	CHL(mg)	%FAT
Crackers, Whole Wheat	2	70	1.0	15	-	12.9
Wheatmeal Biscuits	2	70	1.0	15	-	12.9

☞**Devonsheer**	S. S.	CAL	FAT(g)	SOD(mg)	CHL(mg)	%FAT
Melba Rounds, Garlic	5	56	1.2	132	0	19.5
Melba Rounds, Honey Bran	5	52	0.9	98	0	15.6
Melba Rounds, Onion	5	51	0.6	120	0	10.5
Melba Rounds, Plain, Unsalted	5	52	0.6	<5	0	10.3
Melba Rounds, Rye	5	53	0.6	130	0	10.2
Melba Rounds, Sesame	5	57	1.8	131	0	28.6
Melba Toast, Honey Bran	1	16	0.4	25	0	22.5
Melba Toast, Plain	1	16	0.4	30	0	22.5
Melba Toast, Plain, Unsalted	1	16	0.4	5	0	22.5
Melba Toast, Sesame	1	16	0.5	25	0	28.1
Melba Toast, Whole Wheat	1	16	0.4	30	0	22.5

☞**Finn Crisp**	S. S.	CAL	FAT(g)	SOD(mg)	CHL(mg)	%FAT
Crispbread, Dark	2	38	<1.0	130	0	<23.7
Crispbread, Dark w/ Caraway	2	38	<1.0	130	0	<23.7
Crispbread, Rye, Light, Hi-Fiber	1	35	1.0	60	0	25.7
Crispbread, Rye, Original, Hi-Fiber	1	40	0.0	95	0	0.0
Rye Crackers	1 oz.	120	4.0	200	-	30.0

CRACKERS

☞ Finn Crisp	S. S.	CAL	FAT(g)	SOD(mg)	CHL(mg)	%FAT
Rye Crackers, No Salt Added	1 oz.	120	4.0	10	-	30.0

☞ J. J. Flats	S. S.	CAL	FAT(g)	SOD(mg)	CHL(mg)	%FAT
Bread Flats, Caraway and Salt	1 slice	51	0.8	213	0	14.2
Bread Flats, Cinnamon	1 slice	53	0.7	126	0	12.0
Bread Flats, Flavorall	1 slice	52	0.9	139	0	15.5
Bread Flats, Garlic	1 slice	52	0.7	127	0	12.0
Bread Flats, Oat Bran	1 slice	49	0.9	141	0	16.6
Bread Flats, Plain	1 slice	53	0.8	143	0	13.5
Bread Flats, Poppy	1 slice	53	1.1	126	0	18.5
Bread Flats, Sesame	1 slice	55	1.5	124	0	24.5

☞ Kavli Norwegian	S. S.	CAL	FAT(g)	SOD(mg)	CHL(mg)	%FAT
Crispbread, Thick	1	35	0.3	32	0	7.7
Crispbread, Thin	2	40	0.3	65	0	6.8

☞ Keebler	S. S.	CAL	FAT(g)	SOD(mg)	CHL(mg)	%FAT
Zesta, Unsalted Tops	5	60	2.0	85	0	30.0
Zesta, Low Salt	5	60	2.0	95	0	30.0
Zesta, Original	5	60	2.0	190	0	30.0
Zesta, soup crackers	39	60	2.0	150	0	30.0
Zesta, Wheat	5	60	2.0	190	0	30.0
Grahams, Cinnamon Crisp	4	70	2.0	85	0	25.7
Grahams, Regular	4	60	2.0	70	0	30.0

☞ Manischewitz	S. S.	CAL	FAT(g)	SOD(mg)	CHL(mg)	%FAT
Crackers, Whole Wheat	10	90	1.0	<10	0	10.0

☞ Manischewitz	S. S.	CAL	FAT(g)	SOD(mg)	CHL(mg)	%FAT
Matzo Cracker Miniatures	10	90	1.0	<10	0	10.0
Matzo Crackers, Passover Egg	10	108	2.0	<10	20	16.7
Matzos, American	1 board	115	1.9	-	-	14.9
Matzos, Dietetic Thins	1 board	91	0.4	<1	0	4.0
Matzos, Egg 'n Onion	1 board	112	1.0	180	15	7.6
Matzos, Passover	1 board	129	0.4	<5	0	2.5
Matzos, Passover Egg	1 board	132	2.0	<5	25	13.6
Matzos, Thin Salted	1 board	100	0.3	-	0	2.6
Matzos, Thin Tea	1 board	103	0.3	<1	0	2.5
Matzos, Unsalted	1 board	110	0.3	<1	0	2.6
Matzos, Whole Wheat with Bran	1 board	110	0.6	<1	0	4.8

☞ Nabisco	S. S.	CAL	FAT(g)	SOD(mg)	CHL(mg)	%FAT
Crown Pilot	1	70	2.0	70	0	25.7
Harvest Crisps, 5 Grain	6	60	2.0	135	0	30.0
Harvest Crisps, Oat	6	60	2.0	135	0	30.0
Harvest Crisps, Rice	6	60	2.0	135	0	30.0
Mr. Phipps Pretzel Chips, Lightly Salted	8	60	1.0	200	0	15.0
Mr. Phipps Pretzel Chips, Original	8	60	1.0	310	0	15.0
Mr. Phipps Pretzel Chips, Sesame	8	60	2.0	250	0	30.0
Mr. Phipps Tater Crisps, Bar-B-Que	11	60	2.0	160	0	30.0
Mr. Phipps Tater Crisps, Original	11	60	2.0	130	0	30.0
Mr. Phipps Tater Crips, Sour Cream 'N Onion	11	60	2.0	150	0	30.0
Oysterettes, Soup & Oyster	18	60	1.0	140	0	15.0
Premium Plus Saltine, Whole Wheat	5	60	2.0	130	0	30.0
Premium Saltine	5	60	2.0	180	0	30.0
Premium Saltine, Fat Free	5	50	0.0	115	0	0.0
Premium Saltine, Low Salt	5	60	2.0	115	0	30.0
Premium Saltine, Unsalted Tops	5	60	2.0	135	0	30.0
Premium Soup and Oyster Crackers	20	60	1.0	210	0	15.0
Royal Lunch	1	60	2.0	80	<2	30.0
Snackwell's Cheese Crackers	18	60	1.0	160	0	15.0
Snackwell's Wheat Crackers	5	50	0.0	160	0	0.0

CRACKERS

☞ **Nabisco**	S. S.	CAL	FAT(g)	SOD(mg)	CHL(mg)	%FAT
Triscuit Bits Wafers	8	60	2.0	75	0	30.0
Triscuit Wafers	3	60	2.0	75	0	30.0
Triscuit Wafers, Deli Style Rye	3	60	2.0	80	0	30.0
Triscuit Wafers, Low Salt	3	60	2.0	35	0	30.0
Triscuit Wafers, Wheat'n Bran	3	60	2.0	75	0	30.0
Uneeda Biscuits, Unsalted Tops	2	60	2.0	100	0	30.0
Zwieback Toast	2	60	1.0	20	<2	15.0

☞ **Oat Bran Krisp**	S. S.	CAL	FAT(g)	SOD(mg)	CHL(mg)	%FAT
Crackers	2	60	2.0	140	0	30.0

☞ **Old London**	S. S.	CAL	FAT(g)	SOD(mg)	CHL(mg)	%FAT
Melba Toast, Rye	3	52	0.7	132	0	12.1
Melba Toast, Sesame	3	55	1.8	148	0	29.7
Melba Toast, Sesame, Unsalted	3	55	1.8	5	0	29.7
Melba Toast, Whole Grain, Unsalted	3	53	1.0	4	0	17.0
Rounds, Bacon	5	53	1.0	126	0	17.0
Rounds, Garlic	5	56	1.2	132	0	19.3
Rounds, Onion	5	52	0.8	121	0	13.8
Rounds, Rye	5	52	0.7	132	0	12.2
Rounds, Sesame	5	56	1.8	149	0	28.7
Rounds, White	5	48	0.6	111	0	11.2
Rounds, Whole Grain	5	54	1.2	102	0	20.1

☞ **Peek Freans**	S. S.	CAL	FAT(g)	SOD(mg)	CHL(mg)	%FAT
Biscuits for Cheese, Cream	3.7	91	3.0	86	-	29.4
Biscuits for Cheese, Dixie	3.7	91	3.0	86	-	29.4
Biscuits for Cheese, Oyster	4.8	91	3.0	86	-	29.4
Biscuits for Cheese, Table	3.8	91	3.0	86	-	29.4

☞ Peek Freans	S. S.	CAL	FAT(g)	SOD(mg)	CHL(mg)	%FAT
Biscuits for Cheese, Water	2.6	83	1.2	102	-	13.0
Cream Crackers	3.7	91	3.0	86	-	29.4

☞ Pepperidge Farm	S. S.	CAL	FAT(g)	SOD(mg)	CHL(mg)	%FAT
Cheddar Cheese Goldfish	1 oz.	120	4.0	230	5	30.0
English Water Biscuits	4	70	1.0	100	0	12.9
Low Salt Cheddar Cheese Goldfish	1 oz.	120	4.0	130	5	30.0
Parmesan Cheese Goldfish	1 oz.	120	4.0	330	<5	30.0
Pretzel Goldfish	1 oz.	110	3.0	160	0	24.5
Pretzel Snack Sticks	8	120	3.0	430	0	22.5
Wholesome Crackers, Garden Vegetable	5	70	2.0	130	0	25.7
Wholesome Crackers, Multi Grain	4	70	2.0	130	0	25.7

☞ R.W. Frookie	S. S.	CAL	FAT(g)	SOD(mg)	CHL(mg)	%FAT
Gourmet Cracked Pepper Crackers	4	35	0.0	120	0	0.0
Gourmet Herb and Garlic Crackers	4	35	0.0	40	0	0.0
Gourmet Water Crackers	4	35	0.0	60	0	0.0

☞ Red Oval Farms	S. S.	CAL	FAT(g)	SOD(mg)	CHL(mg)	%FAT
Stoned Corn Thins	4	55	1.5	105	-	24.5
Stoned Rye Thins	4	54	1.3	104	-	21.7
Stoned Wheat Thins	4	56	1.3	97	-	20.9
Stoned Wheat Thins Lower Salt	4	57	1.3	80	-	20.5

☞ Rykrisp	S. S.	CAL	FAT(g)	SOD(mg)	CHL(mg)	%FAT
Crackers, Natural	2	40	0.0	75	0	0.0
Crackers, Seasoned	2	45	1.0	105	0	20.0

CRACKERS

☞Ryvita	S. S.	CAL	FAT(g)	SOD(mg)	CHL(mg)	%FAT
Crisp Bread, Rye, Dark	1	26	<1.0	35	0	-
Crisp Bread, Rye, Sesame, Toasted	1	31	<1.0	10	0	<29.0
Crisp Bread, High Fiber	1	23	<1.0	10	0	-
Crisp Bread, Rye, Light	1	26	< 1.0	20	0	-
Snack Bread, High Fiber	1	14	< 1.0	25	0	-
Snack Bread, Original Wheat	1	20	<1.0	20	0	-

☞Sunshine	S. S.	CAL	FAT(g)	SOD(mg)	CHL(mg)	%FAT
Krispy, Saltine	5	60	1.0	210	0	15.0
Krispy, Saltine, Whole Wheat	5	60	1.0	210	0	15.0
Krispy, Unsalted Tops	5	60	1.0	120	0	15.0
Oyster & Soup Crackers	16	60	1.0	190	0	15.0

☞Venus	S. S.	CAL	FAT(g)	SOD(mg)	CHL(mg)	%FAT
Cracker Bread, Armenian	5	60	1.0	90	0	15.0
Wafers, Bran, Salt Free	8	90	1.0	0	0	10.0
Wafers, Corn, Salt Free	8	100	2.0	0	0	18.0
Wafers, Oat Bran	8	100	2.0	170	0	18.0
Wafers, Oat Bran, Salt Free	8	100	2.0	0	0	18.0
Wafers, Rye, Salt Free	8	100	1.0	0	0	9.0
Wafers, Wheat	8	100	2.0	180	-	18.0
Wafers, Wheat, Cracked, Salt Free	8	100	2.0	0	0	18.0
Wafers, Wheat, Salt Free	8	100	2.0	0	0	18.0

☞Wasa	S. S.	CAL	FAT(g)	SOD(mg)	CHL(mg)	%FAT
Crispbread, Breakfast	1	50	1.0	65	0	18.0
Crispbread, Extra Crisp	1	25	0.0	40	0	0.0
Crispbread, Fiber Plus	1	35	1.0	65	0	25.7
Crispbread, Rye, Falue	1	30	0.0	60	0	0.0

☞ Wasa	S. S.	CAL	FAT(g)	SOD(mg)	CHL(mg)	%FAT
Crispbread, Rye, Golden	1	35	0.0	55	0	0.0
Crispbread, Rye, Hearty	1	45	0.0	70	0	0.0
Crispbread, Rye, Light	1	25	0.0	49	0	0.0
Crispbread, Rye, Sesame	1	30	1.0	45	0	30.0
Crispbread, Sesame, Savory	1	30	1.0	40	0	30.0
Crispbread, Wheat, Sesame	1	60	2.0	65	0	30.0
Crispbread, Whole Grain	1	30	1.0	40	0	30.0

DAIRY CASE

CHEESE

☞Alpine Lace Free N' Lean	S. S.	CAL	FAT(g)	SOD(mg)	CHL(mg)	%FAT
American, Fat Free, Low Cholesterol	1 oz.	35	0.0	290	5	0.0
Cheddar, Fat Free, Low Cholesterol	1 oz.	35	0.0	290	5	0.0
Cream Cheese Product, Fat Free	1 oz.	30	0.0	180	5	0.0
Mozzarella, Natural, Fat Free, Low Cholesterol	1 oz.	40	0.0	120	5	0.0
Mozzarella, Past. Proc., Fat Free, Low Cholesterol	1 oz.	35	0.0	290	5	0.0

☞Cabot	S. S.	CAL	FAT(g)	SOD(mg)	CHL(mg)	%FAT
Cheddar, Reduced Fat	1 oz.	60	2.0	200	10	30.0

☞Friendship	S. S.	CAL	FAT(g)	SOD(mg)	CHL(mg)	%FAT
Hoop Cheese	4 oz.	84	1.0	10	8	10.7

☞Frigo	S. S.	CAL	FAT(g)	SOD(mg)	CHL(mg)	%FAT
Mozzarella, Lite, Part Skim	1 oz.	60	2.0	140	8	30.0
String, Lite	1 oz.	60	2.0	140	8	30.0

☞Kraft Free	S. S.	CAL	FAT(g)	SOD(mg)	CHL(mg)	%FAT
Cheese Product, Singles, Nonfat	1 oz.	45	0.0	420	5	0.0

DAIRY CASE

☞ Lifetime	S. S.	CAL	FAT(g)	SOD(mg)	CHL(mg)	%FAT
Processed Cheese, Garden Vegetable, Fat Free	1 oz.	40	0.0	200	3	0.0
Processed Cheese, Cheddar, Fat Free	1 oz.	40	0.0	200	3	0.0
Processed Cheese, Mild Mexican, Fat Free	1 oz.	40	0.0	200	3	0.0
Processed Cheese, Swiss, Fat Free	1 oz.	40	0.0	200	3	0.0

☞ Polly-O Free	S. S.	CAL	FAT(g)	SOD(mg)	CHL(mg)	%FAT
Mozzarella, Nonfat	1 oz.	40	0.0	240	5	0.0

☞ Sargento	S. S.	CAL	FAT(g)	SOD(mg)	CHL(mg)	%FAT
Pot Cheese	1 oz.	26	0.2	1	-	6.9

☞ Weight Watchers	S. S.	CAL	FAT(g)	SOD(mg)	CHL(mg)	%FAT
American Slices	2 slices	35	1.0	270	5	25.7

COTTAGE CHEESE

☞ Breakstone's	S. S.	CAL	FAT(g)	SOD(mg)	CHL(mg)	%FAT
Cottage Cheese, 2% Milkfat	4 oz.	100	2.0	510	15	18.0
Cottage Cheese, Dry Curd	4 oz.	90	0.0	65	10	0.0

☞ Cabot	S. S.	CAL	FAT(g)	SOD(mg)	CHL(mg)	%FAT
Cottage Cheese, Light	4 oz.	90	1.0	360	5	10.0

☞ **Friendship**	S. S.	CAL	FAT(g)	SOD(mg)	CHL(mg)	%FAT
Cottage Cheese, Lowfat, Lactose Reduced, 1% Milkfat	4 oz.	90	1.0	350	5	10.0
Cottage Cheese, Lowfat, No Salt Added, 1% Milkfat	4 oz.	90	1.0	31	5	10.0
Cottage Cheese, Nonfat	4 oz.	70	0.0	350	0	0.0
Cottage Cheese, Pot Style Lowfat, 2% Milkfat	4 oz.	100	2.0	405	9	18.0
Cottage Cheese, Whipped, 1% Milkfat	4 oz.	90	1.0	350	5	10.0
Cottage Cheese, with Pineapple, 4% Milkfat	4 oz.	140	4.0	300	17	25.7
Cottage Cheese, with Pineapple, Lowfat, 1% Milkfat	4 oz.	110	1.0	300	5	8.2

☞ **Hood**	S. S.	CAL	FAT(g)	SOD(mg)	CHL(mg)	%FAT
Cottage Cheese, Nonfat	4 oz.	70	0.0	290	0	0.0
Nuform Cottage Cheese, Low-Fat, 1% Milkfat	4 oz.	90	1.0	370	5	10.0
Cottage Cheese, Nonfat, with Pineapple	4 oz.	90	0.0	230	0	0.0

☞ **Knudsen**	S. S.	CAL	FAT(g)	SOD(mg)	CHL(mg)	%FAT
Cottage Cheese, 2% Milkfat	4 oz.	100	2.0	370	15	18.0
Cottage Cheese, 2% Milkfat, with Fruit Cocktail	4 oz.	130	2.0	330	10	13.8
Cottage Cheese, 2% Milkfat, with Mandarin Orange	4 oz.	110	2.0	320	10	16.4
Cottage Cheese, 2% Milkfat, with Peach	6 oz.	170	2.0	270	15	10.6
Cottage Cheese, 2% Milkfat, with Pear	4 oz.	110	2.0	320	10	16.4
Cottage Cheese, 2% Milkfat, with Pineapple	6 oz.	170	2.0	300	15	10.6
Cottage Cheese, 2% Milkfat, with Spiced Apple	6 oz.	180	2.0	280	15	10.0
Cottage Cheese, 2% Milkfat, with Strawberry	6 oz.	170	2.0	320	15	10.6
Cottage Cheese, Nonfat	4 oz.	70	0.0	420	5	0.0

DAIRY CASE

DAIRY CASE

🖙 Light N' Lively	S. S.	CAL	FAT(g)	SOD(mg)	CHL(mg)	%FAT
Cottage Cheese, Nonfat	4 oz.	90	0.0	400	10	0.0
Cottage Cheese, 1% Milkfat	4 oz.	80	2.0	370	10	22.5
Cottage Cheese, 1% Milkfat, Garden Salad	4 oz.	80	2.0	350	10	22.5
Cottage Cheese, 1% Milkfat, with Peach and Pineapple	4 oz.	100	1.0	320	10	9.0

🖙 Sealtest	S. S.	CAL	FAT(g)	SOD(mg)	CHL(mg)	%FAT
Cottage Cheese, 2% Milkfat	4 oz.	100	2.0	340	15	18.0

🖙 Weight Watchers	S. S.	CAL	FAT(g)	SOD(mg)	CHL(mg)	%FAT
Cottage Cheese, 1% Milkfat	1/2 cup	90	1.0	460	-	10.0
Cottage Cheese, 2% Milkfat	1/2 cup	100	2.0	460	-	18.0

DAIRY DESSERTS

🖙 Hershey's	S. S.	CAL	FAT(g)	SOD(mg)	CHL(mg)	%FAT
Chocolate Bar Flavored Puddings, Hershey's Caramello	4 oz.	180	6.0	180	-	30.0
Chocolate Bar Flavored Puddings, Hershey's Chocolate	4 oz.	180	6.0	240	-	30.0
Chocolate Bar Flavored Puddings, Hershey's Chocolate & Almond	4 oz.	180	6.0	180	-	30.0
Chocolate Bar Flavored Puddings, Hershey's Kisses Chocolate & Vanilla	4 oz.	180	6.0	170	-	30.0
Chocolate Bar Flavored Puddings, Hershey's Special Dark	4 oz.	170	4.0	180	-	21.2
Chocolate Bar Flavored Puddings, Hershey's York Peppermint Pattie	4 oz.	180	6.0	190	-	30.0

☞ Jell-O	S. S.	CAL	FAT(g)	SOD(mg)	CHL(mg)	%FAT
Pudding Snacks, Butterscotch/ Chocolate/Vanilla Swirl	4 oz.	180	6.0	140	0	30.0
Pudding Snacks, Vanilla/ Chocolate Swirl	4 oz.	180	6.0	140	0	30.0
Light Pudding Snacks, Chocolate	4 oz.	100	2.0	125	5	18.0
Light Pudding Snacks, Chocolate Fudge	4 oz.	100	1.0	125	5	9.0
Light Pudding Snacks, Chocolate Vanilla Combo	4 oz.	100	2.0	125	5	18.0
Light Pudding Snacks, Vanilla	4 oz.	100	2.0	130	5	18.0

☞ Swiss Miss	S. S.	CAL	FAT(g)	SOD(mg)	CHL(mg)	%FAT
Pudding Sundae, Chocolate	4 oz.	220	7.0	140	1	28.6
Pudding Sundae, Vanilla	4 oz.	220	7.0	180	1	28.6
Light Pudding, Vanilla	4 oz.	100	1.0	105	<1	9.0
Light Pudding, Chocolate	4 oz.	100	1.0	120	1	9.0
Pudding, Chocolate	4 oz.	180	6.0	160	1	30.0
Pudding, Chocolate Fudge	4 oz.	220	6.0	180	1	24.5
Parfait, Vanilla	4 oz.	180	6.0	150	1	30.0
Pudding, Tapioca	4 oz.	160	5.0	170	1	28.1
Pudding, Butterscotch	4 oz.	180	6.0	135	1	30.0
Pudding, Custard	4 oz.	190	6.0	190	5	28.4

☞ Yoplait	S. S.	CAL	FAT(g)	SOD(mg)	CHL(mg)	%FAT
Pudding, Double Chocolate	4 oz.	180	4.0	95	10	20.0
Pudding, Milk Chocolate	4 oz.	180	4.0	105	10	20.0
Pudding, Vanilla	4 oz.	180	3.0	105	10	20.0

MILK

☞ Generic	S. S.	CAL	FAT(g)	SOD(mg)	CHL(mg)	%FAT
Buttermilk, Cultured	8 fl. oz.	99	2.2	257	9	20.0

DAIRY CASE

☞ Generic	S. S.	CAL	FAT(g)	SOD(mg)	CHL(mg)	%FAT
Calcimilk	8 fl. oz.	102	3.0	123	10	26.5
Milk, Chocolate, 1% Milkfat	8 fl oz.	158	2.5	152	7	14.2
Lactaid	8 fl oz.	102	3.0	123	10	26.5
Milk, Lowfat, 1% Milkfat	8 fl oz.	102	2.6	123	10	22.9
Milk, Nonfat (Skim)	8 fl oz.	86	0.4	126	4	4.2

RICOTTA CHEESE

☞ Dragone	S. S.	CAL	FAT(g)	SOD(mg)	CHL(mg)	%FAT
Ricotta, Lite	1 oz.	30	1.0	10	0	30.0

☞ Frigo	S. S.	CAL	FAT(g)	SOD(mg)	CHL(mg)	%FAT
Ricotta, Low Fat/Low Salt	1 oz.	30	1.0	10	5	30.0

☞ Polly-O	S. S.	CAL	FAT(g)	SOD(mg)	CHL(mg)	%FAT
Ricotta Cheese, Lite Reduced Fat	1 oz.	35	1.0	20	5	25.7
Ricotta Cheese, Nonfat, Free	1 oz.	25	0.0	35	0	0.0

☞ Sargento	S. S.	CAL	FAT(g)	SOD(mg)	CHL(mg)	%FAT
Ricotta, Lite	1 oz.	24	0.8	23	4	30.0

SOUR CREAM

☞ Hood	S. S.	CAL	FAT(g)	SOD(mg)	CHL(mg)	%FAT
Hood Free Sour Cream Alternative, Nonfat	2 Tbsp.	25	0.0	50	0	0.0

☞Light N' Lively Free	S. S.	CAL	FAT(g)	SOD(mg)	CHL(mg)	%FAT
Sour Cream Alternative, Nonfat	1 Tbsp.	10	0.0	10	0	0.0

YOGURT

☞Breyers	S. S.	CAL	FAT(g)	SOD(mg)	CHL(mg)	%FAT
Yogurt, Lowfat, 1% Milkfat, Black Cherry	8 oz.	260	3.0	120	10	10.4
Yogurt, Lowfat, 1% Milkfat, Blueberry	8 oz.	250	2.0	120	10	7.2
Yogurt, Lowfat, 1% Milkfat, Mixed Berry	8 oz.	250	2.0	120	10	7.2
Yogurt, Lowfat, 1% Milkfat, Pineapple	8 oz.	250	2.0	120	10	7.2
Yogurt, Lowfat, 1% Milkfat, Red Raspberry	8 oz.	250	2.0	120	10	7.2
Yogurt, Lowfat, 1% Milkfat, Strawberry	8 oz.	250	2.0	120	10	7.2
Yogurt, Lowfat, 1% Milkfat, Strawberry Banana	8 oz.	250	2.0	120	10	7.2
Yogurt, Lowfat, 1.5% Milkfat, Plain	8 oz.	140	3.0	170	20	19.3
Yogurt, Lowfat, 1.5% Milkfat, Vanilla Bean	8 oz.	230	3.0	150	20	11.7

☞Continental	S. S.	CAL	FAT(g)	SOD(mg)	CHL(mg)	%FAT
Yogurt, Boysenberry	1 cup	200	<1.0	105	-	<4.5
Yogurt, Cappuccino	1 cup	200	<1.0	105	-	<4.5
Yogurt, Honey Nut	1 cup	200	<1.0	105	-	<4.5
Yogurt, Lemon	1 cup	190	<1.0	120	<5	<4.7
Yogurt, Lowfat, Plain	1 cup	170	5.0	-	-	26.5
Yogurt, Nonfat, Plain	1 cup	140	<1.0	115	<5	<6.4
Yogurt, Peach	1 cup	200	<1.0	105	-	<4.5
Yogurt, Raspberry	1 cup	200	<1.0	105	-	< 4.5
Yogurt, Strawberry	1 cup	200	<1.0	105	-	<4.5
Yogurt, Strawberry Banana	1 cup	190	<1.0	120	<5	<4.7
Yogurt, Strawberry Peach	1 cup	190	<1.0	120	<5	<4.7
Yogurt, Wildberry	1 cup	200	<1.0	105	-	<4.5

DAIRY CASE

☞ Colombo	S. S.	CAL	FAT(g)	SOD(mg)	CHL(mg)	%FAT
Yogurt, Nonfat Fruit On-The-Bottom, All Flavors	1 cup	190	<1.0	140	5	<4.7
Yogurt, Classic Fruit On-The-Bottom, All Flavors	1 cup	230	4.0	115	-	15.7
Yogurt, Nonfat Lite Vanilla	1 cup	160	<1.0	140	5	<5.6
Yogurt, Classic French Vanilla	1 cup	190	4.0	130	-	18.9
Yogurt, Classic Strawberry	1 cup	180	4.0	130	-	20.0
Yogurt, Nonfat Lite Plain	1 cup	110	<1.0	160	5	<8.2
Yogurt, Classic Plain	1 cup	130	4.0	150	-	27.7
Yogurt, Nonfat Lite Mini Pack	4.4 oz.	100	0.0	70	-	0.0

☞ Dannon	S. S.	CAL	FAT(g)	SOD(mg)	CHL(mg)	%FAT
Yogurt, Lowfat Blended, Peach	4 oz.	110	2.0	55	5	16.4
Yogurt, Lowfat Blended, Raspberry	4 oz.	110	2.0	55	5	16.4
Yogurt, Lowfat Blended, Strawberry	4 oz.	110	2.0	55	5	16.4
Yogurt, Lowfat Blended, Strawberry-Banana	4 oz.	110	2.0	55	5	16.4
Yogurt, Lowfat Flavored, Blueberry	8 oz.	200	4.0	160	-	18.0
Yogurt, Lowfat Flavored, Coffee	8 oz.	200	3.0	120	10	13.5
Yogurt, Lowfat Flavored, Lemon	8 oz.	200	3.0	120	10	13.5
Yogurt, Lowfat Flavored, Raspberry	8 oz.	200	4.0	160	-	18.0
Yogurt, Lowfat Flavored, Strawberry	8 oz.	200	4.0	160	-	18.0
Yogurt, Lowfat Flavored, Strawberry-Banana	8 oz.	200	4.0	160	-	18.0
Yogurt, Lowfat Flavored, Vanilla	8 oz.	200	3.0	120	10	13.5
Yogurt, Lowfat Fruit on the Bottom, Banana	8 oz.	240	3.0	120	10	11.3
Yogurt, Lowfat Fruit on the Bottom, Blueberry	8 oz.	240	3.0	120	10	11.3
Yogurt, Lowfat Fruit on the Bottom, Boysenberry	8 oz.	240	3.0	120	10	11.3
Yogurt, Lowfat Fruit on the Bottom, Dutch Apple	8 oz.	240	3.0	120	10	11.3

☞ **Dannon**	S. S.	CAL	FAT(g)	SOD(mg)	CHL(mg)	%FAT
Yogurt, Lowfat Fruit on the Bottom, Exotic Fruit	8 oz.	240	3.0	120	-	11.3
Yogurt, Lowfat Fruit on the Bottom, Mixed Berries	8 oz.	240	3.0	120	10	11.3
Yogurt, Lowfat Fruit on the Bottom, Peach	8 oz.	240	3.0	120	10	11.3
Yogurt, Lowfat Fruit on the Bottom, Piña-Colada	8 oz.	240	3.0	120	10	11.3
Yogurt, Lowfat Fruit on the Bottom, Raspberry	8 oz.	240	3.0	120	10	11.3
Yogurt, Lowfat Fruit on the Bottom, Strawberry	8 oz.	240	3.0	120	10	11.3
Yogurt, Lowfat Fruit on the Bottom, Strawberry-Banana	8 oz.	240	3.0	120	10	11.3
Yogurt, Nonfat Blended, Strawberry-Banana	6 oz.	140	0.0	105	<5	0.0
Yogurt, Nonfat Blended, Blueberry	6 oz.	140	0.0	105	<5	0.0
Yogurt, Nonfat Blended, Peach	6 oz.	140	0.0	105	<5	0.0
Yogurt, Nonfat Blended, Raspberry	6 oz.	140	0.0	105	<5	0.0
Yogurt, Nonfat Blended, Strawberry	6 oz.	140	0.0	105	<5	0.0
Yogurt, Nonfat Light, Blueberry	8 oz.	100	0.0	130	<5	0.0
Yogurt, Nonfat Light, Cherry Vanilla	8 oz.	100	0.0	130	<5	0.0
Yogurt, Nonfat Light, Peach	8 oz.	100	0.0	130	<5	0.0
Yogurt, Nonfat Light, Raspberry	8 oz.	100	0.0	130	<5	0.0
Yogurt, Nonfat Light, Strawberry	8 oz.	100	0.0	130	<5	0.0
Yogurt, Nonfat Light, Strawberry Fruit Cup	8 oz.	100	0.0	130	<5	0.0
Yogurt, Nonfat Light, Strawberry-Banana	8 oz.	100	0.0	130	<5	0.0
Yogurt, Nonfat Light, Vanilla	8 oz.	100	0.0	130	<5	0.0
Yogurt, Nonfat, Plain	8 oz.	110	0.0	140	5	0.0

☞ **Friendship**	S. S.	CAL	FAT(g)	SOD(mg)	CHL(mg)	%FAT
Yogurt, Lowfat, Plain	8 oz.	150	3.0	190	14	18.0
Yorgurt, Lowfat, Vanilla & Coffee	8 oz.	210	3.0	125	14	12.9

DAIRY CASE

☞ **Knudsen**	S. S.	CAL	FAT(g)	SOD(mg)	CHL(mg)	%FAT
Yogurt, Cal 70 Nonfat, Black Cherry	6 oz.	70	0.0	75	5	0.0
Yogurt, Cal 70 Nonfat, Blueberry	6 oz.	70	0.0	80	5	0.0
Yogurt, Cal 70 Nonfat, Lemon	6 oz.	70	0.0	125	0	0.0
Yogurt, Cal 70 Nonfat, Peach	6 oz.	70	0.0	95	0	0.0
Yogurt, Cal 70 Nonfat, Pineapple	6 oz.	70	0.0	125	0	0.0
Yogurt, Cal 70 Nonfat, Red Raspberry	6 oz.	70	0.0	80	5	0.0
Yogurt, Cal 70 Nonfat, Strawberry	6 oz.	70	0.0	85	0	0.0
Yogurt, Cal 70 Nonfat, Strawberry Banana	6 oz.	70	0.0	80	0	0.0
Yogurt, Cal 70 Nonfat, Strawberry Fruit Basket	6 oz.	70	0.0	75	5	0.0
Yogurt, Cal 70 Nonfat, Vanilla	6 oz.	70	0.0	90	0	0.0
Yogurt, Lowfat, 1.5% Milkfat, Boysenberry	8 oz.	240	4.0	135	15	15.0
Yogurt, Lowfat, 1.5% Milkfat, Cherry	8 oz.	240	4.0	135	15	15.0
Yogurt, Lowfat, 1.5% Milkfat, Lemon	8 oz.	240	4.0	135	15	15.0
Yogurt, Lowfat, 1.5% Milkfat, Lime	8 oz.	240	4.0	135	15	15.0
Yogurt, Lowfat, 1.5% Milkfat, Peach	8 oz.	240	4.0	135	15	15.0
Yogurt, Lowfat, 1.5% Milkfat, Raspberry	8 oz.	240	4.0	135	15	15.0
Yogurt, Lowfat, 1.5% Milkfat, Strawberry	8 oz.	250	4.0	135	15	14.4
Yogurt, Lowfat, 1.5% Milkfat, Strawberry-Banana	8 oz.	240	4.0	135	15	15.0
Yogurt, Lowfat, 1.5% Milkfat, Vanilla	8 oz.	240	4.0	135	15	15.0
Yogurt, Lowfat, 2% Milkfat, Plain	8 oz.	160	5.0	180	25	28.1

☞ **Light N' Lively**	S. S.	CAL	FAT(g)	SOD(mg)	CHL(mg)	%FAT
Yogurt, 100 Calorie Nonfat, Black Cherry	8 oz.	100	0.0	100	0	0.0
Yogurt, 100 Calorie Nonfat, Blueberry	8 oz.	90	0.0	110	0	0.0
Yogurt, 100 Calorie Nonfat, Lemon	8 oz.	100	0.0	150	5	0.0

☞ Light N' Lively	S. S.	CAL	FAT(g)	SOD(mg)	CHL(mg)	%FAT
Yogurt, 100 Calorie Nonfat, Peach	8 oz.	100	0.0	115	5	0.0
Yogurt, 100 Calorie Nonfat, Red Raspberry	8 oz.	90	0.0	105	0	0.0
Yogurt, 100 Calorie Nonfat, Strawberry	8 oz.	90	0.0	105	5	0.0
Yogurt, 100 Calorie Nonfat, Strawberry Banana	8 oz.	100	0.0	105	0	0.0
Yogurt, 100 Calorie Nonfat, Strawberry Fruit Cup	8 oz.	90	0.0	100	0	0.0
Yogurt, Lowfat, 1% Milkfat, Black Cherry	8 oz.	230	2.0	125	15	7.8
Yogurt, Lowfat, 1% Milkfat, Blueberry	8 oz.	240	2.0	130	10	7.5
Yogurt, Lowfat, 1% Milkfat, Peach	8 oz.	240	2.0	120	15	7.5
Yogurt, Lowfat, 1% Milkfat, Pineapple	8 oz.	230	2.0	120	10	7.8
Yogurt, Lowfat, 1% Milkfat, Red Raspberry	8 oz.	230	2.0	130	10	7.8
Yogurt, Lowfat, 1% Milkfat, Strawberry	8 oz.	240	2.0	130	15	7.5
Yogurt, Lowfat, 1% Milkfat, Strawberry Banana	8 oz.	260	2..0	120	10	6.9
Yogurt, Lowfat, 1% Milkfat, Strawberry Fruit Cup	8 oz.	240	2.0	120	15	7.5

☞ Light N' Lively Free	S. S.	CAL	FAT(g)	SOD(mg)	CHL(mg)	%FAT
Yogurt, Nonfat, Blueberry	4.4 oz.	50	0.0	60	0	0.0
Yogurt, Nonfat, Red Raspberry	4.4 oz.	50	0.0	60	0	0.0
Yogurt, Nonfat, Strawberry	4.4 oz.	50	0.0	60	0	0.0
Yogurt, Nonfat, Strawberry Banana	4.4 oz.	50	0.0	60	0	0.0
Yogurt, Nonfat, Strawberry Fruit Cup	4.4 oz.	50	0.0	55	0	0.0

☞ Stonyfield Farm	S. S.	CAL	FAT(g)	SOD(mg)	CHL(mg)	%FAT
Yogurt, Nonfat, Plain	8 oz.	110	0.0	145	0	0.0
Yogurt, Nonfat, Ftuited/ Fiavored, All Varieties	8 oz.	160	0.0	115	0	0.0

DAIRY CASE

☞ Stonyfield Farm	S. S.	CAL	FAT(g)	SOD(mg)	CHL(mg)	%FAT
Yogurt, Whole Milk, Fuited/ Flavored, All Varieties	8 oz.	210	7.0	130	-	30.0

☞ Yoplait	S. S.	CAL	FAT(g)	SOD(mg)	CHL(mg)	%FAT
Yogurt, Custard Style, Banana	6 oz.	190	4.0	95	20	18.9
Yogurt, Custard Style, Blueberry	6 oz.	190	4.0	95	20	18.9
Yogurt, Custard Style, Cherry	6 oz.	180	4.0	95	20	20.0
Yogurt, Custard Style, Lemon	6 oz.	190	4.0	95	20	18.9
Yogurt, Custard Style, Mixed Berry	6 oz.	180	4.0	95	20	20.0
Yogurt, Custard Style, Raspberry	6 oz.	190	4.0	95	20	18.9
Yogurt, Custard Style, Strawberry	6 oz.	190	4.0	95	20	18.9
Yogurt, Custard Style, Strawberry-Banana	6 oz.	190	4.0	95	20	18.9
Yogurt, Custard Style, Vanilla	6 oz.	180	4.0	110	20	20.0
Yogurt, Fat Free, All Fruit Flavors	6 oz.	150	0.0	95	5	0.0
Yogurt, Light, All Fruit Flavors	6 oz.	90	0.0	100	<5	0.0
Yogurt, Nonfat, Plain	8 oz.	120	0.0	160	5	0.0
Yogurt, Nonfat, Vanilla	8 oz.	180	0.0	140	5	0.0
Yogurt, Original, All Fruit Flavors	6 oz.	190	3.0	110	10	14.2
Yogurt, Plain	6 oz.	130	3.0	140	15	20.8
Yogurt, Vanilla	6 oz.	180	3.0	120	10	15.0

DAIRY CASE

FREEZER CASE

FROZEN BAKERY, BREAKFAST

☞ Aunt Jemima	S. S.	CAL	FAT(g)	SOD(mg)	CHL(mg)	%FAT
French Toast, Original and Cinnamon	2 slices	220	7.0	290	90	28.6
Microwave Pancakes, Original	3	210	4.0	700	-	17.1
Waffles, Homestyle	1	90	3.0	220	-	30.0
Waffles, Homestyle Blueberry	1	90	3.0	280	-	30.0
Waffles, Lite Healthy	1	60	1.0	240	0	15.0

☞ Downeyflake/ Roman Meal	S. S.	CAL	FAT(g)	SOD(mg)	CHL(mg)	%FAT
Pancakes, Blueberry	3	290	9.0	920	-	27.9
Pancakes, Buttermilk	3	280	9.0	920	-	27.9
Pancakes, Regular	3	280	9.0	920	-	28.9
Waffles, Blueberry	2	180	4.0	570	0	20.0
Waffles, Buttermilk	2	190	5.0	750	0	23.7
Waffles, Hot-N-Buttery	2	180	6.0	620	-	30.0
Waffles, Regular	2	120	3.0	420	0	22.5
Waffles, Regular, Jumbo	2	170	4.0	570	0	21.2

☞ Hungry Jack	S. S.	CAL	FAT(g)	SOD(mg)	CHL(mg)	%FAT
Microwave Pancakes, Blueberry	3	230	4.0	550	10	15.7
Microwave Pancakes, Buttermilk	3	260	4.0	590	10	13.8
Microwave Pancakes, Oat Bran	3	230	4.0	580	10	15.7
Microwave Pancakes, Original	3	240	4.0	560	10	15.0
Microwave Pancakes, Harvest Wheat	3	230	4.0	560	10	15.7

FREEZER CASE

☞ Healthy Choice

	S.S.	CAL	FAT(g)	SOD(mg)	CHL(mg)	%FAT
Breakfast, Apple Spice Muffin	2.5 oz.	190	4.0	90	0	18.9
Breakfast, Banana Nut Muffin	2.5 oz.	180	6.0	80	0	30.0
Breakfast, Blueberry Muffin	2.5 oz.	190	4.0	110	0	18.9
Breakfast, English Muffin Sandwich	4.25 oz.	200	3.0	510	20	13.5
Breakfast, Turkey Sausage Omlet on English Muffin	4.75 oz.	210	4.0	470	20	17.1
Breakfast, Western Style Omlet on English Muffin	4.75 oz.	200	3.0	480	15	13.5

☞ Krusteaz

	S.S.	CAL	FAT(g)	SOD(mg)	CHL(mg)	%FAT
Microwave French Toast, Cinnamon Sugar	2	270	5.0	370	135	16.7
Microwave French Toast, Regular	2	260	6.0	370	130	20.8
Microwave Pancakes, Blueberry	1	100	2.0	370	11	18.0
Microwave Pancakes, Buttermilk	1	96	2.0	370	18	18.8
Microwave Pancakes, Whole Wheat	1	83	1.0	330	11	10.8
Pancakes, Blueberry	3	205	4.0	660	14	17.6
Pancakes, Buckwheat	3	215	3.0	770	20	12.6
Pancakes, Buttermilk	3	200	3.0	770	20	13.5
Pancakes, Whole Wheat	3	215	1.0	630	14	4.2

☞ Weight Watchers

	S.S.	CAL	FAT(g)	SOD(mg)	CHL(mg)	%FAT
Bagel Sandwich, Ham and Cheese	1	210	6.0	460	15	25.7
Belgian Waffles, Multi-Grain	1	120	4.0	200	5	30.0
Cinnamon Rolls	1	180	5.0	170	5	25.0
Coffee Cake, Cinnamon Streusel	1	160	4.0	-	-	22.5
French Toast with Cinnamon	2	160	4.0	280	5	22.5
Muffins, Banana Nut	1	170	5.0	-	-	26.5
Muffins, Blueberry	1	170	5.0	220	10	26.5
Omlette Sandwich, Garden Vegetable	1	210	6.0	-	-	25.7
Omlette, Ham and Cheese	1	180	5.0	-	-	25.0
Pancakes, Buttermilk	2	140	3.0	270	10	19.3

☞Weight Watchers	S. S.	CAL	FAT(g)	SOD(mg)	CHL(mg)	%FAT
Sweet Rolls, Cheese	1	180	4.0	-	-	20.0

FROZEN BAKERY, SWEET

☞Lean Cuisine	S. S.	CAL	FAT(g)	SOD(mg)	CHL(mg)	%FAT
Carrot Cake	1	180	4.0	300	150	20.0
Cherry Parfait Cake	1	170	5.0	280	15	26.5
Chocolate Cream Cheese Brownie	1	160	4.0	250	15	22.5
Lemon Swirl Cake	1	180	5.0	160	20	25.0
Strawberry Cheesecake	1	190	6.0	220	20	28.4

☞Pepperidge Farm	S. S.	CAL	FAT(g)	SOD(mg)	CHL(mg)	%FAT
American Collection Desserts, Berkshire Apple Crisp	1	250	8.0	130	4.3	28.8
American Collection Desserts, Charleston Peach Melba Shortcake	1	220	5.0	170	41	20.5
American Collection Desserts, Manhattan Strawberry Cheesecake	1	300	9.0	250	49	27.0
Dessert Lights, Apple 'n Spice Bake	4.25 oz.	170	2.0	105	10	10.6
Dessert Lights, Cherries Supreme	3.25 oz.	170	2.0	35	80	10.6
Dessert Lights, Lemon Cake Supreme	2.75 oz.	170	5.0	100	50	26.5
Dessert Lights, Peach Parfait	4.25 oz.	150	5.0	70	10	30.0
Dessert Lights, Raspberry Vanilla Swirl	3.25 oz.	160	5.0	140	15	28.1
Dessert Lights, Strawberry Shortcake	3 oz.	170	5.0	50	70	26.5
Old Fashioned Muffins, Cinnamon Swirl	1 muffin	190	6.0	170	35	28.4
Pound Cake, 98% Fat Free, Chocolate	1 oz.	70	1.0	85	0	13.0
Pound Cake, 98% Fat Free, Golden	1 oz.	70	0.0	80	0	0.0
Supreme Cakes, Peach Melba	3.13 oz.	270	7.0	135	35	23.3

FREEZER CASE

☞ Sara Lee	S. S.	CAL	FAT(g)	SOD(mg)	CHL(mg)	%FAT
Apple Streusel Pie Free & Light	1 slice	170	2.0	140	0	10.6
Free & Light, Apple Danish	1 slice	130	0.0	120	0	0.0
Free & Light, Blueberry Muffin	1 muffin	120	0.0	140	0	0.0
Free & Light, Cherry Streusel	1 slice	160	2.0	140	0	11.3
Free & Light, Chocolate Cake	1 slice	110	0.0	140	0	0.0
Free & Light, Pound Cake	1 slice	70	0.0	105	0	0.0
Free & Light, Strawberry Yogurt Dessert	1 slice	121	1.0	90	0	7.5
Lights, Apple Crisp Cake	1	150	2.0	130	5	12.0
Lights, Black Forest Cake	1	170	5.0	85	10	26.5
Lights, Carrot Cake	1	170	4.0	75	5	21.2
Lights, Double Chocolate Cake	1	150	5.0	85	10	30.0
Lights, French Cheesecake	1	150	4.0	90	15	24.0
Lights, Lemon Cream Cake	1	180	6.0	60	10	30.0
Lights, Strawberry French Cake	1	150	2.0	65	5	12.0
Muffin, Apple Oat Bran	1	190	6.0	300	0	28.4
Muffin, Raisin Bran	1	220	7.0	400	0	28.6

☞ Weight Watchers	S. S.	CAL	FAT(g)	SOD(mg)	CHL(mg)	%FAT
Apple Crisp	1/2 pkg.	190	5.0	190	0	23.7
Apple Pie	1/2 pkg.	165	4.0	90	0	21.8
Brownie Ala Mode	1/2 pkg.	180	4.0	150	5	20.0
Brownie Cheesecake	1/2 pkg.	200	5.0	260	10	22.5
Cherries and Cream Cake	1/2 pkg.	150	2.0	200	5	12.0
Chocolate Brownie	1/2 pkg.	100	3.0	150	5	27.0
Chocolate Cake	1/2 pkg.	180	5.0	250	5	25.0
Chocolate Eclaire	1/3 pkg.	120	4.0	110	15	30.0
Chocolate Mocha Pie	1/2 pkg.	180	4.0	150	5	20.0
Chocolate Mousse	1/2 pkg.	160	3.0	160	5	16.9
Double Fudge Cake	1/2 pkg.	190	4.0	150	5	18.9
Mint Frosted Brownie	1/3 pkg.	100	2.0	130	5	18.0
Praline Pecan Mousse	1/2 pkg.	180	4.0	180	20	20.0
Strawberry Cheesecake	1/2 pkg.	180	4.0	210	20	20.0

FROZEN BAKERY, NONSWEET

☞ Lender's	S.S.	CAL	FAT(g)	SOD(mg)	CHL(mg)	%FAT
Bagels, Big 'n Crusty Cinnamon 'n Raisin	1	250	2.0	370	0	7.2
Bagels, Big 'n Crusty Egg	1	250	2.0	380	15	7.2
Bagels, Big 'n Crusty Garlic	1	250	1.0	530	0	3.6
Bagels, Big 'n Crusty Onion	1	230	1.0	480	0	3.9
Bagels, Big 'n Crusty Plain	1	240	1.0	450	0	3.8
Bagels, Blueberry	1	190	1.0	250	0	4.7
Bagels, Cinnamon 'n Raisin	1	200	1.0	310	0	4.5
Bagels, Cranberry and Raisin	1	200	3.0	320	0	13.5
Bagels, Egg	1	150	1.0	360	5	6.0
Bagels, Garlic	1	160	1.0	340	0	5.6
Bagels, Multi Grain	1	200	2.0	410	0	9.0
Bagels, Oat Bran	1	170	2.0	290	0	10.6
Bagels, Onion	1	160	1.0	290	0	5.6
Bagels, Peach and Raisin	1	220	3.0	400	0	12.3
Bagels, Plain	1	150	1.0	320	0	6.0
Bagels, Poppy	1	160	1.0	370	0	5.6
Bagels, Pumpernickel	1	160	1.0	330	0	5.6
Bagels, Raisin Bran	1	220	3.0	360	0	12.3
Bagels, Rye	1	150	1.0	310	0	6.0
Bagels, Sesame	1	160	1.0	320	0	5.6
Bagels, Soft	1	210	3.0	350	10	12.9
Bagels, Soft Onion	1	200	3.0	380	0	13.5
Bagels, Wheat 'n Raisin	1	190	1.0	310	0	4.7

☞ Sara Lee	S.S.	CAL	FAT(g)	SOD(mg)	CHL(mg)	%FAT
Bagels, Cinnamon Raisin	1 small	200	2.0	230	0	9.0
Bagels, Cinnamon Raisin	1 large	240	2.0	280	0	7.5
Bagels, Egg	1 small	200	2.0	360	15	9.0
Bagels, Egg	1 large	250	2.0	450	20	7.2
Bagels, Oat Bran	1 small	180	1.0	360	0	5.0
Bagels, Oat Bran	1 large	220	1.0	450	0	4.1
Bagels, Onion	1 small	190	1.0	450	0	4.7

☞Sara Lee	S. S.	CAL	FAT(g)	SOD(mg)	CHL(mg)	%FAT
Bagels, Onion	1 large	230	1.0	560	0	3.9
Bagels, Plain	1 small	190	1.0	460	0	4.7
Bagels, Plain	1 large	230	1.0	580	0	3.9
Bagels, Poppy Seed	1 small	190	1.0	450	0	4.7
Bagels, Poppy Seed	1 large	230	1.0	560	0	3.9
Bagels, Sesame Seed	1 small	190	1.0	440	0	4.7
Bagels, Sesame Seed	1 large	240	2.0	550	0	7.5

☞Super Pretzel	S. S.	CAL	FAT(g)	SOD(mg)	CHL(mg)	%FAT
Soft Pretzel	2.25 oz.	170	0.0	140	0	0.0

FROZEN DOUGH

☞Fillo	S. S.	CAL	FAT(g)	SOD(mg)	CHL(mg)	%FAT
Dough Leaves	1 oz.	80	0.0	100	0	0.0

☞Goodhue's	S. S.	CAL	FAT(g)	SOD(mg)	CHL(mg)	%FAT
White Frozen Dough, Multi-Purpose	1 oz.	70	1.0	140	0	12.9

☞J.J. Nissen	S. S.	CAL	FAT(g)	SOD(mg)	CHL(mg)	%FAT
Italian Bread Dough	1 oz.	70	<1.0	130	0	<12.9

☞Rich's	S. S.	CAL	FAT(g)	SOD(mg)	CHL(mg)	%FAT
White Bread Dough, Enriched	2 slices	120	1.0	250	0	7.5

FREEZER CASE

☞ Rhodes	S. S.	CAL	FAT(g)	SOD(mg)	CHL(mg)	%FAT
Honey Wheat Bread	28 grams	69	1.2	117	0	15.7
Texas Wheat Roll	50 grams	129	1.4	193	0	9.8
Texas White Roll	50 grams	150	3.5	227	0	21.0
White Bread	25 grams	67	1.0	117	0	13.4
White Dinner Roll	28 grams	154	3.2	246	0	18.7

FROZEN ICE CREAM/SORBET/YOGURT

☞ Bonjour	S. S.	CAL	FAT(g)	SOD(mg)	CHL(mg)	%FAT
Frozen Yogurt, Nonfat	4 fl. oz.	100	0.0	60	0	0.0

☞ Borden	S. S.	CAL	FAT(g)	SOD(mg)	CHL(mg)	%FAT
Ice Milk, Chocolate	1/2 cup	100	2.0	80	-	18.0
Ice Milk, Strawberry	1/2 cup	90	2.0	65	-	20.0
Ice Milk, Vanilla	1/2 cup	90	2.0	65	-	20.0
Orange Sherbet	1/2 cup	110	1.0	40	-	8.2

☞ Breyers Light	S. S.	CAL	FAT(g)	SOD(mg)	CHL(mg)	%FAT
Ice Milk, Chocolate	4 fl. oz.	120	4.0	55	15	30.0
Ice Milk, Chocolate Fudge Twirl	4 fl. oz.	130	4.0	60	10	27.7
Ice Milk, Heavenly Hash	4 fl. oz.	150	5.0	55	10	30.0
Ice Milk, Strawberry	4 fl. oz.	110	3.0	50	15	24.5
Ice Milk, Vanilla	4 fl. oz.	120	4.0	60	10	30.0
Ice Milk, Vanilla Red Raspberry Parfait	4 fl. oz.	130	3.0	50	15	20.8
Ice Milk, Vanilla-Chocolate-trawberry	4 fl. oz.	120	4.0	55	15	30.0

☞ Colombo

	S.S.	CAL	FAT(g)	SOD(mg)	CHL(mg)	%FAT
Frozen Yogurt, Lowfat (All Flavors)	4 fl. oz.	110	2.0	50	7	16.4
Frozen Yogurt, Nonfat	4 fl. oz.	100	0.0	60	0	0.0
Frozen Yogurt, Sugar Free, Nonfat (All Flavors)	4 fl. oz.	60	0.0	60	0	0.0

☞ Dannon

	S.S.	CAL	FAT(g)	SOD(mg)	CHL(mg)	%FAT
Frozen Yogurt, Lowfat Soft, Blueberry	4 fl. oz.	110	2.0	65	5	16.4
Frozen Yogurt, Lowfat Soft, Butter Pecan	4 fl. oz.	110	2.0	65	10	16.4
Frozen Yogurt, Lowfat Soft, Cappuccino	4 fl. oz.	110	2.0	65	5	16.4
Frozen Yogurt, Lowfat Soft, Cheesecake	4 fl. oz.	110	2.0	65	5	16.4
Frozen Yogurt, Lowfat Soft, Chocolate	4 fl. oz.	140	2.0	65	5	12.9
Frozen Yogurt, Lowfat Soft, Lemon Meringue	4 fl. oz.	110	2.0	65	5	16.4
Frozen Yogurt, Lowfat Soft, Peach	4 fl. oz.	110	2.0	65	5	16.4
Frozen Yogurt, Lowfat Soft, Peanut Butter	4 fl. oz.	130	3.0	70	5	20.8
Frozen Yogurt, Lowfat Soft, Piña-Colada	4 fl. oz.	110	2.0	65	5	16.4
Frozen Yogurt, Lowfat Soft, Plain	4 fl. oz.	90	1.0	60	5	10.0
Frozen Yogurt, Lowfat Soft, Raspberry	4 fl. oz.	110	2.0	65	5	16.4
Frozen Yogurt, Lowfat Soft, Strawberry	4 fl. oz.	110	2.0	65	5	16.4
Frozen Yogurt, Lowfat Soft, Strawberry-Banana	4 fl. oz.	110	2.0	65	5	16.4
Frozen Yogurt, Lowfat Soft, Vanilla	4 fl. oz.	110	2.0	65	5	16.4
Frozen Yogurt, Nonfat Soft, Golden Vanilla	4 fl. oz.	100	0.0	65	0	0.0
Frozen Yogurt, Nonfat Soft, Red Raspberry	4 fl. oz.	100	0.0	60	0	0.0
Frozen Yogurt, Nonfat Soft, Rum Raisin	4 fl. oz.	100	0.0	65	0	0.0

FREEZER CASE

☞ **Dole**	S. S.	CAL	FAT(g)	SOD(mg)	CHL(mg)	%FAT
Sorbet, Mandarin Orange	4 oz.	110	<1.0	10	0	<8.2
Sorbet, Peach	4 oz.	110	<1.0	10	0	<8.0
Sorbet, Pineapple	4 oz.	110	<1.0	10	0	<8.0
Sorbet, Raspberry	4 oz.	110	<1.0	10	0	<8.2
Sorbet, Strawberry	4 oz.	100	<1.0	10	0	<9.0

☞ **Dreyer's**	S. S.	CAL	FAT(g)	SOD(mg)	CHL(mg)	%FAT
American Dream, Chocolate	3 fl. oz.	90	1.0	55	0	10.0
American Dream, Chocolate Chip	3 fl. oz.	100	1.0	55	0	9.0
American Dream, Cookies 'N' Cream	3 fl. oz.	100	1.0	55	0	9.0
American Dream, Mocha Almond Fudge	3 fl. zo.	110	1.0	55	0	8.2
American Dream, Rocky Road	3 fl. zo.	110	1.0	55	0	8.2
American Dream, Strawberry	3 fl. oz.	70	0.0	50	0	0.0
American Dream, Toasted Almond	3 fl. oz.	110	1.0	55	0	8.2
American Dream, Vanilla	3 fl. oz.	80	1.0	55	0	11.3
American Dream, Vanilla-hocolate-Strawberry	3 fl. oz.	80	0.0	55	0	0.0
Frozen Yogurt Inspirations, Banana-Strawberry	3 fl. oz.	80	1.0	40	5	11.3
Frozen Yogurt Inspirations, Blueberry	3 fl. oz.	80	1.0	40	5	11.3
Frozen Yogurt Inspirations, Cherry	3 fl. oz.	80	1.0	40	5	11.3
Frozen Yogurt Inspirations, Chocolate	3 fl. oz.	80	1.0	40	5	11.3
Frozen Yogurt Inspirations, Chocolate Chip	3 fl. oz.	100	1.0	55	5	9.0
Frozen Yogurt Inspirations, Citrus Heights	3 fl. oz.	80	1.0	40	5	11.3
Frozen Yogurt Inspirations, Cookies 'N' Cream	3 fl. oz.	100	1.0	55	5	9.0
Frozen Yogurt Inspirations, Marble Fudge	3 fl. oz.	100	1.0	55	5	9.0
Frozen Yogurt Inspirations, Nonfat, Cherry	3 fl. oz.	70	0.0	40	0	0.0
Frozen Yogurt Inspirations, Nonfat, Chocolate	3 fl. oz.	80	0.0	40	0	0.0

FREEZER CASE

☞ Dreyer's

	S. S.	CAL	FAT(g)	SOD(mg)	CHL(mg)	%FAT
Frozen Yogurt Inspirations, Nonfat, Mixed Berry	3 fl. oz.	70	0.0	40	0	0.0
Frozen Yogurt Inspirations, Nonfat, Mocha	3 fl. oz.	80	0.0	40	0	0.0
Frozen Yogurt Inspirations, Nonfat, Raspberry	3 fl. oz.	70	0.0	40	0	0.0
Frozen Yogurt Inspirations, Nonfat, Strawberry	3 fl. oz.	70	0.0	40	0	0.0
Frozen Yogurt Inspirations, Nonfat, Vanilla	3 fl. oz.	80	0.0	40	0	0.0
Frozen Yogurt Inspirations, Perfectly Peach	3 fl. oz.	80	1.0	40	5	11.3
Frozen Yogurt Inspirations, Raspberry	3 fl. oz.	80	1.0	40	5	11.3
Frozen Yogurt Inspirations, Raspberry-Vanilla Swirl	3 fl. oz.	80	1.0	45	5	11.3
Frozen Yogurt Inspirations, Strawberry	3 fl. oz.	80	1.0	40	5	11.3
Frozen Yogurt Inspirations, Vanilla	3 fl. oz.	80	1.0	50	5	11.3

☞ Dreyer's & Edy's

	S. S.	CAL	FAT(g)	SOD(mg)	CHL(mg)	%FAT
Frozen Dietary Dairy Dessert, Chocolate	3 fl. oz.	110	3.0	45	10	24.5
Frozen Dietary Dairy Dessert, Marble Fudge	3 fl. oz.	120	3.0	45	10	22.5
Frozen Dietary Dairy Dessert, Strawberry	3 fl. oz.	90	3.0	40	10	30.0
Frozen Dietary Dairy Dessert, Vanilla	3 fl. oz.	100	3.0	45	10	27.0

☞ Frusen Gladje

	S. S.	CAL	FAT(g)	SOD(mg)	CHL(mg)	%FAT
Sorbet, Raspberry	4 fl. oz.	140	0.0	10	0	0.0

☞ Haagen-Dazs

	S. S.	CAL	FAT(g)	SOD(mg)	CHL(mg)	%FAT
Frozen Yogurt, Chocolate	3 fl. oz.	130	3.0	40	25	20.8

☞ Haagen-Dazs	S. S.	CAL	FAT(g)	SOD(mg)	CHL(mg)	%FAT
Frozen Yogurt, Peach	3 fl. oz.	120	3.0	30	31	22.5
Frozen Yogurt, Strawberry	3 fl. oz.	120	3.0	30	29	22.5
Frozen Yogurt, Vanilla	3 fl. oz.	130	3.0	40	36	20.8
Frozen Yogurt, Vanilla Almond Crunch	3 fl. oz.	150	5.0	65	33	30.0

☞ Healthy Choice	S. S.	CAL	FAT(g)	SOD(mg)	CHL(mg)	%FAT
Frozen Dairy Dessert, Bordeaux Cherry	4 oz.	120	2.0	50	5	15.0
Frozen Dairy Dessert, Chocolate	4 oz.	130	2.0	70	5	13.8
Frozen Dairy Dessert, Cookies N' Cream	4 oz.	130	2.0	80	5	13.8
Frozen Dairy Dessert, Neapolitan	4 oz.	120	2.0	60	5	15.0
Frozen Dairy Dessert, Old Fashioned Vanilla	4 oz.	120	2.0	60	5	15.0
Frozen Dairy Dessert, Praline & Caramel	4 oz.	130	2.0	70	5	13.8
Frozen Dairy Dessert, Rocky Road	4 oz.	160	2.0	70	5	11.3
Frozen Dairy Dessert, Strawberry	4 oz.	120	2.0	50	5	15.0
Frozen Dairy Dessert, Vanilla	4 oz.	120	2.0	60	5	15.0
Frozen Dairy Dessert, Wild Berry Swirl	4 oz.	120	2.0	60	5	15.0

☞ Light N' Lively	S. S.	CAL	FAT(g)	SOD(mg)	CHL(mg)	%FAT
Ice Milk, Carmel Nut	4 fl. oz.	120	4.0	85	10	30.0
Ice Milk, Chocolate Chip	4 fl. oz.	120	4.0	35	10	30.0
Ice Milk, Coffee Ice	4 fl. oz.	100	3.0	40	10	27.0
Ice Milk, Cookies n' Cream	4 fl. oz.	110	3.0	65	10	24.5
Ice Milk, Heavenly Hash	4 fl. oz.	120	4.0	35	10	30.0
Ice Milk, Vanilla	4 fl. oz.	100	3.0	40	10	27.0
Ice Milk, Vanilla Fudge Twirl	4 fl. oz.	110	3.0	45	10	24.5
Ice Milk, Vanilla with Chocolate Covered Almonds	4 fl. oz.	120	4.0	45	10	30.0
Ice Milk, Vanilla with Red Raspberry Swirl	4 fl. oz.	110	3.0	35	10	24.5

FREEZER CASE

☞ Light N' Lively	S. S.	CAL	FAT(g)	SOD(mg)	CHL(mg)	%FAT
Ice Milk, Vanilla-Chocolate-Strawberry	4 fl. oz.	100	3.0	35	10	27.0

☞ Sealtest	S. S.	CAL	FAT(g)	SOD(mg)	CHL(mg)	%FAT
Cubic Scoops, Vanilla with Orange Sherbet	4 fl. oz.	130	4.0	40	15	27.7
Cubic Scoops, Vanilla with Red Raspberry Sherbet	4 fl. oz.	130	4.0	40	15	27.7

☞ Sealtest Free	S. S.	CAL	FAT(g)	SOD(mg)	CHL(mg)	%FAT
Nonfat Frozen Dessert Bars, Chocolate Fudge Swirl	1 bar	90	0.0	30	0	0.0
Nonfat Frozen Dessert Bars, Vanilla Fudge Swirl	1 bar	80	0.0	30	0	0.0
Nonfat Frozen Dessert Bars, Vanilla Strawberry Swirl	1 bar	80	0.0	40	0	0.0
Nonfat Frozen Dessert, Black Cherry	4 fl. oz.	100	0.0	45	0	0.0
Nonfat Frozen Dessert, Chocolate	4 fl. oz.	100	0.0	50	0	0.0
Nonfat Frozen Dessert, Peach	4 fl. oz.	100	0.0	45	0	0.0
Nonfat Frozen Dessert, Strawberry	4 fl. oz.	100	0.0	40	0	0.0
Nonfat Frozen Dessert, Vanilla	4 fl. oz.	100	0.0	45	0	0.0
Nonfat Frozen Dessert, Vanilla Fudge Royale	4 fl. oz.	100	0.0	50	0	0.0
Nonfat Frozen Dessert, Vanilla Strawberry Royale	4 fl. oz.	100	0.0	35	0	0.0
Nonfat Frozen Dessert, Vanilla-Chocolate-Strawberry	4 fl. oz.	100	0.0	40	0	0.0
Nonfat Frozen Yogurt, Black Cherry	4 fl. oz.	110	0.0	50	0	0.0
Nonfat Frozen Yogurt, Chocolate	4 fl. oz.	110	0.0	55	0	0.0
Nonfat Frozen Yogurt, Peach	4 fl. oz.	100	0.0	35	0	0.0
Nonfat Frozen Yogurt, Red Raspberry	4 fl. oz.	100	0.0	40	0	0.0
Nonfat Frozen Yogurt, Strawberry	4 fl. oz.	100	0.0	35	0	0.0
Nonfat Frozen Yogurt, Vanilla	4 fl. oz.	100	0.0	45	0	0.0
Sherbet, Lime	4 fl. oz.	130	1.0	30	5	6.9

☞**Sealtest Free**	S. S.	CAL	FAT(g)	SOD(mg)	CHL(mg)	%FAT
Sherbet, Orange	4 fl. oz.	130	1.0	30	5	6.9
Sherbet, Rainbow	4 fl. oz.	130	1.0	30	5	6.9
Sherbet, Red Raspberry	4 fl. oz.	130	1.0	30	5	6.9

☞**Simple Pleasures Light**	S. S.	CAL	FAT(g)	SOD(mg)	CHL(mg)	%FAT
Frozen Dairy Dessert, Chocolate	1/2 cup	130	<1.0	55	10	<6.4
Frozen Dairy Dessert, Chocolate Chip	1/2 cup	140	3.0	50	15	19.3
Frozen Dairy Dessert, Coffee	1/2 cup	120	<1.0	65	15	<7.5
Frozen Dairy Dessert, Cookies ' N Cream	1/2 cup	150	2.0	852	10	12.0
Frozen Dairy Dessert, Mint Chocolate Chocolate Chip	1/2 cup	140	2.0	50	5	12.9
Frozen Dairy Dessert, Peach	1/2 cup	120	<1.0	65	10	<7.5
Frozen Dairy Dessert, Pecan Pralien	1/2 cup	140	2.0	60	5	12.9
Frozen Dairy Dessert, Rum Raisin	1/2 cup	130	<1.0	85	15	<6.9
Frozen Dairy Dessert, Strawberry	1/2 cup	110	<1.0	50	15	<8.2
Frozen Dairy Dessert, Toffee Crunch	1/2 cup	130	<1.0	80	5	<6.9
Frozen Dairy Dessert, Vanilla	1/2 cup	120	<1.0	50	15	<7.5
No Sugar Added Frozen Dairy Dessert, Chocolate	1/2 cup	80	<1.0	80	10	<11.3
No Sugar Added Frozen Dairy Dessert, Chocolate Carmel Sundae	1/2 cup	90	<1.0	90	10	<10.0
No Sugar Added Frozen Dairy Dessert, Vanilla	1/2 cup	80	<1.0	80	10	<11.3
No Sugar Added Frozen Dairy Dessert, Vanilla Fudge Swirl	1/2 cup	90	<1.0	90	10	<10.0

☞**Stonyfield Farm**	S. S.	CAL	FAT(g)	SOD(mg)	CHL(mg)	%FAT
Frozen Yogurt, Non-Fat, Apricot Mango	1/2 cup	140	0.0	66	0	0.0
Frozen Yogurt, Non-Fat, Double Raspberry	1/2 cup	155	0.0	62	0	0.0
Frozen Yogurt, Non-Fat, Double Strawberry	1/2 cup	135	0.0	64	0	0.0

☞ Stonyfield Farm	S. S.	CAL	FAT(g)	SOD(mg)	CHL(mg)	%FAT
Frozen Yogurt, Non-Fat, Dutch Chocolate	1/2 cup	140	0.0	80	0	0.0
Frozen Yogurt, Non-Fat, Mocha Fudge Swirl	1/2 cup	152	0.0	83	0	0.0
Frozen Yogurt, Non-Fat, Peach Melba	1/2 cup	148	0.0	89	0	0.0
Frozen Yogurt, Non-Fat, Strawberry Banana	1/2 cup	132	0.0	63	0	0.0
Frozen Yogurt, Non-Fat, Vanilla Fudge	1/2 cup	152	0.0	85	0	0.0
Frozen Yogurt, Non-Fat, Very Vanilla	1/2 cup	140	0.0	82	0	0.0

☞ Tofutti	S. S.	CAL	FAT(g)	SOD(mg)	CHL(mg)	%FAT
Land of the Free Nondairy Frozen Dessert, Three Berry	1/2 cup	90	0.0	90	0	0.0
Land of the Free Nondairy Frozen Dessert, Vanilla Apple Orchard	1/2 cup	90	0.0	90	0	0.0
Lite Lite Nondairy Frozen Dessert, Deep Chocolate Fudge	1/2 cup	100	<1.0	160	0	<9.0
Lite Lite Nondairy Frozen Dessert, Special Strawberry	1/2 cup	90	<1.0	155	0	<10.0
Lite Lite Nondairy Frozen Dessert, Swiss Coffee Mocha	1/2 cup	90	<1.0	175	0	<10.0
Lite Lite Nondairy Frozen Dessert, Vanilla Chocolate Strawberry	1/2 cup	90	<1.0	180	0	<10.0

☞ Weight Watchers	S. S.	CAL	FAT(g)	SOD(mg)	CHL(mg)	%FAT
Grand Collection, Chocolate Chip Ice Milk	1/2 cup	120	4.0	80	10	30.0
Grand Collection, Chocolate Fat Free Frozen Dessert	1/2 cup	80	0.0	75	5	0.0
Grand Collection, Chocolate Swirl Fat Free Frozen Dessert	1/2 cup	90	0.0	75	5	0.0
Grand Collection, Neapolitan Fat Free Frozen Dessert	1/2 cup	80	0.0	75	5	0.0
Grand Collection, Pecan Pralines 'n Cream Ice Milk	1/2 cup	130	4.0	90	10	27.7
Grand Collection, Vanilla Fat Free Frozen Dessert	1/2 cup	80	0.0	75	5	0.0

FREEZER CASE

☞**Weight Watchers**	S. S.	CAL	FAT(g)	SOD(mg)	CHL(mg)	%FAT
One-ders, Brownies 'n Creme	4 oz.	130	4.0	115	10	27.7
One-ders, Chocolate Chip	4 oz.	120	4.0	80	10	30.0
One-ders, Heavenly Hash	4 oz.	130	3.0	90	10	20.8
One-ders, Pralines 'n Cream	4 oz.	130	4.0	75	10	27.7
One-ders, Strawberry	4 oz.	110	3.0	75	10	24.5

☞**Wells' Blue Bunny**	S. S.	CAL	FAT(g)	SOD(mg)	CHL(mg)	%FAT
Lite Sugar Free Lowfat Frozen Yogurt, Burgundy Cherry	3 fl. oz.	50	1.0	40	5	18.0
Lite Sugar Free Lowfat Frozen Yogurt, Chocolate	3 fl, oz.	60	1.0	65	5	15.0
Lite Sugar Free Lowfat Frozen Yogurt, Peach	3 fl. oz.	50	1.0	40	5	18.0
Lite Sugar Free Lowfat Frozen Yogurt, Strawberry	3 fl. oz.	50	1.0	40	5	18.0
Lite Sugar Free Lowfat Frozen Yogurt, Vanilla	3 fl. oz.	60	1.0	45	5	15.0
Frozen Yogurt, Burgundy Cherry	4 fl. oz.	120	3.0	50	-	22.5
Frozen Yogurt, Chocolate	4 fl. oz.	120	3.0	55	-	22.5
Frozen Yogurt, Neapolitan	4 fl. oz.	110	3.0	55	-	24.5
Frozen Yogurt, Peach	4 fl. oz.	120	3.0	60	-	22.5
Frozen Yogurt, Strawberry	4 fl. oz.	110	3.0	60	-	24.5
Hi Lite Ice Milk, Cherry Nut	3 fl. oz.	90	2.0	50	-	20.0
Hi Lite Ice Milk, Chocolate Almond	3 fl. oz.	90	3.0	50	-	30.0
Hi Lite Ice Milk, Chocolate Chip	3 fl. oz.	90	3.0	50	-	30.0
Hi Lite Ice Milk, Cookies and Cream	3 fl. oz.	110	3.0	50	-	24.5
Hi Lite Ice Milk, Dutch Chocolate	3 fl. oz.	90	2.0	50	-	20.0
Hi Lite Ice Milk, English Toffe	3 fl. oz.	90	2.0	60	-	20.0
Hi Lite Ice Milk, Fresh Peach	3 fl. oz.	90	2.0	50	-	20.0
Hi Lite Ice Milk, Fudge Nut Sundae	3 fl. oz.	100	3.0	60	-	27.0
Hi Lite Ice Milk, Neapolitan	3 fl. oz.	90	2.0	50	-	20.0
Hi Lite Ice Milk, Strawberry Cheesecake	3 fl. oz	90	2.0	50	-	20.0
Hi Lite Ice Milk, Vanilla	3 fl. oz.	90	3.0	50	-	30.0
Natural Lite Dairy Dessert, Chunky Cherry Nut	3 fl. oz.	90	3.0	50	-	30.0

FREEZER CASE

☞ Wells' Blue Bunny	S. S.	CAL	FAT(g)	SOD(mg)	CHL(mg)	%FAT
Natural Lite Dairy Dessert, French Vanilla	3 fl. oz.	90	3.0	50	-	30.0
Natural Lite Dairy Dessert, Fresh Strawberry	3 fl. oz.	80	2.0	40	-	22.5
Natural Lite Dairy Dessert, Vanilla	3 fl. oz.	80	2.0	50	-	22.5
Nonfat Dairy Dessert, Burgundy Cherry	3 fl. oz.	70	0.0	35	0	0.0
Nonfat Dairy Dessert, Chocolate	3 fl. oz.	70	0.0	45	0	0.0
Nonfat Dairy Dessert, Neapolitan	3 fl. oz.	70	0.0	45	0	0.0
Nonfat Dairy Dessert, Peach	3 fl. oz.	70	0.0	35	0	0.0
Nonfat Dairy Dessert, Strawberry	3 fl. oz.	70	0.0	35	0	0.0
Nonfat Dairy Dessert, Vanilla	3 fl. oz.	70	0.0	45	0	0.0
Nonfat Frozen Dessert, Chocolate	3 fl. oz.	50	0.0	60	0	0.0
Nonfat Frozen Dessert, Raspberry	3 fl. oz.	50	0.0	50	0	0.0
Nonfat Frozen Dessert, Strawberry	3 fl. oz.	50	0.0	50	0	0.0
Nonfat Frozen Dessert, Vanilla	3 fl. oz.	50	0.0	50	0	0.0
Nonfat Frozen Yogurt, Burgundy Cherry	3 fl. oz.	60	0.0	45	0	0.0
Nonfat Frozen Yogurt, Chocolate	3 fl. oz.	60	0.0	50	0	0.0
Nonfat Frozen Yogurt, Peach	3 fl. oz.	60	0.0	45	0	0.0
Nonfat Frozen Yogurt, Strawberry	3 fl. oz.	60	0.0	45	0	0.0
Nonfat Frozen Yogurt, Vanilla	3 fl. oz.	60	0.0	45	0	0.0
Sherbet, All Natural Lime	4 fl. oz.	120	1.0	35	-	7.5
Sherbet, All Natural Orange	4 fl. oz.	120	1.0	35	-	7.5
Sherbet, All Natural Pineapple	4 fl. oz.	140	1.0	35	-	6.4
Sherbet, All Natural Rainbow	4 fl. oz.	120	1.0	35	-	7.5
Sherbet, Raspberry	4 fl. oz.	130	1.0	35	-	6.9
Sherbet, Strawberry	4 fl. oz.	125	1.0	35	-	7.2

☞ Yoplait	S. S.	CAL	FAT(g)	SOD(mg)	CHL(mg)	%FAT
Soft Frozen Yogurt, All Other Flavors	3 fl. oz.	90	2.0	40	5	20.0
Soft Frozen Yogurt, Vanilla Chocolate Chip	3 fl. oz.	100	2.0	40	5	18.0

FROZEN NOVELTIES

☞ **Chilly Things**	S. S.	CAL	FAT(g)	SOD(mg)	CHL(mg)	%FAT
Chilly Pop	1 bar	40	0.0	5	0	0.0
Light Pops	1 bar	12	0.0	5	0	0.0

☞ **Creamsicle**	S. S.	CAL	FAT(g)	SOD(mg)	CHL(mg)	%FAT
Cream Pops. All Flavors	1.75 fl. oz.	60	0.0	15	-	0.0

☞ **Crystal Light**	S. S.	CAL	FAT(g)	SOD(mg)	CHL(mg)	%FAT
Bars, All Flavors, Average Values	1 bar	14	0.0	10	0	0.0
Cool N' Creamy Bars, Amaretto Chocolate Swirl	1 bar	60	2.0	60	0	30.0
Cool N' Creamy Bars, Orange Vanilla	1 bar	30	1.0	25	0	30.0

☞ **Disney**	S. S.	CAL	FAT(g)	SOD(mg)	CHL(mg)	%FAT
Ice Pops, All Flavors	2 fl. oz.	60	0.0	0	-	0.0
Ice Pops, Paradise Pops	2 fl. oz.	50	0.0	0	-	0.0

☞ **Dole**	S. S.	CAL	FAT(g)	SOD(mg)	CHL(mg)	%FAT
Fresh Lites, Chocolate Chip	1 bar	60	1.0	30	-	15.0
Fruit N' Cream Bars, Peach	1 bar	90	1.0	20	5	10.0
Fruit N' Cream Bars, Raspberry	1 bar	90	1.0	15	5	10.0
Fruit N' Cream Bars, Strawberry	1 bar	90	1.0	20	5	10.0
Fruit N' Juice Bars, Peach Passion Fruit	1 bar	70	<1.0	10	0	<12.9
Fruit N' Juice Bars, Pine-Orange Banana	1 bar	70	<1.0	10	0	<12.9
Fruit N' Juice Bars, Pineapple	1 bar	70	<1.0	5	0	<12.9
Fruit N' Juice Bars, Raspberry	1 bar	60	<1.0	15	0	<15.0

FREEZER CASE

☞ **Dole**	S. S.	CAL	FAT(g)	SOD(mg)	CHL(mg)	%FAT
Fruit N' Juice Bars, Strawberry	1 bar	70	<1.0	10	0	<12.9
Sun Tops, Grape	1 bar	40	<1.0	5	0	<22.5
Sun Tops, Lemonade	1 bar	40	<1.0	5	0	<22.5
Sun Tops, Orange	1 bar	40	<1.0	5	0	<22.5
Sun Tops, Punch	1 bar	40	<1.0	5	0	<22.5
Yogurt Bars, Chocolate	1 bar	70	<1.0	50	-	<12.5
Yogurt Bars, Strawberry	1 bar	70	<1.0	25	2	<12.9
Yogurt Bars, Strawberry-Banana	1 bar	60	<1.0	15	2	<15.0

☞ **Fudgesicle**	S. S.	CAL	FAT(g)	SOD(mg)	CHL(mg)	%FAT
Fat Free Fudgsicle, All Flavors	1.75 fl. oz.	70	0.0	45	0	0.0
Fudgesicle Bar	1.75 fl. oz.	70	1.0	70	-	12.9
Fudgesicle Bar Wheel Cool	1.75 fl. oz.	70	1.0	70	-	12.9
Sugar Free Fudgsicle, All Flavors	1.75 fl oz.	35	1.0	50	5	25.7

☞ **Gold Bond**	S. S.	CAL	FAT(g)	SOD(mg)	CHL(mg)	%FAT
Citrus Bites, Orange, Raspberry, Lime	1.75 fl. oz.	50	0.0	0	-	0.0
Fudge Bar	2.25 fl. oz.	100	0.0	100	-	0.0
Fun Box of Fudge	1.75 fl .oz.	80	0.0	80	-	0.0
Insulated Cup, Chocolate	4 fl. oz.	110	3.0	65	-	24.5
Insulated Cup, Strawberry	4 fl. oz.	100	3.0	50	-	27.0
Sundae Cup, Chocolate	4 fl. oz.	120	2.0	60	-	15.0
Sundae Cup, Vanilla	4 fl. oz.	110	3.0	50	-	24.5
Twin Pop, All Flavors	2.5 fl .oz	60	0.0	0	-	0.0

☞ **Good Humor**	S. S.	CAL	FAT(g)	SOD(mg)	CHL(mg)	%FAT
Calippo, Cherry Ice	4.5 fl. oz.	120	0.0	0	-	0.0
Calippo, Lemon Ice	4.5 fl. oz.	130	0.0	0	-	0.0
Calippo, Orange Ice	4.5 fl. oz.	120	0.0	0	-	0.0

☞ Good Humor	S. S.	CAL	FAT(g)	SOD(mg)	CHL(mg)	%FAT
Cherry Italian Ice	6 fl. oz.	140	0.0	0	-	0.0
Cool Shark	3.0 fl. oz.	60	0.0	5	-	0.0
Finger Bar	2.5 fl. oz.	50	0.0	0	-	0.0
Fudge Bar	2.5 fl. oz.	130	0.0	90	-	0.0
Jumbo Jet	4.5 fl. oz.	80	0.0	0	-	0.0
Milky Pop, Vanilla, Strawberry	1.5 fl. oz.	45	0.0	25	-	0.0
Strawberry King Cone	5 fl. oz.	230	5.0	100	-	19.6
Sunkist Lemonade Bar	4 fl. oz.	90	0.0	5	-	0.0
Sunkist Orange Juice Bar	4 fl. oz.	100	0.0	0	-	0.0
Sunkist Strawberry and Cream	4 fl. oz.	90	1.0	30	-	10.0
Sunkist Wildberry Bar	4 fl. oz.	140	0.0	15	-	0.0

☞ Great American	S. S.	CAL	FAT(g)	SOD(mg)	CHL(mg)	%FAT
Chilly Pops	2 fl. oz.	40	0.0	5	0	0.0

☞ Jell-O	S. S.	CAL	FAT(g)	SOD(mg)	CHL(mg)	%FAT
Gelatin Pops, All Flavors, Average Values	1 bar	35	0.0	25	0	0.0
Pudding Pops, Chocolate Fudge	1 bar	80	2.0	90	0	22.5
Pudding Pops, Chocolate/ Vanilla Swirl	1 bar	80	2.0	70	0	22.5
Pudding Pops, Double Chocolate Swirl	1 bar	80	2.0	90	0	22.5
Pudding Pops, Milk Chocolate	1 bar	80	2.0	90	0	22.5
Pudding Pops, Vanilla	1 bar	80	2.0	55	0	22.5
Pudding Pops, Chocolate	1 bar	80	2.0	85	0	22.5
Snowburst Bars, Lemon	1 bar	45	0.0	10	0	0.0
Snowburst Bars, Orange	1 bar	45	0.0	10	0	0.0

☞ Juicy Pickin's	S. S.	CAL	FAT(g)	SOD(mg)	CHL(mg)	%FAT
Frozen Dessert, All Flavors	3 fl. oz.	60	0.0	10	0	0.0

FREEZER CASE

☞ **Kool-Aid**	S. S.	CAL	FAT(g)	SOD(mg)	CHL(mg)	%FAT
Kool Pops, All Flavors, Average Values	1 bar	40	0.0	10	0	0.0

☞ **Minute Maid**	S. S.	CAL	FAT(g)	SOD(mg)	CHL(mg)	%FAT
Fruit Juicee, Cherry	2.25 fl. oz.	60	0.0	10	-	0.0
Fruit Juicee, Grape	2.25 fl. oz.	60	0.0	0	-	0.0
Fruit Juicee, Orange	2.25 fl. oz.	60	0.0	0	-	0.0
Fruit Juicee, Strawberry	2.25 fl. oz.	60	0.0	5	-	0.0

☞ **Popsicle**	S. S.	CAL	FAT(g)	SOD(mg)	CHL(mg)	%FAT
All Natural, All Flavors	1.75 fl. oz.	40	0.0	10	0	0.0
Big Stick Ice Pop, All Flavors	3.5 fl. oz.	80	0.0	20	0	0.0
Ice Cream Sandwich	2.5 fl. oz.	150	3.0	180	-	18.0
Sugar Free Bar	1.75 fl. oz.	18	0	10	0	0.0
Supersicle Firecracker	4.5 fl. oz.	100	0,0	0	0	0.0
Supersicle Rainbow	4.5 fl. oz.	100	0.0	0	0	0.0
Supersicle, Cherry, Banana	4.5 fl. oz.	100	0.0	0	0	0.0
Water Ice, All Flavors	1.75 fl oz.	50	0.0	10	0	0.0
Water Ice, Orange, Cherry, Grape	2.5 fl. oz.	70	0.0	15	0	0.0

☞ **Push Ups**	S. S.	CAL	FAT(g)	SOD(mg)	CHL(mg)	%FAT
Orange Sherbet	1 bar	90	1.0	25	<5	10.0

☞ **Weight Watchers**	S. S.	CAL	FAT(g)	SOD(mg)	CHL(mg)	%FAT
Chocolate Treat Bars, Fat Free	1 bar	90	0.0	75	0	0.0
Double Fudge Bars	1 bar	60	1.0	50	5	15.0
Sugar Free Chocolate Mousse Bars	1 bar	35	<1.0	30	5	<25.7

☞**Weight Watchers**	S. S.	CAL	FAT(g)	SOD(mg)	CHL(mg)	%FAT
Sugar Free Orange Vanilla Treat Bars, Fat Free	1 bar	30	0.0	40	0	0.0
Vanilla Sandwich Bars, Fat Free	1 bar	130	0.0	170	0	0.0

☞**Welch's**	S. S.	CAL	FAT(g)	SOD(mg)	CHL(mg)	%FAT
Fruit Juice Bars, Grape	3 fl. oz.	80	0.0	0	0	0.0
Fruit Juice Bars, Grape	1.75 fl. oz.	45	0.0	0	0	0.0
Fruit Juice Bars, Raspberry	3 fl. oz.	80	0.0	0	0	0.0
Fruit Juice Bars, Raspberry	1.75 fl. oz.	45	0.0	0	0	0.0
Fruit Juice Bars, Strawberry	3 fl. oz.	80	0.0	0	0	0.0
Fruit Juice Bars, Strawberry	1.75 fl. oz.	45	0.0	0	0	0.0
No Sugar Added Juice Bars, Grape	3 fl. oz.	25	0.0	0	0	0.0
No Sugar Added Juice Bars, Raspberry	3 fl. oz.	25	0.0	0	0	0.0
No Sugar Added Juice Bars, Strawberry	3 fl. oz.	25	0.0	0	0	0.0

☞**Wells' Blue Bunny**	S. S.	CAL	FAT(g)	SOD(mg)	CHL(mg)	%FAT
Frozen Dessert Bars, Deluxe Rainbow Sticks	1 bar	50	1.0	25	-	18.0
Frozen Dessert Bars, Frozen Yogurt and Fruit Snacks	1 bar	50	1.0	20	-	18.0
Frozen Dessert Bars, Fudge Sticks	1 bar	100	0.0	90	-	0.0
Frozen Dessert Bars, NutraSweet Citrus Bars	1 bar	160	0.0	10	-	0.0
Frozen Dessert Bars, NutraSweet Sugar Free	1 bar	8	0.0	10	-	0.0
Frozen Dessert Bars, Polar Pops	1 bar	40	0.0	5	-	0.0
Frozen Dessert Bars, Twin Pop Sticks	1 bar	70	0.0	5	-	0.0

FROZEN DINNERS

☞Armour Classics Lite	S. S.	CAL	FAT(g)	SOD(mg)	CHL(mg)	%FAT
Beef Pepper Steak	1 pkg.	220	4.0	970	35	16.4
Beef Stroganoff	1 pkg.	250	6.0	510	55	21.6
Chicken Ala King	1 pkg.	290	7.0	630	55	21.7
Chicken Burgundy	1 pkg.	210	2.0	780	45	8.6
Chicken Marsala	1 pkg.	250	7.0	930	80	25.2
Chicken Oriental	1 pkg.	180	1.0	660	35	5.0
Shrimp Creole	1 pkg.	260	2.0	900	45	6.9
Sweet and Sour Chicken	1 pkg.	240	2.0	820	35	7.5

☞Banquet	S. S.	CAL	FAT(g)	SOD(mg)	CHL(mg)	%FAT
Casseroles, Spaghetti with Meat Sauce	1 pkg.	270	8.0	1250	-	26.7
Cookin' Bags, Chicken & Vegetables Prima Vera	1 pkg.	100	2.0	-	-	18.0
Cookin' Bags, Turkey Chili	1 pkg.	80	2.0	740	15	22.5

☞Booth	S. S.	CAL	FAT(g)	SOD(mg)	CHL(mg)	%FAT
Filet Entrees, Au Gratin	1 pkg.	280	8.0	780	72	25.7
Filet Entrees, Florentine	1 pkg.	260	8.0	670	82	27.7
Filet Entrees, Parmigiana	1 pkg.	273	5.0	930	88	16.5
Filet Entrees, with Mushroom Sauce	1 pkg.	280	9.0	750	58	28.9
Shrimp Entrees, Fettucini Alfredo	1 pkg.	260	80	620	138	27.7
Shrimp Entrees, New Orleans	1 pkg.	230	5.0	950	91	19.6
Shrimp Entrees, Oriental	1 pkg.	190	3.0	950	91	14.2
Shrimp Entrees, Prima Vera with Fettuccine	1 pkg.	200	3.0	760	90	13.5

☞Budget Gourmet	S. S.	CAL	FAT(g)	SOD(mg)	CHL(mg)	%FAT
Entrees, Chicken Marsala	1 pkg.	260	8.0	730	90	27.2

FREEZER CASE

☞ Budget Gourmet	S. S.	CAL	FAT(g)	SOD(mg)	CHL(mg)	%FAT
Entrees, Pepper Steak with Rice	1 pkg.	320	9.0	590	30	25.3
Entrees, Sweet and Sour Chicken	1 pkg.	340	5.0	630	30	13.2
Light and Healthy Dinners, Chicken Breast Parmigiana	1 pkg.	260	8.0	420	50	27.7
Light and Healthy Dinners, Herb Chicken Breast with Fettucini	1 pkg.	240	7.0	430	55	26.3
Light and Healthy Dinners, Sirloin of Beef in Wine Sauce	1 pkg.	270	8.0	520	30	26.7
Light and Healthy Dinners, Stuffed Turkey Breast	1 pkg.	230	6.0	520	40	23.5
Light Dinners, Teriyaki Chicken Breast	1 pkg.	270	6.0	460	30	20.0
Light Entrees, Cheese Lasagna with Vegetables	1 pkg.	290	9.0	780	15	27.9
Light Entrees, Glazed Turkey	1 pkg.	270	5.0	760	40	16.7
Light Entrees, Mandarin Chicken	1 pkg.	300	7.0	670	40	21.0
Light Entrees, Orange Glazed Chicken	1 pkg.	250	3.0	1044	10	10.8
Light Entrees, Oriental Beef	1 pkg.	290	9.0	810	30	27.9
Light Entrees, Vegetable Lasagna	1 pkg.	290	9.0	780	15	27.9
Three Dish Dinners, Scallop and Shrimp Marinara	1 pkg.	330	9.0	730	70	24.5

☞ Cajun Cookin'	S. S.	CAL	FAT(g)	SOD(mg)	CHL(mg)	%FAT
Crawfish Etouffee	1 pkg.	390	10.0	1110	-	23.1
Seafood Gumbo	1 pkg.	330	7.0	1330	-	19.1
Shrimp Creole	1 pkg.	390	11.0	1130	-	25.4
Shrimp Etouffee	1 pkg.	360	9.0	1170	-	22.5

☞ Chun King	S. S.	CAL	FAT(g)	SOD(mg)	CHL(mg)	%FAT
Egg Rolls, Pork, Restaurant Style	3	180	6.0	450	25	30.0
Egg Rolls, Shrimp	3.6	200	6.0	480	20	27.0
Entrees, Beef Pepper Oriental	1 pkg.	310	3.0	1300	40	8.7
Entrees, Chicken Chow Mein	1 pkg.	370	6.0	1560	85	14.6
Entrees, Crunchy Walnut Chicken	1 pkg.	310	5.0	1700	45	14.5

FREEZER CASE

☞ Chun King

	S.S.	CAL	FAT(g)	SOD(mg)	CHL(mg)	%FAT
Entrees, Imperial Chicken	1 pkg.	300	1.0	1540	30	3.0
Entrees, Sweet and Sour Pork	1 pkg.	400	5.0	1460	25	11.3
Side Dishes, Fried Rice with Chicken	1 pkg.	260	4.0	1460	75	13.8
Side Dishes, Fried Rice with Pork	1 pkg.	270	6.0	1210	55	20.0

☞ Dining Lite

	S.S.	CAL	FAT(g)	SOD(mg)	CHL(mg)	%FAT
Cheese Cannelloni	1 pkg.	310	9.0	650	70	26.1
Cheese Lasagna	1 pkg.	260	6.0	800	30	20.8
Chicken Ala King	1 pkg.	240	7.0	780	40	26.3
Chicken Chow Mein	1 pkg.	180	2.0	650	30	10.0
Chicken with Noodles	1 pkg.	240	7.0	570	50	26.3
Lasagna with Meat Sauce	1 pkg.	240	5.0	800	25	18.8

☞ Healthy Choice

	S.S.	CAL	FAT(g)	SOD(mg)	CHL(mg)	%FAT
Breakfast, Apple Spice Muffin	2.5 oz.	190	4.0	90	0	18.9
Breakfast, Banana Nut Muffin	2.5 oz.	180	6.0	80	0	30.0
Breakfast, Blueberry Muffin	2.5 oz.	190	4.0	110	0	18.9
Breakfast, English Muffin Sandwich	4.25 oz.	200	3.0	510	20	13.5
Breakfast, Turkey Sausage Omlet on English Muffin	4.75 oz.	210	4.0	470	20	17.1
Breakfast, Western Style Omlet on English Muffin	4.75 oz.	200	3.0	480	15	13.5
Dinner, Baked Potato with Broccoli & Cheese Sauce	1 pkg.	240	5.0	510	15	18.8
Dinner, Beef Enchiladas	1 pkg.	350	7.0	430	30	18.0
Dinner, Beef Pepper Steak	1 pkg.	290	6.0	530	65	18.6
Dinner, Beef Sirloin Tips	1 pkg.	280	8.0	370	65	25.7
Dinner, Breast of Turkey	1 pkg.	290	5.0	420	45	15.5
Dinner, Chicken and Pasta Divan	1 pkg.	310	4.0	510	60	11.6
Dinner, Chicken Dijon	1 pkg.	260	3.0	420	45	10.4
Dinner, Chicken Enchiladas	1 pkg.	280	6.0	510	30	19.3
Dinner, Chicken Oriental	1 pkg.	230	1.0	460	45	3.9
Dinner, Chicken Parmigiana	1 pkg.	270	3.0	240	50	10.0

☞ Healthy Choice	S. S.	CAL	FAT(g)	SOD(mg)	CHL(mg)	%FAT
Dinner, Herb Roasted Chicken	1 pkg.	290	4.0	430	50	12.4
Dinner, Macaroni and Cheese	1 pkg.	280	6.0	520	20	16.1
Dinner, Mesquite Chicken	1 pkg.	340	1.0	290	45	2.6
Dinner, Pasta Primavera	1 pkg.	280	3.0	360	15	9.6
Dinner, Salisbury Steak	1 pkg.	300	7.0	480	50	21.0
Dinner, Salsa Chicken	1 pkg.	240	2.0	450	50	7.5
Dinner, Shrimp Creole	1 pkg.	230	2.0	430	60	7.8
Dinner, Shrimp Marinara	1 pkg.	260	1.0	320	60	3.5
Dinner, Sirloin Beef with Barbecue Sauce	1 pkg.	300	6.0	320	50	18.0
Dinner, Sole au Gratin	1 pkg.	270	5.0	470	55	16.7
Dinner, Sweet and Sour Chicken	1 pkg.	280	2.0	260	50	6.4
Dinner, Turkey Tetrazzini	1 pkg.	340	6.0	490	40	15.9
Dinner, Yankee Pot Roast	1 pkg.	250	4.0	360	50	14.4
Entree, Baked Cheese Ravioli	1 pkg.	240	2.0	460	30	7.5
Entree, Beef Fajitas	1 pkg.	210	4.0	250	35	17.1
Entree, Beef Pepper Steak	1 pkg.	250	4.0	340	40	14.4
Entree, Cheese Manicotti	1 pkg.	230	4.0	450	25	15.7
Entree, Chicken A L'Orange	1 pkg.	240	2.0	220	45	7.5
Entree, Chicken and Vegetables	1pkg.	210	1.0	490	35	4.3
Entree, Chicken Chow Mein	1 pkg.	220	3.0	440	45	12.3
Entree, Chicken Fajitas	1 pkg.	200	3.0	310	35	13.5
Entree, Chicken Fettucini	1 pkg.	240	4.0	370	45	15.0
Entree, Fettucini Alfredo	1 pkg.	240	7.0	370	45	26.3
Entree, Glazed Chicken	1 pkg.	220	3.0	390	45	12.3
Entree, Lasagna with Meat Sauce	1 pkg.	260	5.0	420	20	17.3
Entree, Linguini with Shrimp	1 pkg.	230	2.0	420	60	7.8
Entree, Mandarin Chicken	1 pkg.	260	2.0	400	50	6.9
Entree, Rigatoni in Meat Sauce	1 pkg.	240	4.0	470	20	15.0
Entree, Roasted Turkey and Mushrooms in Gravy	1 pkg.	200	3.0	380	40	13.5
Entree, Seafood Newburg	1 pkg.	200	3.0	440	55	13.5
Entree, Sole with Lemon Butter Sauce	1 pkg.	230	4.0	430	45	15.7
Entree, Spaghetti with Meat Sauce	1 pkg.	280	6.0	480	20	19.3
Entree, Zucchini Lasagna	1 pkg.	240	3.0	390	15	11.3
French Bread Pizza, Cheese	1 pkg.	300	3.0	500	20	9.0

FREEZER CASE

☞Healthy Choice	S. S.	CAL	FAT(g)	SOD(mg)	CHL(mg)	%FAT
French Bread Pizza, Deluxe	1 pkg.	330	8.0	490	35	21.8
French Bread Pizza, Italian Turkey Sausage	1 pkg.	320	7.0	440	30	19.7
French Bread Pizza, Pepperoni	1 pkg.	320	8.0	490	30	22.5
Homestyle and Pasta Classics, Barbecue Beef Ribs	1 pkg.	330	6.0	530	70	16.4
Homestyle and Pasta Classics, Cacciatore Chicken	1 pkg.	310	3.0	430	35	8.7
Homestyle and Pasta Classics, Fettucini	1 pkg.	350	6.0	480	-	15.4
Homestyle and Pasta Classics, Pasta with Shrimp	1 pkg.	270	4.0	490	50	13.3
Homestyle and Pasta Classics, Rigatoni with Chicken	1 pkg.	360	4.0	430	60	10.0
Homestyle and Pasta Classics, Salisbury Steak	1 pkg.	280	6.0	500	55	19.3
Homestyle and Pasta Classics, Sliced Turkey	1 pkg.	270	4.0	530	50	13.3
Homestyle and Pasta Classics, Stuffed Pasta Shells	1 pkg.	310	3.0	470	35	8.7
Homestyle and Pasta Classics, Teriyaki Pasta	1 pkg.	350	3.0	370	45	7.7
Homestyle and Pasta Classics, Zesty Tomato Sauce over Ziti	1 pkg.	350	5.0	530	30	12.9

☞Kid Cuisine	S. S.	CAL	FAT(g)	SOD(mg)	CHL(mg)	%FAT
Cheese Pizza	1 pkg.	380	12.0	550	25	28.4
Hamburger Pizza	1 pkg.	330	12.0	700	15	27.3
Mexican Style	1 pkg.	290	8.0	610	20	24.8
Mini Cheese Ravioli	1 pkg.	290	8.0	780	15	24.8
Spaghetti with Meat Sauce	1 pkg.	310	8.0	760	30	23.2

☞Kraft	S. S.	CAL	FAT(g)	SOD(mg)	CHL(mg)	%FAT
Eating Right, Beef Sirloin Tips and Noodles	1 pkg.	250	8.0	340	70	28.8
Eating Right, Chicken Breast and Vegetables	1 pkg.	200	4.0	570	30	18.0

☞Kraft

☞Kraft	S. S.	CAL	FAT(g)	SOD(mg)	CHL(mg)	%FAT
Eating Right, Chicken Breast Parmesan	1 pkg.	300	10.0	540	50	30.0
Eating Right, Fettucini Alfredo	1 pkg.	220	7.0	410	20	28.6
Eating Right, Glazed Chicken Breast	1 pkg.	240	4.0	560	35	15.0
Eating Right, Lasagna with Meat Sauce	1 pkg.	270	7.0	440	30	23.3
Eating Right, Macaroni & Cheese	1 pkg.	270	8.0	590	15	26.7
Eating Right, Shrimp Vegetable Stir Fry	1 pkg.	150	4.0	400	50	24.0
Eating Right, Sliced Turkey Breast	1 pkg.	250	7.0	560	50	25.2
Eating Right, Swedish Meatballs	1 pkg.	290	7.0	470	55	21.7
Turkey and Dressing	1 pkg.	320	10.0	1210	35	28.1

☞Lean Cuisine

☞Lean Cuisine	S. S.	CAL	FAT(g)	SOD(mg)	CHL(mg)	%FAT
Baked Cheese Ravioli	1 pkg.	240	8.0	590	55	30.0
Beef and Bean Enchanadas	1 pkg.	240	6.0	480	45	22.5
Beef Cannelloni with Mornay Sauce	1 pkg.	210	4.0	590	25	17.1
Beefsteak Ranchero	1 pkg.	270	9.0	530	30	30.0
Breast of Chicken Marsala with Vegetables	1 pkg.	190	5.0	450	5	23.7
Breast of Chicken Parmesan	1 pkg.	270	9.0	450	35	30.0
Broccoli and Cheddar Baked Potato	1 pkg.	290	9.0	590	20	27.9
Cheese Cannelloni with Tomato Sauce	1 pkg.	270	8.0	590	25	26.7
Cheese Pizza	1 pkg.	300	9.0	590	15	27.0
Chicken and Vegetables with Vermicelli	1 pkg.	280	7.0	480	35	22.5
Chicken à l'Orange with Almond Rice	1 pkg.	280	4.0	290	55	12.9
Chicken Cacciatore with Vermicelli	1 pkg.	280	7.0	570	45	22.5
Chicken Chow Mein with Rice	1 pkg.	240	5.0	530	30	18.8
Chicken Enchanadas	1 pkg.	290	9.0	500	55	27.9
Chicken Fettucini	1 pkg.	280	8.0	530	45	25.7
Chicken in Barbecue Sauce	1 pkg.	260	6.0	500	50	20.8
Chicken Italiano	1 pkg.	290	8.0	490	45	24.8
Chicken Oriental	1 pkg.	250	7.0	570	45	25.2

FREEZER CASE

☞ Lean Cuisine	S. S.	CAL	FAT(g)	SOD(mg)	CHL(mg)	%FAT
Chicken Tenderloins in Herb Cream Sauce	1 pkg.	240	5.0	490	60	18.8
Chicken Tenderloins in Peanut Sauce	1 pkg.	290	7.0	530	45	21.7
Fiesta Chicken	1 pkg.	240	5.0	560	40	18.8
Filet of Fish Divan	1 pkg.	210	5.0	490	65	21.4
Filet of Fish Florentine	1 pkg.	220	7.0	590	65	28.6
Glazed Chicken with Vegetable Rice	1 pkg.	260	8.0	570	55	27.7
Homestyle Turkey with Vegetables and Pasta	1 pkg.	230	5.0	550	50	19.6
Lasagna with Meat and Sauce	1 pkg.	260	5.0	590	25	17.3
Linguini with Clam Sauce	1 pkg.	280	8.0	560	30	25.7
Macaroni and beef in Tomato Sauce	1 pkg.	240	6.0	590	40	22.5
Macaroni and Cheese	1 pkg.	290	9.0	550	30	27.9
Oriental Beef with Vegetables and Rice	1 pkg.	290	9.0	590	40	27.9
Rigatoni Bake with Meat Sauce Cheese	1 pkg.	250	8.0	430	25	28.8
Salisbury Steak with Gravy and Scalloped Potatoes	1 pkg.	240	7.0	580	45	26.3
Sausage Pizza	1 pkg.	330	9.0	860	40	24.5
Sliced Turkey Breast in Mushroom Sauce	1 pkg.	220	6.0	550	40	24.5
Sliced Turkey Breast in Mushroom Sauce	1 pkg.	220	6.0	550	40	24.5
Sliced Turkey Breast with Dressing	1 pkg.	200	5.0	590	25	22.5
Spaghetti with Meat Sauce	1 pkg.	290	6.0	500	20	18.6
Spaghetti with Meatballs	1 pkg.	280	7.0	490	35	22.5
Stuffed Cabbage with Meat in Tomato Sauce	1 pkg.	210	6.0	560	40	25.7
Swedish Meatballs in Gravy with Pasta	1 pkg.	290	8.0	590	50	24.8
Tuna Lasagna with Spinach Noodles and Vegetables	1 pkg.	240	7.0	520	20	26.3
Turkey Dijon	1 pkg.	230	5.0	590	45	19.6
Zucchini Lasagna	1 pkg.	260	5.0	550	20	17.3

☞ LeMenu	S. S.	CAL	FAT(g)	SOD(mg)	CHL(mg)	%FAT
Healthy Dinners, Cheese Tortellini	1 pkg.	230	6.0	460	15	23.5

☞ LeMenu	S. S.	CAL	FAT(g)	SOD(mg)	CHL(mg)	%FAT
Healthy Dinners, Glazed Chicken	1 pkg.	230	3.0	480	55	11.7
Healthy Dinners, Herb Roasted Chicken	1 pkg.	240	7.0	400	70	26.3
Healthy Dinners, Salisbury Steak	1 pkg.	280	9.0	400	35	28.9
Healthy Dinners, Sliced Turkey	1 pkg.	210	5.0	540	30	21.4
Healthy Dinners, Stuffed Shells	1 pkg.	280	8.0	690	25	25.7
Healthy Dinners, Sweet & Sour Chicken	1 pkg.	250	7.0	530	40	25.2
Healthy Dinners, Turkey Divan	1 pkg.	260	7.0	420	60	24.2
Healthy Dinners, Veal Marsala	1 pkg.	230	3.0	700	75	11.7
Healthy Entrees, Cheese Tortellini	1 pkg.	250	8.0	480	15	28.8
Healthy Entrees, Chicken a la King	1 pkg.	240	5.0	670	30	18.8
Healthy Entrees, Chicken Dijon	1 pkg.	240	7.0	500	40	26.3
Healthy Entrees, Chicken Enchilada	1 pkg.	280	8.0	530	35	25.7
Healthy Entrees, Empresse Chicken	1 pkg.	210	5.0	690	30	21.4
Healthy Entrees, Glazed Turkey	1 pkg.	260	6.0	720	35	20.8
Healthy Entrees, Herb Roasted Chicken	1 pkg.	260	6.0	500	45	20.8
Healthy Entrees, Lasagna with Meat Sauce	1 pkg.	290	8.0	510	30	24.8
Healthy Entrees, Spaghetti with Meat Sauce	1 pkg.	280	6.0	450	15	19.3
Healthy Entrees, Swedish Meatballs	1 pkg.	260	8.0	700	40	27.7
Healthy Entrees, Traditional Turkey	1 pkg.	200	5.0	610	25	22.5
Healthy Entrees, Vegetable Lasagna	1 pkg.	260	8.0	500	25	27.7
Light Style Dinners, 3-Cheese Stuffed Shells	1 pkg.	280	8.0	720	-	25.7
Light Style Dinners, Chicken Cacciatore	1 pkg.	270	8.0	640	-	26.7
Light Style Dinners, Chicken Cannelloni	1 pkg.	270	5.0	590	-	16.7
Light Style Dinners, Chicken Chow Mein	1 pkg.	260	4.0	830	-	13.8
Light Style Dinners, Glazed Chicken Breast	1 pkg.	270	6.0	770	-	20.0
Light Style Dinners, Herb Roasted Chicken	1 pkg.	220	6.0	610	-	24.5
Light Style Dinners, Salisbury Steak	1 pkg.	220	7.0	830	-	28.6
Light Style Dinners, Turkey Divan	1 pkg.	280	9.0	840	-	28.9
Light Style Dinners, Veal Marsala	1 pkg.	260	6.0	800	-	20.8

FREEZER CASE

☞ Looney Tunes Meals

	S. S.	CAL	FAT(g)	SOD(mg)	CHL(mg)	%FAT
Daffy Duck Spaghetti & Meatballs	1 pkg.	340	10.0	570	-	26.5
Elmer Fudd Turkey & Dressing	1 pkg.	260	7.0	510	-	24.2
Foghorn Leghorn Pepperoni Pizza	1 pkg.	400	13.0	610	-	29.3
Tweety Macaroni & Cheese	1 pkg.	340	10	650	-	26.5

☞ Morton Dinners

	S. S.	CAL	FAT(g)	SOD(mg)	CHL(mg)	%FAT
Chili Gravy with Beef Enchilada and Tamale	1 pkg.	300	10.0	1390	20	30.0
Glazed Ham	1 pkg.	230	3.0	1120	35	11.7
Spaghetti & Meat Sauce	1 pkg.	170	2.0	930	10	10.6
Veal Parmagian	1 pkg.	230	7.0	1330	30	27.4

☞ Mrs. Paul's

	S. S.	CAL	FAT(g)	SOD(mg)	CHL(mg)	%FAT
Light Seafood Entree, Fish Dijon	1 pkg.	200	5.0	650	60	22.5
Light Seafood Entree, Seafood Lasagna	1 pkg.	290	8.0	750	57	24.8
Light Seafood Entree, Seafood Rotini	1 pkg.	240	6.0	570	25	22.5
Light Seafood Entree, Shrimp and Clams with Linguini	1 pkg.	240	5.0	750	40	18.8

☞ Old El Paso

	S. S.	CAL	FAT(g)	SOD(mg)	CHL(mg)	%FAT
Bean and Cheese Burrito	1 pkg.	330	11.0	740	-	30.0

☞ Stouffer's

	S. S.	CAL	FAT(g)	SOD(mg)	CHL(mg)	%FAT
Baked Chicken Breast & Vegetable Medley	1 pkg.	190	6.0	560	-	28.4
Chicken à la King with Rice	1 pkg.	290	9.0	890	-	27.9
Chicken Chow Mein without Noodles	1 pkg.	190	4.0	1080	-	27.7

☞ **Stouffer's**	S. S.	CAL	FAT(g)	SOD(mg)	CHL(mg)	%FAT
Green Pepper Steak with Rice	1 pkg.	330	11.0	1440	-	30.0
Homestyle Beef and Noodles & Vegetable Medley	1 pkg.	230	7.0	720	-	27.4
Spaghetti with Meat Sauce	1 pkg.	370	11.0	1510	-	26.8

☞ **Swanson**	S. S.	CAL	FAT(g)	SOD(mg)	CHL(mg)	%FAT
3-Compartment Dinners, Noodles and Chicken	1 pkg.	280	8.0	740	-	25.7
4-Compartment Dinners, Beef	1 pkg.	310	6.0	770	-	17.4
4-Compartment Dinners, Swiss Steak	1 pkg.	350	11.0	700	-	28.3
4-Compartment Dinners, Turkey	1 pkg.	350	11.0	1090	-	28.3
Homestyle Recipe Entrees, Chicken Cacciatore	1 pkg.	260	8.0	1030	-	27.7
Homestyle Recipe Entrees, Seafood Creole with Rice	1 pkg.	240	6.0	810	-	22.5
Homestyle Recipe Entrees, Sirloin Tips in Burgundy Sauce	1 pkg.	160	5.0	550	-	28.1
Hungry Man Dinners, Sliced Beef	1 pkg.	450	12.0	1060	-	24.0
Hungry Man Dinners, Turkey	1 pkg.	550	18.0	1810	-	29.5

☞ **Tyson**	S. S.	CAL	FAT(g)	SOD(mg)	CHL(mg)	%FAT
Gourmet Selection Dinners, A L'Orange	1 pkg.	300	8.0	670	-	24.0
Gourmet Selection Dinners, Chicken with Gravy	1 pkg.	230	6.0	480	50	23.5
Gourmet Selection Dinners, Glazed Chicken	1 pkg.	240	4.0	930	45	15.0
Gourmet Selection Dinners, Grilled Chicken	1 pkg.	220	3.0	520	55	12.3
Gourmet Selection Dinners, Marsala	1 pkg.	200	4.0	670	52	18.0
Gourmet Selection Dinners, Mesquite	1 pkg.	320	8.0	660	-	22.5
Gourmet Selection Dinners, Sweet & Sour	1 pkg.	440	8.0	850	-	16.4
Gourmet Selection Dinners, Turkey	1 pkg.	380	11.0	1350	-	26.1

FREEZER CASE

☞ Ultra Slim Fast

	S. S.	CAL	FAT(g)	SOD(mg)	CHL(mg)	%FAT
Beef Pepper Steak and Parsleyed Rice	1 pkg.	270	4.0	690	45	13.3
Cheese Ravioli	1 pkg.	330	3.0	770	40	8.2
Chicken & Vegetables	1 pkg.	290	3.0	850	30	9.3
Chicken Chow Mein	1 pkg.	320	6.0	580	60	16.9
Chicken Fettucini	1 pkg.	380	12.0	980	65	28.4
Country Style Vegetables & Beef Tips	1 pkg.	230	5.0	960	45	19.6
Glazed Turkey with Dressing	1 pkg.	340	5.0	570	50	13.2
Lasagna with Meat Sauce	1 pkg.	330	9.0	980	55	24.5
Mesquite Chicken	1 pkg.	360	1.0	300	65	2.5
Mushroom Gravy Over Salisbury Steak	1 pkg.	290	5.0	830	35	15.5
Roasted Chicken in Mushroom Sauce	1 pkg.	280	6.0	830	80	19.3
Shrimp Creole	1 pkg.	240	4.0	730	80	15.0
Shrimp Marinara	1 pkg.	290	3.0	880	70	9.3
Spaghetti with Beef & Mushroom Sauce	1 pkg.	370	10.0	990	25	24.3
Sweet & Sour Chicken	1 pkg.	330	2.0	160	35	5.5
Tomato Sauce Over Meatloaf	1 pkg.	340	9.0	780	35	23.8
Turkey Medallions in Herb Sauce	1 pkg.	280	6.0	950	40	19.3
Vegetable Lasagna	1 pkg.	240	4.0	730	15	15.0

☞ Weight Watchers

	S. S.	CAL	FAT(g)	SOD(mg)	CHL(mg)	%FAT
Angel Hair Pasta	1 pkg.	200	4.0	330	10	18.0
Baked Cheese Ravioli	1 pkg.	240	6.0	370	30	22.5
Beef Sirloin Tips & Mushrooms in Wine Sauce	1 pkg.	210	6.0	560	30	25.7
Beef Stroganoff	1 pkg.	280	9.0	590	30	28.9
Broccoli & Cheese Baked Potato	1 pkg.	270	6.0	570	5	20.0
Cheese Manicotti	1 pkg.	260	8.0	510	25	27.7
Cheese Tortellini	1 pkg.	310	6.0	570	15	17.4
Chicken Ala King	1 pkg.	230	4.0	460	30	15.7
Chicken Divan Baked Potato	1 pkg.	280	7.0	480	30	22.5
Chicken Fajitas	1 pkg.	210	5.0	490	25	21.4
Chicken Fettucini	1 pkg.	280	9.0	590	40	28.9

☞Weight Watchers	S. S.	CAL	FAT(g)	SOD(mg)	CHL(mg)	%FAT
Homestyle Chicken & Noodles	1 pkg.	240	7.0	450	30	26.3
Homestyle Turkey Baked Potato	1 pkg.	250	7.0	510	60	25.2
Imperial Chicken	1 pkg.	210	4.0	420	25	17.1
Lasagna	1 pkg.	270	6.0	510	5	20.0
Lasagna, Garden	1 pkg.	260	7.0	430	15	24.2
Lasagna, Italian Cheese	1 pkg.	290	7.0	510	20	21.7
London Broil in Mushroom Sauce	1 pkg.	110	3.0	320	25	24.5
Oven Baked Fish	1 pkg.	150	4.0	260	10	24.0
Pizza, Cheese	1 pkg.	300	7.0	310	10	21.0
Pizza, Deluxe Combination	1 pkg.	320	9.0	370	10	25.3
Pizza, Pepperoni	1 pkg.	320	8.0	550	15	22.5
Pizza, Sausage	1 pkg.	340	10.0	380	10	26.5
Spaghetti with Meat Sauce	1 pkg.	240	7.0	490	5	26.3
Veal Patty Parmigiana	1 pkg.	190	6.0	650	55	28.4

FROZEN PASTA

☞Angy's	S. S.	CAL	FAT(g)	SOD(mg)	CHL(mg)	%FAT
Ravioli with Cheese	8	120	4.0	170	20	30.0
Ravioli with Meat	8	140	2.0	180	10	12.9
Tortellini with Cheese	14	130	2.0	140	6	13.8
Tortellini with Meat	19	160	2.0	210	9	11.3

☞Celentano	S. S.	CAL	FAT(g)	SOD(mg)	CHL(mg)	%FAT
Baked Pasta and Cheese	6 oz.	280	7.0	390	35	22.5
Cannelloni Florentine	12 oz.	350	8.0	620	81	20.6
Cavatelli	3.2 oz.	250	1.0	5	2	3.6
Chicken Primavera	11.5 oz.	260	7.0	620	30	24.2
Mini Ravioli	4 oz.	250	5.0	210	50	18.0
Stuffed Shells, 16 oz.	8 oz.	330	11.0	680	74	30.0

FREEZER CASE

☞ Louisa

	S. S.	CAL	FAT(g)	SOD(mg)	CHL(mg)	%FAT
Ravioli, Beef	4 oz.	269	8.0	355	60	26.8
Ravioli, Cheese	4 oz.	254	8.0	262	69	28.3
Ravioli, Breaded	4.8 oz.	311	8.0	788	48	23.2
Tortellini	3 oz.	237	5.0	201	-	19.0

☞ Mama Rosie's

	S. S.	CAL	FAT(g)	SOD(mg)	CHL(mg)	%FAT
Ravioli, Cheese	6	185	5.0	165	-	24.3

FROZEN PIZZA

☞ Celentano

	S. S.	CAL	FAT(g)	SOD(mg)	CHL(mg)	%FAT
9-Slice Pizza	2.7 oz.	150	4.0	390	8	24.0

☞ Healthy Choice

	S. S.	CAL	FAT(g)	SOD(mg)	CHL(mg)	%FAT
French Bread Pizza, Cheese	1 pkg.	300	3.0	500	20	9.0
French Bread Pizza, Deluxe	1 pkg.	330	8.0	490	35	21.8
French Bread Pizza, Italian Turkey Sausage	1 pkg.	320	7.0	440	30	19.7
French Bread Pizza, Pepperoni	1 pkg.	320	8.0	490	30	22.5

☞ Jeno's

	S. S.	CAL	FAT(g)	SOD(mg)	CHL(mg)	%FAT
Pizza Rolls, Cheese	3 oz.	200	5.0	370	20	22.5
Pizza Rolls, Sausage	3 oz.	210	7.0	340	15	30.0

☞ Lean Cuisine

	S. S.	CAL	FAT(g)	SOD(mg)	CHL(mg)	%FAT
French Bread Pizza, Cheese	5.5 oz.	320	10.0	700	15	28.1
French Bread Pizza, Sausage	6 oz.	350	11.0	960	40	28.3

☞ **McCain Ellio's**	S. S.	CAL	FAT(g)	SOD(mg)	CHL(mg)	%FAT
Ellio's Healthy Slice Pizza, Cheese	2.67 oz.	160	2.0	390	5	11.3
Ellio's Healthy Slice Pizza, Garden Style	3.03 oz.	150	2.0	370	5	12.0
Ellio's Healthy Slice Pizza, Mixed Vegetable	3.10 oz.	150	2.0	370	5	12.0

☞ **Pappalo's**	S. S.	CAL	FAT(g)	SOD(mg)	CHL(mg)	%FAT
9" Pizza, Three Cheese	1/2	350	11.0	640	30	28.3
12" Pizza, Pepperoni	1/4	350	11.0	700	45	28.3
12" Pizza, Three Cheese	1/4	310	7.0	440	30	20.3
Pan Pizza, Pepperoni	1/5	350	11.0	720	50	28.3
Pan Pizza, Sausage	1/5	350	11.0	530	40	28.3
Pan Pizza, Sausage & Pepperoni	1/5	360	12.0	630	45	30.0
Pan Pizza, Three Cheese	1/5	310	8.0	490	30	23.2

☞ **Tombstone**	S. S.	CAL	FAT(g)	SOD(mg)	CHL(mg)	%FAT
Light Pizza, Chicken	1/2	240	9.0	540	25	30.0
Light Pizza, Italian Sausage, 12"	1/5	240	8.0	590	15	30.0
Light Pizza, Vegetable	1/2	240	8.0	500	10	30.0

☞ **Weight Watchers**	S. S.	CAL	FAT(g)	SOD(mg)	CHL(mg)	%FAT
Pizza, Cheese	1 pkg.	300	7.0	310	10	21.0
Pizza, Pepperoni	1 pkg.	320	8.0	550	15	22.5
Pizza, Sausage	1 pkg.	340	10.0	380	10	26.5
Pizza, Deluxe Combination	1 pkg.	320	9.0	370	10	25.3

FROZEN POULTRY

☞ Tyson	S. S.	CAL	FAT(g)	SOD(mg)	CHL(mg)	%FAT
Breast Filet, Barbecue	3 oz.	110	3.0	310	35	24.5
Breast Filet, Grilled	2.75 oz.	100	3.0	410	45	27.0
Breast Filet, Lemon Pepper	2.75 oz.	100	3.0	380	40	27.0
Breast Strips, Grilled	2.75 oz.	100	3.0	410	45	27.0
Breast Strips, Oriental	2.75 oz.	110	3.0	250	40	24.5
Breast Tenders, Hot & Spicy	2.75 oz.	110	3.0	490	35	24.5
Breast Tenders, Mesquite	2.75 oz.	110	3.0	420	45	24.5
Diced Meat	3.0 oz.	130	3.0	40	70	20.8
Marinated Breast Filets, Barbecue	3.75 oz.	120	3.0	400	-	22.5
Marinated Breast Filets, Italian	3.75 oz.	120	3.0	430	-	22.5
Marinated Breast Filets, Lemon Pepper	3.75 oz.	130	3.0	210	-	20.8
Marinated Breast Filets, Teriyaki	3.75 oz.	130	3.0	290	-	20.8
Microwave BBQ Beef Sandwich	1 sandwich	200	2.7	600	30	12.2
Sandwich, Grilled Chicken	3.5 oz.	200	5.0	470	32	22.5
Sandwich, Microwave BBQ Chicken	4.0 oz.	230	6.0	600	50	23.5
Sandwich, Microwave Mini	3.5 oz.	230	5.0	540	-	19.6

☞ Weaver	S. S.	CAL	FAT(g)	SOD(mg)	CHL(mg)	%FAT
Breast, Hickory Smoked	1 slice	26	0.8	195	-	27.7
Breast, Oven Roasted	1 slice	25	0.5	185	-	18.0
Breast, Turkey	1 slice	20	0.4	136	-	18.0

FROZEN SEAFOOD

☞ Booth	S. S.	CAL	FAT(g)	SOD(mg)	CHL(mg)	%FAT
Filets-Block, Cod	4 oz.	89	1.0	80	49	10.1
Filets-Block, Flounder	4 oz.	90	1.0	90	54	10.0
Filets-Block, Haddock	4 oz.	90	1.0	70	-	10.0
Filets-Block, Ocean Perch	4 oz.	100	1.0	90	48	9.0
Filets-Block, Sole	4 oz.	90	1.0	90	54	10.0
Filets-Block, Whiting	4 oz.	100	1.0	90	76	9.0

FREEZER CASE

☞**Booth**	S. S.	CAL	FAT(g)	SOD(mg)	CHL(mg)	%FAT
Low Salt Filets, Cod	4 oz.	90	1.0	80	49	10.0
Low Salt Filets, Flounder	4 oz.	90	0.0	90	54	0.0
Low Salt Filets, Haddock	4 oz.	90	0.0	70	65	0.0
Low Salt Filets, Perch	4 oz.	100	1.0	90	48	9.0
Low Salt Filets, Sole	4 oz.	90	0.0	90	54	0.0
Low Salt Filets, Whiting	4 oz.	80	1.0	85	76	11.3

☞**Gorton's**	S. S.	CAL	FAT(g)	SOD(mg)	CHL(mg)	%FAT
Butterfly Shrimp	4 oz.	160	<1.0	540	-	<5.6
Fishmarket Fresh, Cod	5 oz.	110	1.0	90	-	8.2
Fishmarket Fresh, Flounder	5 oz.	110	1.0	170	-	8.2
Fishmarket Fresh, Haddock	5 oz.	110	1.0	120	-	8.2
Fishmarket Fresh, Ocean Perch	5 oz.	140	3.0	100	-	19.3
Fishmarket Fresh, Sole	5 oz.	110	1.0	140	-	8.2

☞**Healthy Choice**	S. S.	CAL	FAT(g)	SOD(mg)	CHL(mg)	%FAT
Breaded Fish Filets (2 Filets)	1 Filet	160	5.0	350	30	28.1
Breaded Fish Filets (4 Filets)	1 Filet	140	4.0	300	25	25.7
Breaded Fish Filets (8 Filets)	1 Filet	120	4.0	250	20	30.0
Breaded Fish Sticks	3 Sticks	120	4.0	350	20	30.0

☞**Mrs. Paul's**	S. S.	CAL	FAT(g)	SOD(mg)	CHL(mg)	%FAT
Filet, Haddock, Crunchy Batter	2	190	5.0	580	25	23.7
Healthy Treasures Breaded Fish Filets, 8 oz. package	1 Filet	170	3.0	290	25	15.9
Healthy Treasures Breaded Fish Filets, 12 oz. package	1 Filet	130	3.0	210	20	20.8
Healthy Treasures Breaded Fish Sticks	3 Sticks	110	3.0	270	15	24.5

☞Van de Kamp's	S. S.	CAL	FAT(g)	SOD(mg)	CHL(mg)	%FAT
Natural Filets, Cod	4 oz.	90	1.0	90	25	10.0
Natural Filets, Flounder	4 oz.	100	2.0	100	35	18.0
Natural Filets, Haddock	4 oz.	90	1.0	125	20	10.0
Natural Filets, Sole	4 oz.	100	2.0	105	35	18.0
Crisp and Healthy Breaded Fish Sticks	4 sticks	120	2.0	330	15	15.0
Crisp and Healthy Breaded Fish Filets	2 filets	150	3.0	350	25	18.0

FROZEN SOUPS

☞Kettle Ready	S. S.	CAL	FAT(g)	SOD(mg)	CHL(mg)	%FAT
Frozen Soup, Chicken Noodle	3/4 cup	94	2.9	600	-	27.9
Frozen Soup, Garden Vegetable	3/4 cup	85	2.8	461	-	29.7
Frozen Soup, Hearty Beef Vegetable	3/4 cup	85	2.8	354	-	29.6
Frozen Soup, Savory Bean with Ham	3/4 cup	113	3.6	404	-	28.7
Frozen Soup, Split Pea with Ham	3/4 cup	155	4.4	352	0	25.6

☞Tabatchnick	S. S.	CAL	FAT(g)	SOD(mg)	CHL(mg)	%FAT
Soup, Frozen Fresh, Boil 'n' Bag, Barley and Bean	7.5 oz.	130	2.0	217	0	13.8
Soup, Frozen Fresh, Boil 'n' Bag, Cabbage	7.5 oz.	110	2.0	185	0	16.4
Soup, Frozen Fresh, Boil 'n' Bag, Chicken	7.5 oz.	65	2.0	255	0	27.7
Soup, Frozen Fresh, Boil 'n' Bag, Cream of Mushroom	6.0 oz.	75	2.0	325	3	24.0
Soup, Frozen Fresh, Boil 'n' Bag, Cream of Spinach	7.5 oz.	85	2.0	200	4	21.2
Soup, Frozen Fresh, Boil 'n' Bag, Lentil	7.5 oz.	170	2.0	240	0	10.6
Soup, Frozen Fresh, Boil 'n' Bag, Minestrone	7.5 oz.	137	2.0	255	0	13.1
Soup, Frozen Fresh, Boil 'n' Bag, Mushroom Barley	7.5 oz.	92	2.0	234	0	19.6
Soup, Frozen Fresh, Boil 'n' Bag, Mushroom Barley, No Salt	7.5 oz.	97	1.0	77	0	9.3

☞ **Tabatchnick**	S. S.	CAL	FAT(g)	SOD(mg)	CHL(mg)	%FAT
Soup, Frozen Fresh, Boil 'n' Bag, New England	7.5 oz.	98	2.0	255	0	18.4
Soup, Frozen Fresh, Boil 'n' Bag, Northern Bean	7.5 oz.	165	2.0	240	0	10.9
Soup, Frozen Fresh, Boil 'n' Bag, Pea	7.5 oz.	175	1.0	290	0	5.1
Soup, Frozen Fresh, Boil 'n' Bag, Pea, No Salt	7.5 oz.	175	1.0	79	0	5.1
Soup, Frozen Fresh, Boil 'n' Bag, Tomato Rice	6.0 oz.	73	1.0	300	0	12.3
Soup, Frozen Fresh, Boil 'n' Bag, Vegetable	7.5 oz.	97	1.0	190	0	9.3
Soup, Frozen Fresh, Boil 'n' Bag, Vegetable, No Salt	7.5 oz.	92	2.0	77	0	19.6
Soup, Frozen Fresh, Boil 'n' Bag, Zucchini	6.0 oz.	80	2.0	285	3	22.5

FROZEN VEGETABLES

☞ **Birds Eye**	S. S.	CAL	FAT(g)	SOD(mg)	CHL(mg)	%FAT
Butter Sauce Combination Vegetables, Tender Sweet Corn in Butter Sauce	3.3 oz.	90	2.0	250	5	20.0
Custom Cuisine, Chow Mein Vegetables in Oriental Sauce	4.6 oz.	80	2.0	570	0	22.5
Custom Cuisine, Vegetables with Creamy Mushroom Sauce for Beef	4.6 oz.	60	2.0	450	5	30.0
Custom Cuisine, Vegetables with Savory Tomato Basil Sauce for Chicken	4.6 oz.	110	3.0	360	0	24.5
Custom Cuisine, Vegetables with Wild Rice in White Wine Sauce for Chicken	4.6 oz.	100	0.0	510	0	0.0

☞ **Green Giant**	S. S.	CAL	FAT(g)	SOD(mg)	CHL(mg)	%FAT
Butter Sauce Vegetables, Broccoli, Cauliflower and Carrots	1/2 cup	30	1.0	240	5	30.0
Butter Sauce Vegetables, Brussel Sprouts	1/2 cup	40	1.0	280	5	22.5
Butter Sauce Vegetables, Cut Green Beans	1/2 cup	30	1.0	230	5	30.0

FREEZER CASE

☞ **Green Giant**	S. S.	CAL	FAT(g)	SOD(mg)	CHL(mg)	%FAT
Butter Sauce Vegetables, Golden Corn	1/2 cup	100	2.0	310	5	18.0
Butter Sauce Vegetables, Le Sueur Early Peas	1/2 cup	80	2.0	440	5	22.5
Butter Sauce Vegetables, Lima Beans	1/2 cup	100	3.0	390	5	27.0
Butter Sauce Vegetables, Mixed Vegetables	1/2 cup	60	2.0	300	5	30.0
Butter Sauce Vegetables, Sweet Peas	1/2 cup	80	2.0	410	5	22.5
Butter Sauce Vegetables, White Corn	1/2 cup	100	2.0	280	5	18.0
Cheese Sauce Vegetables, Broccoli	1/2 cup	60	2.0	530	2	30.0
Cheese Sauce Vegetables, Broccoli, Cauliflower and Carrots	1/2 cup	60	2.0	490	2	30.0
Cheese Sauce Vegetables, Cauliflower	1/2 cup	60	2.0	500	2	30.0
Cream Sauce Vegetables, Cream Style Corn Shoepeg	1/2 cup	110	1.0	370	0	8.2
Garden Gourmet, Asparagus Pilaf	1 pkg.	190	4.0	610	10	18.9
Garden Gourmet, Tortellini Provencale	1 pkg.	260	6.0	840	15	20.8
One Serve, Broccoli, Carrots and Rotini in Cheese Sauce	5.0 oz.	100	2.0	440	5	18.0
One Serve, Cauliflower in Cheese Sauce	5.5 oz.	80	2.0	640	5	22.5
One Serve, Early Peas in Butter Sauce	4.5 oz.	60	2.0	370	5	30.0
One Serve, Green Beans in Butter Sauce	5.5 oz.	60	2.0	370	5	30.0
One Serve, Niblets Corn in Butter Sauce	4.5 oz.	120	2.0	260	5	15.0
One Serve, Pasta Parmesan with Sweet Peas	5.5 oz.	160	5.0	420	10	28.1
One Serve, Rice 'N Broccoli in Cheese Sauce	5.5 oz.	160	5.0	490	5	28.1
One Serving Vegetables, Pasta & Rice, Broccoli, Cauliflowe & Carrots in Cheese Sauce	1 pkg.	80	2.0	650	5	22.5
One Serving Vegetables, Pasta & Rice, Cut Broccoli in Cheese Sauce	1 pkg.	80	2.0	700	5	22.5
One Serving Vegetables, Pasta & Rice, Potatoes & Broccoli in Cheese Sauce	1 pkg.	130	4.0	580	5	27.7
Pasta Accents, Creamy Cheddar	1 /2 cup	90	3.0	280	5	30.0
Rice Originals, Pilaf	1/2 cup	110	1.0	530	2	8.2
Rice Originals, Rice 'n Broccoli	1/2 cup	120	4.0	400	10	30.0

☞**Green Giant**	S. S.	CAL	FAT(g)	SOD(mg)	CHL(mg)	%FAT
Rice Originals, Rice Florentine	1/2 cup	140	4.0	310	5	25.7
Rice Originals, Rice Medley	1/2 cup	100	1.0	310	5	9.0
Rice Originals, White and Wild Rice	1/2 cup	130	2.0	540	0	13.8

◆ All Frozen Vegetables without butter and sauce are very low fat

MISCELLANEOUS FROZEN FOODS

☞**Chun King**	S. S.	CAL	FAT(g)	SOD(mg)	CHL(mg)	%FAT
Egg Roll, Restaurant Style, Pork	3 oz.	180	6.0	450	25	30.0
Egg Roll, Shrimp	3.6 oz.	200	6.0	480	20	27.0

☞**Fleischmann's**	S. S.	CAL	FAT(g)	SOD(mg)	CHL(mg)	%FAT
Egg Beaters Egg Substitute	1/4 cup	25	0.0	80	0	0.0
Egg Beaters Vegetable Omlette Mix	1/2 cup	50	0.0	170	0	0.0

☞**Healthy Choice**	S. S.	CAL	FAT(g)	SOD(mg)	CHL(mg)	%FAT
Egg Product	1/4 cup	30	<1.0	90	0	<30.0

☞**La Choy**	S. S.	CAL	FAT(g)	SOD(mg)	CHL(mg)	%FAT
Egg Rolls, Almond Chicken	3 oz.	120	3.0	290	5	22.5
Egg Rolls, Sweet & Sour	3 oz.	150	4.0	280	5	24.0
Egg Rolls, Restaurant Style, Pork	3 oz.	150	5.0	480	7	30.0
Egg Rolls, Restaurant Style, Shrimp	3 oz.	130	4.0	260	5	27.7
Snack Egg Rolls, Chicken	1.45 oz.	690	3.0	140	<1	30.0
Snack Egg Rolls, Lobster	1.45 oz.	75	2.0	150	<1	24.0
Snack Egg Rolls, Shrimp	1.45 oz.	75	2.0	120	4	24.0

☞ Lean Pockets	S. S.	CAL	FAT(g)	SOD(mg)	CHL(mg)	%FAT
Beef and Broccoli	1	260	10.0	950	25	34.6
Chicken Deluxe	1	290	11.0	660	30	34.1
Chicken Fajita	1	270	10.0	840	30	33.3
Chicken Oriental	1	260	9.0	830	35	31.2
Chicken Parmesan	1	270	11.0	670	30	36.7
Chicken Supreme	1	260	10.0	760	25	34.6

☞ Mrs. Paul's	S. S.	CAL	FAT(g)	SOD(mg)	CHL(mg)	%FAT
Sweet Potatoes, Candied	4 oz.	170	0.0	40	-	0.0
Sweets 'N Apples, Candied	4 oz.	160	0.0	60	-	0.0

☞ Ore Ida	S. S.	CAL	FAT(g)	SOD(mg)	CHL(mg)	%FAT
French Fries, Country Style Dinner Fries	3 oz.	110	3.0	15	0	24.5
French Fries, Golden Crinkles	3 oz.	120	4.0	25	0	30.0
French Fries, Golden Fries	3 oz.	120	4.0	30	0	30.0
French Fries, Home Style Potato Wedges	3 oz.	110	3.0	25	0	24.5
French Fries, Lites, Crinkle Cuts	3 oz.	90	2.0	35	0	20.0
Hash Browns, Cheddar Browns	3 oz.	80	2.0	420	5	22.5
Hash Browns, Potatoes O'Brien	3 oz.	60	<1.0	25	0	<15.0
Hash Browns, Shredded	3 oz.	70	<1.0	40	0	<12.9
Hash Browns, Southern Style	3 oz.	70	<1.0	30	0	<12.9
Topped Baked Potato, Broccoli and Cheese	5.9 oz.	160	4.0	400	5	22.5

FREEZER CASE

GRAVY, SEASONING & SAUCE MIXES

BUTTER SPRINKLES

☞ **Best O'Butter**	S. S.	CAL	FAT(g)	SOD(mg)	CHL(mg)	%FAT
Cheddar Cheese Flavor	1/2 tsp.	6	<1.0	75	-	-
Original Flavor	1/2 tsp.	4	<1.0	65	-	-
Sour Cream Flavor	1/2 tsp.	4	<1.0	65	-	-

☞ **Butter Buds**	S. S.	CAL	FAT(g)	SOD(mg)	CHL(mg)	%FAT
Liquid	2 tsp.	4	0.0	57	0	0.0
Sprinkles	1/2 tsp.	4	0.0	33	0	0.0

☞ **Molly McButter**	S. S.	CAL	FAT(g)	SOD(mg)	CHL(mg)	%FAT
Sprinkles, Bacon Flavor	1/2 tsp.	4	0.1	62	0	16.6
Sprinkles, Butter Flavor	1/2 tsp.	3	0.0	90	0	12.0
Sprinkles, Cheese Flavor	1/2 tsp.	4	0.2	60	1	45.6
Sprinkles, Sour Cream & Butter Flavor	1/2 tsp.	4	0.1	69	0	23.1

GRAVIES AND GRAVY MIXES

☞ **Durkee**	S. S.	CAL	FAT(g)	SOD(mg)	CHL(mg)	%FAT
Gravy Mix, Au Jus	2 cups	62	0.3	1826	-	3.8
Gravy Mix, Brown w/ Mushrooms	1 cup	59	0.5	1402	-	7.8
Gravy Mix, Brown w/ Onions	1 cup	66	0.5	1356	-	6.7
Gravy Mix, Brown	1 cup	59	0.4	1037	-	5.3
Gravy Mix, Chicken	1 cup	92	1.2	1537	-	11.7
Gravy Mix, Homestyle	1 cup	70	2.0	830	-	25.7
Gravy Mix, Mushroom	1 cup	60	1.0	1170	-	15.0

☞ Durkee	S. S.	CAL	FAT(g)	SOD(mg)	CHL(mg)	%FAT
Gravy Mix, Onion	1 cup	84	0.5	953	-	5.4
Gravy Mix, Pork	1 cup	70	0.5	2175	-	6.8
Gravy Mix, Swiss Steak	1 1/2 cups	68	0.2	2222	-	2.1
Gravy Mix, Turkey	1 cup	87	0.1	1010	-	0.9

☞ Franco-American	S. S.	CAL	FAT(g)	SOD(mg)	CHL(mg)	%FAT
Canned Gravy, Au jus	2 oz.	10	0.0	330	-	0.0

☞ French's*	S. S.	CAL	FAT(g)	SOD(mg)	CHL(mg)	%FAT
Meat Marinade Mix	1/8 pkg.	10	0.0	540	-	0.0

☞ Hain*	S. S.	CAL	FAT(g)	SOD(mg)	CHL(mg)	%FAT
Brown Gravy Mix	1/4 pkg.	16	0.0	600	0	0.0

☞ McCormick/Schilling	S. S.	CAL	FAT(g)	SOD(mg)	CHL(mg)	%FAT
Gravy Mix, Au Jus	1/4 cup	20	0.3	786	-	13.5
Gravy Mix, Chicken	1/4 cu0p	22	0.4	300	-	16.4
Gravy Mix, Herb	1/4 cup	20	0.5	312	-	22.5
Gravy Mix, Homestyle	1/4 cup	24	0.8	295	-	30.0
Gravy Mix, Mushroom	1/4 cup	19	0.5	270	-	23.7
Gravy Mix, Onion	1/4 cup	22	0.6	337	-	24.5
Gravy Mix, Pork	1/4 cup	20	0.6	297	-	27.0
Gravy Mix, Turkey	1/4 cup	22	0.5	353	-	20.5

☞ **Pillsbury**	S. S.	CAL	FAT(g)	SOD(mg)	CHL(mg)	%FAT
Gravy Mix, Brown	1/4 cup	16	0.0	180	0	0.0
Gravy Mix, Chicken	1/4 cup	18	0.0	170	0	0.0
Gravy Mix, Homestyle	1/4 cup	16	0.0	240	0	0.0

SEASONING AND SAUCE PACKETS

☞ **Durkee**	S. S.	CAL	FAT(g)	SOD(mg)	CHL(mg)	%FAT
Dry Sauce Mix, Meat Marinade	1/2 cup	47	0.7	4104	-	13.4
Dry Sauce Mix, Spaghetti Sauce	2 1/2 cups	224	1.0	3937	-	4.0
Dry Sauce Mix, Spaghetti Sauce, Extra Thick & Rich	2 1/4 cups	212	1.4	1873	-	5.8
Dry Sauce Mix, Spaghetti with Mushroom Sauce	2 2/3 cups	208	0.8	3106	-	3.5
Dry Seasoning Mix, Enchilada Sauce	4 cups	229	2.4	385	-	9.4
Dry Seasoning Mix, Fried Rice Seasoning	2 cups	430	1.4	2698	-	2.9
Dry Seasoning Mix, Sweet & Sour Sauce	1 cup	230	5.7	1053	-	22.3
Roastin' Bag w/ Dry Gravy mix, Au jus*	1 plg.	64	1.0	2628	-	14.1
Roastin' Bag w/ Dry Gravy mix, Chicken Gravy*	1 pkg.	122	1.0	3597	-	7.4
Roastin' Bag w/ Dry Gravy mix, Chicken-Italian Style*	1 pkg.	144	1.0	3614	-	6.3
Roastin' Bag w/ Dry Gravy mix, Lemon Butter Seasoning for Fish*	1 pkg.	75	0.7	1347	-	8.4
Roastin' Bag w/ Dry Gravy mix, Meatloaf*	1 pkg.	129	1.0	3472	-	7.0
Roastin' Bag w/ Dry Gravy mix, Onion Pot Roast*	1 pkg.	124	0.1	2864	-	0.7
Roastin' Bag w/ Dry Gravy mix, Pork Gravy*	1 pkg.	130	1.0	2579	-	6.9
Roastin' Bag w/ Dry Gravy mix, Pot Roast and Stew*	1 pkg.	125	1.0	2965	-	7.2
Roastin' Bag w/ Dry Gravy mix, Sparerib Sauce*	1 pkg.	162	2.0	2185	-	11.1
Roastin' Bag w/ Dry Gravy mix, Swiss Steak*	1 pkg.	115	0.9	3008	-	7.0
Sauce Mix, Spaghetti, Italian Style	1 pkg.	35	0.0	770	-	0.0
Sauce Mix, Stroganoff*	1 pkg.	90	0.7	3002	-	7.0
Seasoning Mix, Beef Stew*	1 pkg.	99	0.5	6953	-	4.5

GRAVY, SEASONING AND SAUCE MIXES

☞ Durkee	S. S.	CAL	FAT(g)	SOD(mg)	CHL(mg)	%FAT
Seasoning Mix, Chili Con Carne*	1 pkg.	148	1.6	3239	-	9.7
Seasoning Mix, Chop Suey*	1 pkg.	128	2.1	828	-	14.8
Seasoning Mix, Ground Beef Mix*	1 pkg.	91	0.9	1314	-	8.9
Seasoning Mix, Italian Meatball*	1 pkg.	22	0.7	1755	-	28.6
Seasoning Mix, Sloppy Joe*	1 pkg.	118	0.2	3512	-	1.5
Seasoning Mix, Taco*	1 pkg.	67	1.0	2106	-	13.4

☞ French's*	S. S.	CAL	FAT(g)	SOD(mg)	CHL(mg)	%FAT
Marinade Mix, Meat	1/8 pkg.	10	0.0	540	-	0.0
Microwave Seasoned Coating Mix, Barbecue Chicken	1/4 pkg.	45	1.0	270	-	20.0
Microwave Seasoned Coating Mix, Garlic Butter Chicken	1/4 pkg.	50	1.0	280	-	18.0
Seasoning Mix, Beef Stew	1/6 pkg.	25	0.0	770	-	0.0
Seasoning Mix, Ground Beef with Onion	1/4 pkg.	25	0.0	440	-	0.0
Seasoning Mix, Hamburger	1/4 pkg.	25	0.0	450	-	0.0
Seasoning Mix, Meatball	1/4 pkg.	35	0.0	830	-	0.0
Seasoning Mix, Meatloaf	1/8 pkg.	20	0.0	620	-	0.0
Seasoning Mix, Sloppy Joe	1/8 pkg.	16	0.0	390	-	0.0

☞ Kikkoman*	S. S.	CAL	FAT(g)	SOD(mg)	CHL(mg)	%FAT
Marinade Mix, Meat	1 pkg.	64	0.4	4500	0	4.9
Sauce Mix, Sweet & Sour	1 pkg.	228	0.4	900	0	1.7
Sauce Mix, Teriyaki	1 pkg.	125	0.4	3990	0	3.0
Seasoning Mix, Chow Mein	1 pkg.	98	0.8	2790	1	7.5
Seasoning Mix, Fried Rice	1 pkg.	91	0.2	1760	1	2.4
Seasoning Mix, Stir-Fry	1 pkg.	84	0.4	2650	0	3.8

☞ Knorr	S. S.	CAL	FAT(g)	SOD(mg)	CHL(mg)	%FAT
Sauce Mix, Lemon Dill	1/4 cup	30	1.0	220	-	30.0

☞ Lawry's*	S. S.	CAL	FAT(g)	SOD(mg)	CHL(mg)	%FAT
Seasoning Blend, Beef Stew	1 pkg.	131	0.7	3181	-	4.8
Seasoning Blend, Burrito	1 pkg.	132	1.7	2516	-	11.6
Seasoning Blend, Chili	1 pkg.	143	1.8	2291	-	11.3
Seasoning Blend, Enchilada	1 pkg.	152	1.2	1723	-	7.1
Seasoning Blend, Fajita	1 pkg.	63	0.4	2118	-	5.7
Seasoning Blend, Gravy, Au Jus	1 pkg.	89	2.5	2790	-	25.5
Seasoning Blend, Gravy, Chicken, Microwave	1 pkg.	102	3.1	1675	-	27.5
Seasoning Blend, Gravy, Turkey, Microwave	1 pkg.	98	2.9	1380	-	26.2
Seasoning Blend, Meat Loaf	1 pkg.	355	1.2	6547	-	3.0
Seasoning Blend, Mexican Rice	1 pkg.	94	2.0	3246	-	19.1
Seasoning Blend, Pot Roast	1 pkg.	122	0.7	4008	-	5.2
Seasoning Blend, Salsa Mix	1 pkg.	95	0.5	2042	-	4.7
Seasoning Blend, Sloppy Joe	1 pkg.	126	0.4	3442	-	2.9
Seasoning Blend, Spaghetti Sauce, Garden Style	1 pkg.	96	1.4	779	-	13.1
Seasoning Blend, Spaghetti Sauce, Rich & Thick	1 pkg.	147	2.2	2172	-	13.5
Seasoning Blend, Spaghetti Sauce, with Mushrooms	1 pkg.	143	1.5	2015	-	9.4
Seasoning Blend, Stroganoff	1 pkg.	123	0.3	2814	-	2.2
Seasoning Blend, Taco	1 pkg.	118	1.1	1441	-	8.4
Seasoning Blend, Taco Salad	1 pkg.	124	0.9	1451	-	6.5

☞ McCormick/Shilling	S. S.	CAL	FAT(g)	SOD(mg)	CHL(mg)	%FAT
Bag'n Season, Chicken*	1/4 pkg.	44	0.4	641	-	8.2
Bag'n Season, Italian Herb*	1/4 pkg.	24	0.1	342	-	1.9
Bag'n Season, Pork Chops*	1/4 pkg.	26	0.1	782	-	3.5
Bag'n Season, Pot Roast*	1/4 pkg.	14	0.2	758	-	12.9
Chicken Sauce Blend, Italian Marinade*	1 pkg.	120	0.7	-	-	5.3
Chicken Sauce Blend, Mesquite Marinade*	1 pkg.	132	3.0	2068	0	20.5
Chicken Sauce Blend, Stir Fry*	1 pkg.	124	0.2	-	-	1.5
Chicken Sauce Blend, Sweet & Sour*	1 pkg.	204	0.9	-	-	4.0
Chicken Sauce Blend, Teriyaki*	1 pkg.	172	3.6	1380	0	18.8

GRAVY, SEASONING AND SAUCE MIXES

☞ McCormick/Shilling	S. S.	CAL	FAT(g)	SOD(mg)	CHL(mg)	%FAT
Pasta Prima Sauce Mix, Marinara	1/2 cup	193	6.0	356	-	28.0
Pasta Prima Sauce Mix, Pesto	1/2 cup	329	8.0	432	-	21.9
Seasoning/Sauce Mix, Beef Stew*	1/4 pkg.	33	0.3	3223	-	6.8
Seasoning/Sauce Mix, Beef Stroganoff*	1/4 pkg.	32	0.3	4313	-	7.0
Seasoning/Sauce Mix, Chili*	1/4 pkg.	27	0.5	1158	-	16.7
Seasoning/Sauce Mix, Fajitas*	1/4 pkg.	28	0.5	417	-	16.2
Seasoning/Sauce Mix, Sloppy Joe*	1/4 pkg.	26	0.5	3000	-	17.3
Seasoning/Sauce Mix, Spaghetti	1/4 pkg.	32	0.0	2460	-	0.7
Seasoning/Sauce Mix, Spaghetti Thick & Zesty*	1/4 pkg.	34	0.2	952	-	4.7
Seasoning/Sauce Mix, Taco*	1/4 pkg.	31	0.5	2700	-	14.5

☞ Tio Sancho	S. S.	CAL	FAT(g)	SOD(mg)	CHL(mg)	%FAT
Seasoning Mix, Chili	1.23 oz.	109	2.2	832	-	18.2
Seasoning Mix, Taco	1.51 oz.	132	1.7	2623	-	11.6

*Values for unprepared mix.
  See Cooking Chapter–Changing Manufacturers Directions.

HEALTH/DIETETIC FOODS

☞Barbara's Bakery	S. S.	CAL	FAT(g)	SOD(mg)	CHL(mg)	%FAT
Bread Sticks, Italian Style	1 oz.	120	3.0	-	0	22.5
Bread Sticks, Regular	1 oz.	120	3.0	-	0	22.5
California Lemon & Orange	2	39	1.0	-	-	23.1
Chocolate & Vanilla Crisps	0.5 oz.	70	2.0	-	0	25.7
Fruit & Nut	2	125	2.0	-	0	14.4
Ginger Snaps	2	39	1.0	-	-	23.1
Oatmeal Raisin	2	102	2.0	-	0	17.6
Sesame Sticks	1 oz.	130	4.0	-	-	27.7
Tropical Coconut	2	64	2.0	-	0	28.1

☞Estee	S. S.	CAL	FAT(g)	SOD(mg)	CHL(mg)	%FAT
Cake Mix, Carrot	1/10	100	2.0	65	0	18.0
Cake Mix, Chocolate	1/10	100	2.0	100	0	18.0
Cake Mix, Lemon	1/10	100	2.0	65	0	18.0
Cake Mix, Pound	1/10	100	2.0	65	0	18.0
Cake Mix, White	1/10	100	2.0	65	0	18.0
Carmels, Vanilla or Chocolate	1	30	1.0	15	0	30.0
Catsup	1 Tbsp.	6	0.0	20	0	0.0
Cookies, All Other Flavors	1	30	1.0	0	0	30.0
Cookies, Fudge	1	30	1.0	0	0	30.0
Crackers, Unsalted	4	60	2.0	0	0	30.0
Frosting Mix	1.5 tsp.	50	1.0	0	0	18.0
Gelatin Dessert	1/2 cup	8	0.0	0	0	0.0
Gum Drops	4	25	0.0	0	0	0.0
Gummy Bears	3	20	0.0	0	0	0.0
Hard Candy	2	25	0.0	0	0	0.0
Lollipops	1	25	0.0	0	0	0.0
Pancake Mix	Three 3" pancakes	100	0.0	135	0	0.0
Peanut Brittle	0.25 oz.	35	1.0	30	0	25.7

HEALTH/DIETETIC FOODS

☞ Estee	S. S.	CAL	FAT(g)	SOD(mg)	CHL(mg)	%FAT
Preserves and Jellies	1 tsp.	2	0.0	10	0	0.0
Pretzels, Unsalted	7	50	<12.0	0	0	<18.0
Pudding, Chocolate	1/2 cup	70	1.0	75	2	12.9
Pudding, Vanilla	1/2 cup	70	<1.0	75	2	<12.9
Raisins, Chocolate Coated	10	30	1.0	10	0	30.0
Salad Dressing, Creamy Garlic	1 Tbsp.	2	0.0	10	0	0.0
Salad Dressing, Creamy Italian	1 Tbsp.	40	0.0	15	0	0.0
Salad Dressing, French	1 Tbsp.	4	0.0	10	0	0.0
Salad Dressing, Italian	1 Tbsp.	4	0.0	15	0	0.0
Salad Dressing, Red Wine Vinegar	1 Tbsp.	2	0.0	10	0	0.0
Salad Dressing, Thousand Island	1 Tbsp.	8	0.0	30	0	0.0
Sauce, Spaghetti	4 oz.	60	1.0	30	0	15.0
Sauce, Steak	1 Tbsp.	14	0.0	35	0	0.0
Syrup, Blueberry	1 Tbsp.	8	0.0	25	0	0.0
Syrup, Pancake	1 Tbsp.	8	0.0	35	0	0.0
Wheat Snack	1 oz.	100	<1.0	15	0	<9.0

☞ Hain	S. S.	CAL	FAT(g)	SOD(mg)	CHL(mg)	%FAT
Chicken Vegetable	8 oz.	110	3.0	790	10	24.5
Chicken Vegetable, No Salt Added	8 oz.	100	3.0	85	10	27.0
Creamy Mushroom	9.5 oz.	120	4.0	900	5	30.0
Italian Vege-Pasta	9.5 oz.	160	5.0	910	20	28.1
Italian Vege-Pasta, Low Sodium	9.5 oz.	150	5.0	90	20	30.0
Minestrone	9.5 oz.	170	3.0	930	0	15.9
Minestrone, No Salt Added	9.5 oz.	160	4.0	75	0	22.5
Mushroom Barley	9.5 oz.	80	2.0	780	5	22.5
New England Clam Chowder	9.25 oz.	150	4.0	780	15	24.0
Soup Mix, Lentil Savory	3/4 cup	130	2.0	810	8	13.8
Soup Mix, Minestrone Savory	3/4 cup	110	1.0	870	6	8.2
Soup Mix, Onion Savory	3/4 cup	50	2.0	900	2	36.0
Soup Mix, Onion Savory, No Added Salt	3/4 cup	50	1.0	470	2	18.0
Soup Mix, Vegetable Savory	3/4 cup	80	1.0	730	-	11.3
Soup Mix, Vegetable Savory, No Added Salt	3/4 cup	80	1.0	330	-	11.3

☞ Hain

	S. S.	CAL	FAT(g)	SOD(mg)	CHL(mg)	%FAT
Vegetable Broth	9.5 oz.	45	0.0	600	0	0.0
Vegetable Broth, Low Sodium	9.5 oz.	40	0.0	85	0	0.0
Vegetable Split Pea	9.5 oz.	170	1.0	970	0	5.3
Vegetable Split Pea, No Salt Added	9.5 oz.	170	1.0	70	0	5.3
Vegetarian Lentil	9.5 oz.	160	3.0	690	0	16.9
Vegetarian Lentil, No Salt Added	9.5 oz.	160	3.0	65	0	16.9
Vegetarian Vegetable	9.5 oz.	150	4.0	790	0	24.0
Vegetarian Vegetable, No Salt Added	9.5 oz.	150	5.0	80	0	30.0

☞ Health Valley

	S. S.	CAL	FAT(g)	SOD(mg)	CHL(mg)	%FAT
Beans, Fat Free, Boston Baked Style	7.5 oz.	190	<1.0	290	0	<4.7
Beans, Fat Free, Boston Baked Style, No Salt Added	7.5 oz.	190	<1.0	20	0	<4.7
Beans, Fat Free, Honey Baked Vegetarian	7.5 oz.	180	<1.0	60	0	<5.0
Cereal, 10 Bran, Fat Free, Almond Flavor	1 oz.	90	<1.0	5	0	<10.0
Cereal, 10 Bran, Fat Free, Apple Cinnamon	1 oz.	90	<1.0	5	0	<10.0
Cereal, 10 Bran, Fat Free, Regular	1 oz.	90	<1.0	5	0	<10.0
Cereal, 7 Sprouts, Fat Free, with Bananas & Hawaiian Fruit	1 oz.	90	<1.0	0	0	<10.0
Cereal, 7 Sprouts, Fat Free, with Raisins	1 oz.	90	<1.0	0	0	<10.0
Cereal, Healthy Crunch, Almond Date	1 oz.	90	1.0	10	0	10.0
Cereal, Healthy Crunch, Apple Cinnamon	1 oz.	90	1.0	10	0	10.0
Cereal, Orangeola, Almonds & Dates	1 oz.	90	1.0	2	0	10.0
Cereal, Orangeola, Bananas & Hawaiian Fruit	1 oz.	90	1.0	2	0	10.0
Cereal, Real Oat Bran, Almond Flavored Crunch	1 oz.	90	1.0	2	0	10.0
Cereal, Real Oat Bran, Hawaiian Fruit	1.2 oz.	100	1.0	2	0	9.0
Cereal, Real Oat Bran, Raisin	1.2 oz.	100	1.0	2	0	9.0
Cereal, Swiss Breakfast, Raisin	1 oz.	80	1.0	5	0	11.3
Cereal, Swiss Breakfast, Tropical Fruit	1 oz.	80	1.0	5	0	11.3

HEALTH/DIETETIC FOODS

☞ Health Valley	S. S.	CAL	FAT(g)	SOD(mg)	CHL(mg)	%FAT
Chili, Fat Free, Vegetarian with Black Beans, Mild	5 oz.	140	<1.0	290	0	<6.4
Chili, Fat Free, Vegetarian with Black Beans, Mild	5 oz.	90	<1.0	180	0	<10.0
Chili, Fat Free, Vegetarian with Black Beans, Spicy	5 oz.	140	<1.0	290	0	<6.4
Cookies, Apple Spice	3	75	<1.0	40	0	<12.0
Cookies, Apricot Delight	3	75	<1.0	40	0	<12.0
Cookies, Date Delight	3	75	<1.0	40	0	<12.0
Cookies, Hawaiian Fruit	3	75	<1.0	40	0	<12.0
Cookies, Jumbo, Apple Raisin	1	70	<1.0	35	0	<12.9
Cookies, Jumbo, Raisin	1	70	<1.0	35	0	<12.9
Cookies, Jumbo, Raspberry	1	70	<1.0	35	0	<12.9
Cookies, Raisin Oatmeal	3	75	<1.0	40	0	<12.0
Fruit Bars, Apple	1	140	<1.0	10	0	<6.4
Fruit Bars, Apricot	1	140	<1.0	10	0	<6.4
Fruit Bars, Date	1	140	<1.0	10	0	<6.4
Fruit Bars, Oat Bran Jumbo, Date & Almond	1	140	2.0	10	0	12.9
Fruit Bars, Oat Bran Jumbo, Fruit & Nut	1	140	2.0	10	0	12.9
Fruit Bars, Oat Bran Jumbo, Raisin Cinnamon	1	140	2.0	10	0	12.9
Fruit Bars, Raisin	1	140	<1.0	10	0	<6.4
Granola, Fat Free, Date & Almond	1 oz.	90	<1.0	20	0	<10.0
Granola, Fat Free, Raisin Cinnamon	1 oz.	90	<1.0	20	0	<10.0
Granola, Fat Free, Tropical Fruit	1 oz.	90	<1.0	20	0	<10.0
Muffins, Fat Free, Apple Spice	1	130	<1.0	110	0	<6.9
Muffins, Fat Free, Banana	1	130	<1.0	110	0	<6.9
Muffins, Fat Free, Raisin Spice	1	140	<1.0	100	0	<6.4
Muffins, Oat Bran, Almond & Date	1	140	<1.0	80	0	<6.4
Muffins, Oat Bran, Blueberry	1	140	<1.0	100	0	<6.4
Muffins, Oat Bran, Raisin	1	140	<1.0	90	0	<6.4
Soup, Fat Free, 14 Garden Vegetable	7.5 oz.	50	<1.0	290	0	<18.0
Soup, Fat Free, 5 Bean	7.5 oz.	70	<1.0	290	0	<12.9
Soup, Fat Free, Black Bean & Vegetable	7.5 oz.	70	<1.0	290	0	<12.9
Soup, Fat Free, Country Corn & Vegetable	7.5 oz.	60	<1.0	290	0	<15.0

☞ Health Valley	S. S.	CAL	FAT(g)	SOD(mg)	CHL(mg)	%FAT
Soup, Fat Free, Lentil & Carrot	7.5 oz.	70	<1.0	290	0	<12.9
Soup, Fat Free, Real Italian Minestrone	7.5 oz.	70	<1.0	290	0	<12.9
Soup, Fat Free, Split Pea & Carrot	7.5 oz.	80	<1.0	290	0	<11.3
Soup, Fat Free, Tomato Vegetable	7.5 oz.	40	<1.0	290	0	<22.5
Soup, Fat Free, Vegetable Barley	7.5 oz.	50	<1.0	290	0	<18.0

☞ Nature's Choice	S. S.	CAL	FAT(g)	SOD(mg)	CHL(mg)	%FAT
Carmel Corn with Peanuts	1.67 oz.	190	2.0	-	-	9.5
Carmel Corn, Original	1.67 oz.	180	1.0	-	-	5.0

☞ Pritikin	S. S.	CAL	FAT(g)	SOD(mg)	CHL(mg)	%FAT
Barbecue Sauce, Original and Hickory	2 Tbsp.	25	0.0	35	0	0.0
Dinner Mix, Cajun	1 cup	210	2.0	110	85	8.6
Dinner Mix, Mexican	1.7 oz.	240	3.0	150	35	11.3
Dinner Mix, Oriental	1.7 oz.	240	3.0	260	35	11.3
Hearty Hot Cereal, Apple Raisin/ Cinnamon	1.64 oz.	160	2.0	0	0	11.3
Hearty Hot Cereal, Multi Grain	1.57 oz.	150	1.0	0	0	6.0
Rice Cakes, Multi-Grain, Sodium-Free	1 cake	35	0.0	0	0	0.0
Rice Cakes, Multi-Grain, Very-Low	1 cake	35	0.0	30	0	0.0
Rice Cakes, Plain, Sodium-Free	1 cake	35	0.0	0	0	0.0
Rice Cakes, Plain, Very-Low	1 cake	35	0.0	35	0	0.0
Rice Cakes, Sesame, Sodium-Free	1 cake	35	0.0	0	0	0.0
Rice Cakes, Sesame, Very-Low	1 cake	35	0.0	35	0	0.0
Rice Mix, Brown Rice Pilaf	1/2 cup	90	<1.0	40	0	<10.0
Rice Mix, Spanish Brown Rice	1/2 cup	90	<1.0	10	0	<10.0
Salad Dressing, French	1 Tbsp.	10	0.0	0	0	0.0
Salad Dressing, Garlic & Herb	1 Tbsp.	6	0.0	0	0	0.0
Salad Dressing, Italian	1 Tbsp.	8	0.0	0	0	0.0
Salad Dressing, Ranch	1 Tbsp.	16	0.0	0	0	0.0
Salad Dressing, Sweet Spicy	1 Tbsp.	18	0.0	0	0	0.0

HEALTH/DIETETIC FOODS

☞ Pritikin	S. S.	CAL	FAT(g)	SOD(mg)	CHL(mg)	%FAT
Salad Dressing, Vinaigrette	1 Tbsp.	8	0.0	0	0	0.0
Salsa	1/4 cup	25	0.0	5	0	0.0
Soup, Chicken	7.25 oz.	80	1.0	170	5	11.3
Soup, Chicken Broth	6.83 oz.	12	0.0	135	0	0.0
Soup, Chicken Gumbo	7.38 oz.	60	1.0	180	5	15.0
Soup, Chicken Vegetable	7.25 oz.	60	1.0	150	5	15.0
Soup, Lentil	7.38 oz.	80	0	160	0	0.0
Soup, Minestrone	7.38 oz.	70	0.0	120	0	0.0
Soup, Navy Bean	7.38 oz.	90	<1.0	160	0	<10.0
Soup, Split Pea	7.5 oz.	120	<1.0	160	0	<7.5
Soup, Tomato	7.25 oz.	70	0.0	135	0	0.0
Soup, Turkey Vegetable	7.38 oz.	50	<1.0	160	5	<18.0
Soup, Vegetable	7.38 oz.	60	0.0	120	0	0.0
Spaghetti Sauce, Chunky Garden	4 oz.	50	0.0	30	0	0.0
Spaghetti Sauce, Original	4 oz.	60	<1.0	35	0	<15.0

☞ Richard Simmons Salad Spray	S. S.	CAL	FAT(g)	SOD(mg)	CHL(mg)	%FAT
Dijon Vinaigrette	1 Tbsp.	14	<1.0	160	0	-
French	1 Tbsp.	14	<1.0	130	0	-
Ranch	1 Tbsp.	17	<1.0	190	0	-
Roma Cheese	1 Tbsp.	14	<1.0	190	1	-

☞ Weight Watchers	S. S.	CAL	FAT(g)	SOD(mg)	CHL(mg)	%FAT
Apple Chips	1 bag	70	0.0	110	0	0.0
Broth Mix, Beef	1 pkg.	8	0.0	910	-	0.0
Broth Mix, Chicken	1 pkg.	8	0.0	900	-	0.0
Cheese Curls	1 bag	70	2.0	45	0	25.7
Cookies, Apple Raisin Bars	1 bar	100	3.0	115	-	27.0
Cookies, Chocolate Chip	2 cookies	90	2.0	65	-	20.0
Cookies, Chocolate Sandwich	2 cookies	90	3.0	90	0	30.0
Cookies, Fruit Filled, Apple	1 bar	80	<1.0	35	0	<11.3
Cookies, Fruit Filled, Raspberry	1 bar	80	<1.0	45	0	<11.3

☞ Weight Watchers	S. S.	CAL	FAT(g)	SOD(mg)	CHL(mg)	%FAT
Cookies, Oatmeal Spice	3 cookies	80	2.0	75	-	22.5
Cookies, Shortbread	3 cookies	80	2.0	95	-	22.5
Corn Snackers	1 bag	60	2.0	230	-	30.0
Corn Snackers, Nacho Cheese	1 bag	60	2.0	270	-	30.0
Crispbread, Garlic Flavored	2 wafers	30	0.0	55	-	0.0
Fruit Snacks, All Flavors	1 pouch	50	<1.0	140	0	<18.0
Hot Cocoa Mix	1 pkg.	60	0.0	160	5	0.0
Instant Pudding, Chocolate	1/2 cup	100	0.0	430	-	0.0
Instant Pudding, Vanilla	1/2 cup	90	0.0	510	-	0.0
New England Clam Chowder	1 tub	90	0.0	450	5	0.0
Popcorn, Microwave	1 bag	100	1.0	5	0	9.0
Popcorn, Ready-to-Eat, Butter Flavored	1 bag	90	3.0	100	-	30.0
Salad Dressing, Caesar	1 Tbsp.	4	0.0	200	-	0.0
Salad Dressing, Caesar, Individual Packets	1 pouch	6	0.0	280	-	0.0
Salad Dressing, Creamy Cucumber	1 Tbsp.	18	0.0	85	-	0.0
Salad Dressing, Creamy Italian	1 Tbsp.	12	0.0	85	-	0.0
Salad Dressing, Creamy Peppercorn	1 Tbsp.	8	0.0	85	-	0.0
Salad Dressing, Creamy Ranch, Individual Packets	1 pouch	35	<1.0	130	-	<25.7
Shake Mix, Chocolate Fudge	1 pkg.	70	<1.0	150	-	<12.9
Shake Mix, Orange Sherbet	1 pkg.	70	<1.0	210	-	<12.9
Soup, Chicken Noodle	1 tub	90	1.0	450	15	10.0
Soup, Chicken Noodle (Can)	1 can	80	2.0	1230	20	22.5
Soup, Cream of Mushroom (Can)	1 can	90	2.0	1250	-	20.0
Soup, Vegetable Beef	1 tub	90	1.0	450	10	10.0
Spaghetti Sauce, Meat	1/3 cup	45	1.0	310	-	20.0
Spaghetti Sauce, Mushroom	1/3 cup	35	0.0	300	0	0.0
Stew, Chunky Beef	1 tub	120	2.0	450	20	15.0
Syrup, Reduced Calorie	1 Tbsp.	25	0.0	40	0	0.0
Tomato Ketchup	2 tsp.	8	0.0	110	-	0.0

ICE CREAM TOPPINGS

ICE CREAM TOPPINGS

☞ **Hershey's**	S. S.	CAL	FAT(g)	SOD(mg)	CHL(mg)	%FAT
Chocolate Flavored Syrup	2 Tbsp.	80	1.0	20	0	11.3

☞ **Nestle's Quik**	S. S.	CAL	FAT(g)	SOD(mg)	CHL(mg)	%FAT
Chocolate Flavored Syrup	1.22 oz.	100	1.0	45	-	9.0

☞ **Smucker's**	S. S.	CAL	FAT(g)	SOD(mg)	CHL(mg)	%FAT
Butterscotch Flavored Topping	2 Tbsp.	140	1.0	75	-	6.4
Caramel Flavored Topping	2 Tbsp.	140	1.0	110	-	6.4
Chocolate Flavored Syrup Topping	2 Tbsp.	130	0.0	35	-	0.0
Chocolate Fudge Topping	2 Tbsp.	130	1.0	50	-	6.9
Fruit Syrups	2 Tbsp.	100	0.0	<10	-	0.0
Hot Carmel Topping	2 Tbsp.	150	4.0	75	-	24.0
Light Hot Fudge Topping	2 Tbsp.	70	<1.0	35	-	<12.9
Marshmallow Topping	2 Tbsp.	120	0.0	0	-	0.0
Peanut Butter-Caramel Topping	2 Tbsp.	150	2.0	120	-	12.0
Pecans In Syrup Topping	2 Tbsp.	130	1.0	0	-	6.9
Pineapple Topping	2 Tbsp.	130	0.0	0	-	0.0
Special Recipe Dark Chocolate Flavored Topping	2 Tbsp.	130	1.0	45	-	6.9
Strawberry Topping	2 Tbsp.	120	0.0	0	-	0.0
Swiss Milk Chocolate Fudge Topping	2 Tbsp.	140	1.0	70	-	6.4
Walnuts In Syrup	2 Tbsp.	130	1.0	0	-	6.9

ICE CREAM CONES

☞ **Keebler**	S. S.	CAL	FAT(g)	SOD(mg)	CHL(mg)	%FAT
Cones, Giant Waffle	1 cone	100	1.0	0	0	9.0
Cones, Sugar	1 cone	45	<1.0	35	0	<20.0
Ice Cream Cups	1 cone	15	<1.0	20	0	-
Ice Cream Cups, Assorted Colors	1 cone	15	<1.0	20	0	-

☞ **Nabisco**	S. S.	CAL	FAT(g)	SOD(mg)	CHL(mg)	%FAT
Comet Cups	1 cone	18	<1.0	5	0	-
Comet Sugar Cones	1 cone	40	<1.0	40	0	<22.5
Comet Waffle Cones	1 cone	70	1.0	30	0	12.9

ICE CREAM TOPPINGS

MEAT CASE

MEATS

☞ **Generic**	S. S.	CAL	FAT(g)	SOD(mg)	CHL(mg)	%FAT
Beef, Bottom Round, Select, Braised	3.6 oz.	192	6.3	51	96	29.5
Beef, Bottom Round, Select, Roasted	3.6 oz.	171	5.4	66	78	28.4
Beef, Chuck, Arm Pot Roast, Select, Braised	3.6 oz.	198	6.3	66	101	28.6
Beef, Eye of Round, Select, Roasted	3.6 oz.	155	3.5	62	69	20.3
Beef, Eye of Round, Choice, Roasted*	3.6 oz.	175	5.7	62	69	29.3
Beef, Tip Round, Select, Roasted	3.6 oz.	170	5.3	65	81	28.1
Beef, Top Round (London Broil), Choice, Braised*	3.6 oz.	207	5.8	45	90	25.2
Beef, Top Round (London Broil), Select, Roasted	3.6 oz.	190	4.0	45	90	18.9
Beef, Top Sirloin, Select, Broiled	3.6 oz.	180	5.6	66	89	28.0
Lamb, Foreshank, Choice, Lean, Braised*	3.6 oz.	187	6.0	74	104	29.0
Pork, Tenderloin, Trimmed, Roasted*	3.5 oz.	166	4.8	67	93	26.0
Veal, Leg (Top Round), Trimmed, Braised*	3.6 oz.	203	5.1	67	135	22.6
Veal, Leg (Top Round), Trimmed, Roasted*	3.6 oz.	150	3.4	68	103	20.3
Veal, Shoulder, Trimmed, Braised*	3.6 oz.	199	6.1	97	130	27.6
Veal, Sirloin, Trimmed, Braised*	3.6 oz.	204	6.5	81	113	28.7
*Most typically found in Supermarkets						

☞ **Healthy Choice**	S. S.	CAL	FAT(g)	SOD(mg)	CHL(mg)	%FAT
Ground Beef, Extra Lean Low-Fat	4 oz.	130	4.0	24	55	27.7

POULTRY

☞ **Generic**	S. S.	CAL	FAT(g)	SOD(mg)	CHL(mg)	%FAT
Chicken, Broilers or Fryers, Breast Meat, Roasted	3.6 oz.	165	3.6	74	85	19.5

MEAT CASE

MEAT CASE

☞ Generic	S. S.	CAL	FAT(g)	SOD(mg)	CHL(mg)	%FAT
Chicken, Broilers or Fryers, Breast Meat, Stewed	3.6 oz.	151	3.0	63	77	18.1
Chicken, Broilers or Fryers, Light Meat, Roasted	3.6 oz.	173	4.5	77	85	23.5
Chicken, Broilers or Fryers, Light Meat, Stewed	3.6 oz.	159	4.0	65	77	22.6
Chicken, Roasting, Light Meat, Roasted	3.6 oz.	153	4.1	51	75	23.9
Turkey Loaf, Breast Meat	3.6 oz.	110	1.6	1431	41	12.9
Turkey, Fryer-Roasters, Back Meat, Roasted	3.6 oz.	170	5.6	74	95	29.9
Turkey, Fryer-Roasters, Breast Meat, Roasted	3.6 oz.	135	0.7	52	83	4.9
Turkey, Fryer-Roasters, Dark Meat, Roasted	3.6 oz.	162	4.3	79	112	23.9
Turkey, Fryer-Roasters, Leg Meat, Roasted	3.6 oz.	159	3.8	81	119	21.3
Turkey, Fryer-Roasters, Light Meat, Roasted	3.6 oz.	140	1.2	56	86	7.6
Turkey, Fryer-Roasters, Roasted	3.6 oz.	150	2.6	67	98	15.8
Turkey, Fryer-Roasters, Wing Meat, Roasted	3.6 oz.	163	3.4	78	102	19.0
Turkey, Light Meat, Roasted	3.6 oz.	157	3.2	64	69	18.5
Turkey, Pre-Basted, Roasted	3.6 oz.	126	3.5	397	42	24.9
Turkey, Roasted	3.6 oz.	170	5.0	70	76	26.3
Turkey, Young Hens, Light Meat, Roasted	3.6 oz.	161	3.7	60	68	20.9
Turkey, Young Hens, Roasted	3.6 oz.	175	5.5	67	73	28.3
Turkey, Young Toms, Light Meat, Roasted	3.6 oz.	154	2.9	68	69	17.1
Turkey, Young Toms, Roasted	3.6 oz.	168	4.7	74	77	25.1

☞ Perdue	S. S.	CAL	FAT(g)	SOD(mg)	CHL(mg)	%FAT
Chicken, Breast, Skinless Split	1 oz.	34	1.1	11	17	29.1
Chicken, Oven Stuffer Roaster, Breasd, Thin-Sliced	1 oz.	31	0.6	9	17	16.1
Fit 'n Easy Chicken, Breast	1 oz.	30	0.6	10	17	18.0
Fit 'n Easy Chiken, Breast and Thighs White Meat	1 oz.	30	0.7	10	17	20.0
Fit 'n Easy Chicken, Breast Tenders	1 oz.	28	0.3	14	17	9.6

☞Perdue	S. S.	CAL	FAT(g)	SOD(mg)	CHL(mg)	%FAT
Fit 'n Easy Chicken, Oven Stuffer Roaster, Breast	1 oz.	31	0.6	9	17	16.1
Fit 'n Easy Turkey, Breast	1 oz.	28	0.2	13	15	6.9
Fit 'n Easy Turkey, Breast Cutlets	1 oz.	28	0.2	13	15	6.9
Fit 'n Easy Turkey, Breast Fillets	1 oz.	28	0.2	13	15	6.9
Fit 'n Easy Turkey, Breast Tenderloins	1 oz.	29	0.3	12	13	10.3
Ground Turkey, Breast Meat	1 oz.	28	0.2	13	15	6.4

☞The Turkey Store	S. S.	CAL	FAT(g)	SOD(mg)	CHL(mg)	%FAT
100% Ground Breast Meat	3.5 oz.	100	1.0	51	56	9.0
Turkey Breast Slices	3.5 oz.	100	1.0	51	60	9.0
Turkey Breast Strips	3.5 oz.	100	1.0	51	60	9.0
Turkey Breast Tenderloins	3.5 oz.	100	1.0	53	60	9.0
Turkey Drumstick Steaks	3.5 oz.	110	3.0	77	69	24.5

PREPARED MEATS–UNCOOKED

☞Country Pride	S. S.	CAL	FAT(g)	SOD(mg)	CHL(mg)	%FAT
Seasoned Chicken Breast Fillet, Barbecue	4 oz.	120	1.0	560	65	7.5
Seasoned Chicken Breast Fillet, Dijon	4 oz.	130	2.0	480	60	13.8
Seasoned Chicken Breast Fillet, Italian Style	4 oz.	120	1.0	640	65	7.5
Seasoned Chicken Breast Fillet, Lemon Butter	4 oz.	110	1.0	480	70	8.2
Seasoned Chicken Breast Fillet, Mesquite Smoke	4 oz.	110	1.0	330	70	8.2
Seasoned Chicken Breast Fillet, Teriyaki	4 oz.	110	1.0	680	65	8.2

☞Hormel	S. S.	CAL	FAT(g)	SOD(mg)	CHL(mg)	%FAT
Chicken By George, Caribbean Grill	5 oz.	200	6.0	610	80	27.0
Chicken By George, Teriyaki	5 oz.	180	5.0	740	70	25.0

MEAT CASE

☞ Hormel	S. S.	CAL	FAT(g)	SOD(mg)	CHL(mg)	%FAT
Turkey By George, Hickory Barbecue	5 oz.	190	5.0	840	65	23.7
Turkey By George, Italian Style Parmesan	5 oz.	170	5.0	860	70	26.5
Turkey By George, Lemon Pepper	5 oz.	160	4.0	830	60	22.5
Turkey By George, Mustard Tarragon	5 oz.	180	6.0	830	80	30.0

☞ Perdue	S. S.	CAL	FAT(g)	SOD(mg)	CHL(mg)	%FAT
Perdue Done It! Chicken, Barbecued, Half, Roasted	1 oz.	40	0.9	110	22	20.0
Perdue Done It! Chicken, Half, Roasted	1 oz.	37	1.1	85	21	27.0
Perdue Done It! Chicken, Whole, Roasted	1 oz.	37	1.1	85	21	27.0

PREPARED SEAFOOD

☞ Seafood Today	S. S.	CAL	FAT(g)	SOD(mg)	CHL(mg)	%FAT
Cajun Style Catfish	5 oz.	158	5.0	392	-	28.5
California Style Cod	5 oz.	100	1.0	118	-	9.0

☞ Louis Kemp	S. S.	CAL	FAT(g)	SOD(mg)	CHL(mg)	%FAT
Crab Delights	2 oz.	90	<1.0	550	10	<15.0
Lobster Delights	2 oz.	60	<1.0	470	10	<15.0

LUNCHEON MEATS

☞ Eckrich	S. S.	CAL	FAT(g)	SOD(mg)	CHL(mg)	%FAT
Lite Oven Roasted Turkey Breast	1 oz.	30	1.0	210	10	30.0
Lite Smoked Chicken Breast	1 oz.	30	1.0	210	20	30.0
Lite Smoked Turkey Breast	1 oz.	30	<1.0	220	10	<30.0

☞ **Hillshire Farm**	S. S.	CAL	FAT(g)	SOD(mg)	CHL(mg)	%FAT
Deli Select, Beef, Oven Roasted Cured	1 oz.	31	0.5	270	-	14.5
Deli Select, Beef, Smoked	1 oz.	31	0.5	270	-	14.5
Deli Select, Chicken Breast, Smoked	1 oz.	31	0.2	290	-	5.8
Deli Select, Corned Beef	1 oz.	31	0.4	230	-	11.6
Deli Select, Ham, Cajun	1 oz.	31	0.9	350	-	26.1
Deli Select, Ham, Honey	1 oz.	31	0.9	270	-	26.1
Deli Select, Ham, Smoked	1 oz.	31	0.9	300	-	26.1
Deli Select, Pastrami	1 oz.	31	0.4	290	-	11.6
Deli Select, Turkey Breast, Oven Roasted	1 oz.	31	0.2	340	-	5.8
Deli Select, Turkey Breast, Smoked	1 oz.	31	0.2	290	-	5.8

☞ **Louis Rich**	S. S.	CAL	FAT(g)	SOD(mg)	CHL(mg)	%FAT
Breast of Turkey, Barbecued	1 oz.	33	0.9	315	12	24.5
Breast of Turkey, Hickory Smoked	1 oz.	33	1.0	3406	13	27.3
Breast of Turkey, Honey Roasted	1 oz.	33	0.8	318	12	21.8
Breast of Turkey, Oven Roasted	1 oz.	31	0.9	296	13	26.1
Chicken Breast, Hickory Smoked	1 oz.	30	0.8	356	14	24.0
Chicken Breast, Oven Roasted, Deluxe	1 oz.	30	0.8	332	14	24.0
Chicken Breast, Oven Roasted, Thin Sliced	1 slice	12	0.3	130	6	22.5
Turkey Breast Roast	1 oz.	42	0.8	20	19	17.1
Turkey Breast Steaks	1 oz.	39	0.5	24	17	11.5
Turkey Breast Tenderloins	1 oz.	39	0.5	24	18	11.5
Turkey Breast, Honey Roasted	1 oz.	32	0.8	315	11	22.5
Turkey Breast, Oven Roasted	1 oz.	31	0.8	323	11	23.2
Turkey Breast, Oven Roasted, Thin Sliced	1 slice	12	0.3	127	4	22.5
Turkey Breast, Sliced	1 slice	21	0.3	211	9	12.9
Turkey Breast, Smoked, Chunk	1 oz.	33	1.0	268	11	27.3
Turkey Breast, Thin Sliced	1 slice	11	0.1	111	5	8.2
Turkey Ham, Honey Cured	1 slice	25	0.7	217	14	25.2
Turkey Ham, Sliced, Square	1 slice	24	0.7	213	14	26.3
Turkey Luncheon Loaf	1 oz.	45	2.8	270	16	56.0
Turkey, Smoked	1 oz.	32	1.0	284	14	28.1

MEAT CASE

☞ **Mr. Turkey**	S. S.	CAL	FAT(g)	SOD(mg)	CHL(mg)	%FAT
Chicken Breast	1 oz.	33	0.9	190	9	24.5
Chicken, Smoked, Deli Sliced	1 oz.	33	0.6	325	15	16.4
Turkey , Oven Prepared, Quarter Breast Chub	1 oz.	32	0.5	232	5	14.1
Turkey Breast	1 oz.	32	0.7	233	10	19.7
Turkey Breast, Honey Smoked	1 oz.	31	0.9	247	10	26.1
Turkey Breast, Smoked	1 oz.	33	0.5	332	10	13.6
Turkey Ham, Deli Sliced	1 oz.	36	1.2	326	22	30.0
Turkey Ham, Hardwood Smoked Ham Chub	1 oz.	36	1.2	324	25	30.0
Turkey Ham, Honey Ham Chub	1 oz.	34	1.1	324	25	29.1
Turkey Pastrami	1 oz.	28	0.9	383	17	28.9
Turkey, BBQ , Quarter Breast Chub	1 oz.	29	0.5	208	5	15.5
Turkey, Smoked, Deli Sliced	1 oz.	2	0.4	306	14	11.3
Turkey, Smoked, Quarter Breast Chub	1 oz.	30	0.5	204	5	15.0

☞ **Oscar Mayer**	S. S.	CAL	FAT(g)	SOD(mg)	CHL(mg)	%FAT
Chicken Breast, Oven Roasted	1 slice	25	0.3	295	12	10.8
Chicken Breast, Smoked	1 slice	25	0.2	279	11	7.2
Deli-Thin, Chicken Breast, Roasted	1 slice	13	0.3	158	7	20.8
Deli-Thin, Ham, Boiled	1 slice	13	0.4	160	7	27.7
Deli-Thin, Ham, Honey	1 slice	13	0.4	152	6	27.7
Deli-Thin, Ham Smoked	1 slice	13	0.4	153	7	27.7
Deli-Thin, Roast Beef	1 slice	14	0.4	121	6	25.7
Deli-Thin, Turkey Breast, Roasted	1 slice	13	0.3	152	5	20.8
Deli-Thin, Turkey Breast, Smoked	1 slice	11	0.1	156	5	8.2
Ham Steaks, Jubilee	1 slice	55	1.8	750	30	29.5
Ham, Baked, Cooked	1 slice	21	0.4	237	11	17.1
Ham, Boiled	1 slice	22	0.6	279	12	24.5
Ham, Breakfast	1 slice	47	1.5	536	21	28.7
Ham, Honey	1 slice	23	0.6	266	11	23.5
Ham, Lower Salt	1 slice	22	0.6	173	10	24.5
Ham, Smoked, Cooked	1 slice	22	0.7	268	11	28.6
Honey Loaf	1 slice	33	.9	378	15	24.5

☞ **Oscar Mayer**	S.S.	CAL	FAT(g)	SOD(mg)	CHL(mg)	%FAT
Healthy Favorites Chicken Breast, Oven Roasted	1 slice	12	0.1	110	5	7.5
Healthy Favorites, Ham, Boiled	1 slice	13	0.3	115	7	9.0
Healthy Favorites, Ham, Cooked	1 slice	22	0.6	173	10	24.5
Healthy Favorites, Ham, Honey	1 slice	13	0.4	113	6	27.7
Healthy Favorites, Ham, Smoked Cooked	1 slice	13	0.3	114	11	20.8
Healthy Favorites, Turkey Breast, Oven Roasted	1 slice	25	0.4	232	8	14.4
Healthy Favorites, Turkey Breast, Oven Roasted, Thin Sliced	1 slice	11	0.1	101	5	8.2
Healthy Favorites, Turkey Breast, Smoked	1 slice	11	0.1	81	5	8.2
Turkey Breast, Smoked	1 slice	19	0.2	273	10	9.5
Turkey breast, Oven Roasted	1 slice	25	0.4	245	8	14.4

HOT DOGS / FRANKS / KIELBASA

☞ **Healthy Choice**	S.S.	CAL	FAT(g)	SOD(mg)	CHL(mg)	%FAT
Frank	1 frank	50	1.0	410	15	18.0
Polska Kielbasa, link	1 link	80	2.0	550	25	22.5
Polska Kielbasa	1 oz.	70	2.0	470	25	25.7

☞ **Hormel**	S.S.	CAL	FAT(g)	SOD(mg)	CHL(mg)	%FAT
Light & Lean Franks	1 frank	45	1.0	350	10	28.0

☞ **Oscar Mayer**	S.S.	CAL	FAT(g)	SOD(mg)	CHL(mg)	%FAT
Healthy Favorites, Hot Dogs	1 link	55	1.7	524	22	27.8

MEAT CASE

MEXICAN SECTION

MEXICAN FOODS

☞ Chi Chi's	S. S.	CAL	FAT(g)	SOD(mg)	CHL(mg)	%FAT
Salsa, Hot	1 oz.	8	0.04	138	0	4.5
Salsa, Medium	1 oz.	8	0.0	130	2.5	0.0
Salsa, Mild	1 oz.	9	0.04	96	0	4.0
Taco Sauce, Hot	1 oz.	17	0.12	247	0	6.4
Taco Sauce, Mild	1 oz.	18	0.07	165	0	3.5
Picante Sauce, Hot	1 oz.	11	0.06	263	0	4.9
Picante Sauce, Mild	1 oz.	11	0.02	191	0	1.6

☞ El Molino	S. S.	CAL	FAT(g)	SOD(mg)	CHL(mg)	%FAT
Green Chili Sauce, Mild	2 Tbsp.	10	0.0	210	-	0.0
Taco Sauce, Red, Mild	2 Tbsp.	10	0.0	170	-	0.0

☞ Gebhardt	S. S.	CAL	FAT(g)	SOD(mg)	CHL(mg)	%FAT
Beans, Chili	4 oz.	115	1.0	580	0	7.8
Beans, Pinto	4 oz.	100	<1.0	600	0	<9.0
Beans, Refried	4 oz.	100	2.0	490	2	18.0
Beans, Refried, Jalapeño	4 oz.	115	2.0	270	2	15.7
Chili Quick Seasoning Mix	1 tsp.	10	<1.0	165	0	-
Hot Sauce	1/2 tsp.	<1	<1.0	55	0	-
Menudo Mix	1 tsp.	5	<1.0	310	0	-

☞ La Victoria	S. S.	CAL	FAT(g)	SOD(mg)	CHL(mg)	%FAT
Chili Dip	1 Tbsp.	6	<1.0	90	-	-
Nacho Jalapenos	1 Tbsp.	2	<1.0	335	-	-
Salsa Brava	1 Tbsp.	6	<1.0	100	-	-

MEXICAN SECTION

☞ La Victoria

	S. S.	CAL	FAT(g)	SOD(mg)	CHL(mg)	%FAT
Salsa Casera	1 Tbsp.	4	<1.0	80	-	-
Salsa Jalapena, Green	1 Tbsp.	4	<1.0	105	-	-
Salsa Jalapena, Red	1 Tbsp.	6	<1.0	95	-	-
Salsa Picante	1 Tbsp.	4	<1.0	80	-	-
Salsa Ranchera	1 Tbsp.	6	<1.0	85	-	-
Salsa Suprema	1 Tbsp.	4	<1.0	95	-	-
Salsa Victoria	1 Tbsp.	4	<1.0	80	-	-
Salsa, Green Chili	1 Tbsp.	3	<1.0	44	-	-
Salsa, Omlette	1 Tbsp.	6	<1.0	95	-	-
Taco Sauce, Green	1 Tbsp.	4	<1.0	85	-	-
Taco Sauce, Red	1 Tbsp.	6	<1.0	85	-	-
Tomatillo Entero	1 Tbsp.	4	<1.0	102	-	-

☞ Lawry's

	S. S.	CAL	FAT(g)	SOD(mg)	CHL(mg)	%FAT
Taco Sauce 'N Seasoner	1/4 cup	40	0.6	636	-	13.5
Taco Sauce, Chunky	1/4 cup	22	0.4	549	-	16.4

☞ Old El Paso

	S. S.	CAL	FAT(g)	SOD(mg)	CHL(mg)	%FAT
Bean Dip, Jalapeno	1 Tbsp.	14	0.0	53	0	0.0
Beans, Garbanzo	1/2 cup	190	<1.0	250	-	<4.7
Beans, Mexe-Beans	1/2 cup	163	1.0	627	0	5.5
Beans, Pinto	1/2 cup	100	0.0	320	0	0.0
Beans, Refried	1/4 cup	55	<1.0	200	1	<16.4
Beans, Refried with Cheese	1/4 cup	36	1.0	280	2	25.0
Beans, Refried with Green Chilies	1/4 cup	49	<1.0	252	-	<18.4
Beans, Refried, Spicy	1/4 cup	35	1.0	280	1	25.7
Beans, Refried, Vegetarian	1/4 cup	70	1.0	590	0	12.9
Chili Salsa, Thick'n Chunky, Green	2 Tbsp.	3	0.0	270	0	0.0
Chilies, Green, Chopped	2 Tbsp.	8	0.0	70	0	0.0
Enchilada Sauce, Green	2 Tbsp.	11	0.0	200	0	0.0
Enchilada Sauce, Hot	1/4 cup	30	1.0	250	0	30.0
Jalapeño Relish	2 Tbsp.	16	0.0	100	0	0.0

☞Old El Paso

☞Old El Paso	S. S.	CAL	FAT(g)	SOD(mg)	CHL(mg)	%FAT
Picante Salsa, Mild, Medium and Hot	2 Tbsp.	10	<1.0	160	0	-
Picante Sauce, Chunky, Mild, Medium and Hot	2 Tbsp.	7	0.0	270	0	0.0
Rice, Mexican	1/2 cup	140	2.0	370	0	12.9
Rice, Spanish	1/2 cup	70	1.0	400	0	12.9
Salsa Verde, Thick'n Chunky	2 Tbsp.	10	<1.0	135	0	-
Salsa, Thick 'n Chunky Green Chili	2 Tbsp.	3	0.0	270	0	0.0
Salsa, Thick'n Chunky, Mild, Medium and Hot	2 Tbsp.	6	<1.0	170	0	-
Taco Sauce, Canned	2 Tbsp.	15	0.0	300	0	0.0
Taco Sauce, Mild, Medium and Hot	2 Tbsp.	10	<1.0	130	0	-
Tomatoes & Green Chilies	1/4 cup	14	<1.0	480	0	-
Tomatoes & Jalapeños	1/4 cup	11	<1.0	150	0	-

☞Ortega	S. S.	CAL	FAT(g)	SOD(mg)	CHL(mg)	%FAT
Salsa, Green Chili, Medium and Hot	1 Tbsp.	6	0.0	190	0	0.0
Salsa, Green Chili, Mild	1 Tbsp.	8	0.0	190	0	0.0
Taco Meat Seasoning Mix, Mild	1 taco	90	1.0	999	0	10.0
Taco Sauce, Hot	1 Tbsp.	8	0.0	105	0	0.0
Taco Sauce, Mild	1 Tbsp.	8	0.0	115	0	0.0

☞Ranch Style	S. S.	CAL	FAT(g)	SOD(mg)	CHL(mg)	%FAT
Spanish Rice	7.5 oz.	160	3.0	1630	-	16.9

☞Rosarita	S. S.	CAL	FAT(g)	SOD(mg)	CHL(mg)	%FAT
Beans, Refried	4 oz.	120	2.0	470	2	15.0
Beans, Refried, Spicy	4 oz.	130	2.0	460	2	13.8
Beans, Refried, Vegetarian	4 oz.	120	2.0	470	0	15.0
Beans, Refried, with Bacon	4 oz.	130	3.0	500	14	20.8
Beans, Refried, with Green Chilies	4 oz.	120	2.0	430	2	15.0

☞Rosarita

	S. S.	CAL	FAT(g)	SOD(mg)	CHL(mg)	%FAT
Beans, Refried, with Nacho Cheese	4 oz.	140	2.0	490	2	12.9
Beans, Refried, with Onions	4 oz.	130	2.0	500	2	13.8
Enchilada Sauce, Hot	3 Tbsp.	15	<1.0	150	0	-
Enchilada Sauce, Mild	3 Tbsp.	15	<1.0	150	0	-
Picante Sauce, Hot Chunky	3 Tbsp.	18	<1.0	515	0	-
Picante Sauce, Medium Chunky	3 Tbsp.	16	<1.0	650	0	-
Picante Sauce, Mild Chunky	3 Tbsp.	25	<1.0	630	0	-
Salsa Dip, Chunky, Mild, Medium and Hot	3 Tbsp.	25	<1.0	340	0	-
Taco Sauce, Medium Chunky	3 Tbsp.	25	<1.0	310	0	-
Taco Sauce, Mild	3 Tbsp.	15	<1.0	310	0	-
Taco Sauce, Mild Chunky	3 Tbsp.	25	<1.0	300	0	-

☞Tio Sancho

	S. S.	CAL	FAT(g)	SOD(mg)	CHL(mg)	%FAT
Refried Beans, Microwave	1 oz.	33	0.5	127	-	13.6
Rice, Mexican, Restaurant Style	1/2 cup	130	1.0	580	-	6.9
Rice, Mexican, with Cheese and Mexican Green Chiles	1/2 cup	130	1.0	560	-	6.9
Rice, Mexican, with Refried Beans	1/2 cup	140	1.0	680	-	6.4
Salsa, Chunky, Mild, Medium and Hot	1/4 cup	22	0.4	549	-	16.4

☞Van Camp's

	S. S.	CAL	FAT(g)	SOD(mg)	CHL(mg)	%FAT
Spanish Rice	1 cup	160	4.0	1270	-	22.5

☞Wise

	S. S.	CAL	FAT(g)	SOD(mg)	CHL(mg)	%FAT
Bean Dip, Jalapeno	2 Tbsp.	25	0.0	100	-	0.0
Picante Sauce	2 Tbsp.	12	0.0	130	-	0.0
Taco Dip	2 Tbsp.	12	0.0	115	-	0.0

TORTILLAS

☞ **Generic**	S. S.	CAL	FAT(g)	SOD(mg)	CHL(mg)	%FAT
Tortillas, Corn	1 tortilla	67	1.1	53	-	14.8

☞ **Azteca**	S. S.	CAL	FAT(g)	SOD(mg)	CHL(mg)	%FAT
Tortillas, Corn	1 tortilla	45	0.0	10	0	0.0
Tortillas, Flour, 7"	1 tortilla	80	2.0	110	0	22.5
Tortillas, Flour, 9"	1 tortilla	130	3.0	180	0	20.8

☞ **El Aguila**	S. S.	CAL	FAT(g)	SOD(mg)	CHL(mg)	%FAT
Tortilla, Corn	1.1 oz.	50	1.0	5	<1	18.0
Tortilla, Corn, Blancas	0.8 oz.	210	3.0	10	0	12.9
Tortilla, Flour, Lite	1.4 oz.	110	2.0	250	<1	16.4

☞ **Mission**	S. S.	CAL	FAT(g)	SOD(mg)	CHL(mg)	%FAT
Tortillas, Corn, For tocos	1 tortilla	45	1.0	25	-	20.0
Tortillas, Corn, for table use	1 tortilla	50	1.0	30	-	18.0
Tortillas, Flour, Fajita Size	1 tortilla	100	2.0	160	0	18.0

☞ **Old El Paso**	S. S.	CAL	FAT(g)	SOD(mg)	CHL(mg)	%FAT
Tortillas, Corn	1 tortilla	60	1.0	170	0	15.0
Tortillas, Flour	1 tortilla	150	3.0	360	0	18.0

☞ **Ramirez & Sons**	S. S.	CAL	FAT(g)	SOD(mg)	CHL(mg)	%FAT
Tortillas, Corn	1 tortilla	35	1.0	20	0	25.7
Tortillas, Flour	1 tortilla	150	5.0	280	0	30.0

☞Tyson	S. S.	CAL	FAT(g)	SOD(mg)	CHL(mg)	%FAT
Tortillas, Corn, Enchilada Style	1 tortilla	54	0.4	4	0	6.7
Tortillas, Flour, Burrito Style	1 tortilla	173	4.0	40	0	20.8
Tortillas, Flour, Fajita Style	1 tortilla	84	2.0	20	0	21.4
Tortillas, Flour, Soft Taco Style	1 tortilla	121	3.0	30	0	22.3

MEXICAN SECTION

ORIENTAL SECTION

ORIENTAL FOODS

☞ Chun King	S. S.	CAL	FAT(g)	SOD(mg)	CHL(mg)	%FAT
Bamboo Shoots	2 oz.	16	0.0	0	0	0.0
Bean Sprouts	4 oz.	40	0.0	5	0	0.0
Chow Mein Vegetables	4 oz.	35	0.0	20	0	0.0
Mustard, Brown	1 tsp.	4	0.0	65	0	0.0
Rice Mix	0.25 oz.	20	0.0	310	0	0.0
Sauce/Glaze Mix for Sweet 'n Sour Entree	3.8 oz.	370	0.0	40	0	0.0
Soy Sauce	1 tsp.	6	0.0	430	0	0.0
Sweet/Sour Sauce	1.8 oz.	60	0.0	240	0	0.0
Water Chesnuts	2 oz.	45	0.0	15	0	0.0

☞ Kikkoman	S. S.	CAL	FAT(g)	SOD(mg)	CHL(mg)	%FAT
Soy Sauce	1 Tbsp.	12	0.0	938	0	0.0
Soy Sauce, Lite	1 Tbsp.	13	0.0	564	0	0.0
Steak Sauce	1 Tbsp.	20	0.0	234	0	1.4
Stir-Fry Sauce	1 Tbsp.	16	0.0	369	1	1.1
Sweet & Sour Sauce	1 Tbsp.	19	0.0	97	0	1.4
Teriyaki Baste & Glaze	1 Tbsp.	24	0.0	310	0	1.1
Teriyaki Sauce	1 Tbsp.	15	0.0	626	0	0.0
Teriyaki Sauce, Lite	1 Tbsp.	14	0.1	298	trace	3.2

☞ La Choy	S. S.	CAL	FAT(g)	SOD(mg)	CHL(mg)	%FAT
Bamboo Shoots	1/4 cup	6	<1.0	2	0	-
Bead Molasses	1/2 tsp.	7	<1.0	1	0	-
Bi-Pack, Beef Chow Mein	3/4 cup	70	1.0	840	20	12.9
Bi-Pack, Beef Pepper	3/4 cup	80	2.0	950	17	22.5
Bi-Pack, Chicken Teriyaki	3/4 cup	85	2.0	850	20	21.2

ORIENTAL SECTION

☞ La Choy	S. S.	CAL	FAT(g)	SOD(mg)	CHL(mg)	%FAT
Bi–Pack, Shrimp Chow Mein	3/4 cup	70	1.0	860	19	12.9
Bi–Pack, Sweet and Sour Chicken	3/4 cup	120	2.0	440	13	15.0
Brown Gravy	1/2 tsp.	15	<1.0	15	0	-
Chinese Fried Rice	3/4 cup	190	1.0	820	0	4.7
Chop Suey Vegetables	1/2 cup	10	<1.0	320	0	-
Dinner Classics, Egg Foo Young*	1/4 pkg.	85	<1.0	1250	0	<10.6
Dinner Classics, Pepper Steak*	1/5 pkg.	35	<1.0	720	0	<25.7
Dinner Classics, Sweet & Sour*	1/4 pkg.	120	<1.0	840	0	<7.5
Entree, Beef Chow Mein	3/4 cup	60	1.0	890	16	15.0
Entree, Chicken Chow Mein	3/4 cup	70	2.0	800	16	25.7
Entree, Shrimp Chow Mein	3/4 cup	35	1.0	940	50	25.7
Entree, Sweet and Sour Chicken	3/4 cup	240	2.0	1420	19	7.5
Entree, Sweet and Sour Pork	3/4 cup	250	4.0	1540	18	14.4
Fancy Mixed Vegetables	1/2 cup	12	<1.0	30	0	-
Fortune Cookies	1 cookie	15	<1.0	1	0	-
Hot & Spicy Szechwan Sauce	1 Tbsp.	25	<1.0	70	0	-
Mandarin Orange Sauce	1 Tbsp.	25	<1.0	40	0	-
Mung Bean Sprouts	2/3 cup	8	<1.0	20	0	-
Soy Sauce	1/2 tsp.	2	<1.0	230	0	-
Soy Sauce, Lite	1/2 tsp.	1	<1.0	110	0	-
Sweet & Sour Duck Sauce	1 Tbsp.	25	<1.0	40	0	-
Sweet & Sour Sauce	1 Tbsp.	25	<1.0	190	0	-
Tangy Plum Sauce	1 Tbsp.	25	<1.0	10	0	-
Teriyaki Sauce	1/2 tsp.	5	<1.0	290	0	-
Teriyaki Sauce, Basting	1/2 tsp.	2	<1.0	110	0	-
Teriyaki Sauce, Lite	1/2 tsp.	5	<1.0	85	0	-
Thick & Rich Teriyaki Sauce	1 Tbsp.	25	<1.0	300	0	-
Water Chestnuts, Sliced	1/4 cup	18	<1.0	3	0	-
Water Chestnuts, Whole	4	14	<1.0	2	0	-

*As packaged

PACKAGED ENTREES & SIDE DISHES
(NON-FROZEN)

MICROWAVE LUNCH BUCKETS

☞Campbell's	S. S.	CAL	FAT(g)	SOD(mg)	CHL(mg)	%FAT
Microwave Soup, Bean with Bacon 'n Ham	1 bucket	230	5.0	830	-	19.6
Microwave Soup, Chilli Beef	1 bucket	190	4.0	870	-	18.9
Microwave Soup, Vegetable Beef	1 bucket	100	2.0	830	-	18.0

☞Chef Boyardee	S. S.	CAL	FAT(g)	SOD(mg)	CHL(mg)	%FAT
ABC's & 123's in Cheese Flavored Sauce	1 bucket	180	1.0	940	3	5.0
Beef Ravioli	1 bucket	190	4.0	1160	15	18.9
Cheese Ravioli in Meat Sauce	1 bucket	200	3.0	1010	10	13.5
Dinosaurs in Cheese Flavored Sauce	1 bucket	180	1.0	880	3	5.0
Lasagna in Garden Vegetable Sauce	1 bucket	170	1.0	940	3	5.3
Main Meals, Beef Ravioli Suprema	1 bucket	290	4.0	1390	10	12.4
Main Meals, Cheese Ravioli Suprema	1 bucket	290	4.0	1360	10	12.4
Main Meals, Lasagna	1 bucket	290	8.0	1000	20	24.8
Main Meals, Noodles with Chicken	1 bucket	170	1.0	1120	20	5.3
Main Meals, Spaghetti Suprema	1 bucket	260	7.0	1000	20	24.2
Main Meals, Zesty Macaroni	1 bucket	290	8.0	1300	25	24.8
Shells in Mushroom Sauce	1 bucket	170	1.0	1080	2	5.3
Tic Tac Toes in Cheese Flavored Sauce	1 bucket	170	1.0	930	2	5.3

☞Dennison's	S. S.	CAL	FAT(g)	SOD(mg)	CHL(mg)	%FAT
Lite Microwave Chicken Chili	1 bucket	180	2.0	840	20	10.0
Lite Microwave Chicken Chili with Beans	1 bucket	180	2.0	880	30	10.0

PACKAGED ENTREES & SIDE DISHES

PACKAGED ENTREES & SIDE DISHES

☞ Healthy Choice	S. S.	CAL	FAT(g)	SOD(mg)	CHL(mg)	%FAT
Microwavable Cups, Beef Stew	1 bucket	140	2.0	540	35	12.9
Microwavable Cups, Chunky Beef Vegetable Soup	1 bucket	110	1.0	490	20	8.2
Microwavable Cups, Chunky Chicken Noodle & Vegetable Soup	1 bucket	160	4.0	500	45	22.5
Microwavable Cups, Lasagna with Meat Sauce	1 bucket	220	5.0	530	25	20.5
Microwavable Cups, Spaghetti Rings	1 bucket	140	0.0	460	0	0.0
Microwavable Cups, Spaghetti with Meat Sauce	1 bucket	150	3.0	390	20	18.0
Microwavable Cups, Spicy Chili with Beans & Ground Turkey	1 bucket	210	5.0	530	40	21.4
Microwavable Cups, Turkey Chili with Beans	1 bucket	200	5.0	560	45	22.5

☞ Hormel	S. S.	CAL	FAT(g)	SOD(mg)	CHL(mg)	%FAT
Micro Cup Entrees, Macaroni & Cheese	1 bucket	190	6.0	900	20	28.4
Micro Cup Entrees, Pork & Beans	1 bucket	250	5.0	650	30	18.0
Micro Cup Hearty Soups, Bean & Ham	1 bucket	190	3.0	670	30	14.2
Micro Cup Hearty Soups, Beef Vegetable	1 bucket	80	1.0	810	9	11.3
Micro Cup Hearty Soups, Chicken Noodle	1 bucket	110	3.0	690	22	24.5
Micro Cup Hearty Soups, Chicken with Rice & Vegetables	1 bucket	110	2.0	890	-	16.4
Micro Cup Hearty Soups, Country Vegetable	1 bucket	90	2.0	770	-	20.0
Micro Cup Hearty Soups, Minestrone	1 bucket	110	2.0	500	-	16.4

☞ Kid's Kitchen	S. S.	CAL	FAT(g)	SOD(mg)	CHL(mg)	%FAT
Micro Cup Entrees, Mac & Beef	1 bucket	200	6.0	780	25	27.0
Micro Cup Entrees, Macaroni and Cheese	1 bucket	220	6.0	830	20	24.5
Micro Cup Entrees, Spaghetti & Mini Meatballs in Tomato Sauce	1 bucket	220	7.0	850	-	28.6

☞ Libby's Diner	S. S.	CAL	FAT(g)	SOD(mg)	CHL(mg)	%FAT
Microwaveable Meals, Beef Ravioli	1 bucket	240	5.0	890	15	18.8
Microwaveable Meals, Lasagna	1 bucket	200	5.0	780	15	22.5
Microwaveable Meals, Macaroni & Beef	1 bucket	230	6.0	670	20	23.5
Microwaveable Meals, Pasta Spirals & Chicken	1 bucket	120	3.0	900	15	22.5
Microwaveable Meals, Spaghetti & Meatballs	1 bucket	190	3.0	870	15	14.2

☞ Light Balance	S. S.	CAL	FAT(g)	SOD(mg)	CHL(mg)	%FAT
Beef & Pasta Bordeaux	1 bucket	180	1.0	660	25	5.0
Beef Americana	1 bucket	170	3.0	700	15	15.9
Chicken Cacciatore	1 bucket	200	1.0	730	25	4.5
Chicken Fiesta	1 bucket	210	3.0	640	15	12.9
Mushroom Stroganoff	1 bucket	180	5.0	620	15	25.0
Pasta & Garden Vegetables	1 bucket	190	1.0	650	0	4.7

☞ Lunch Bucket	S. S.	CAL	FAT(g)	SOD(mg)	CHL(mg)	%FAT
Beef Noodle Soup	1 bucket	120	1.0	950	35	7.5
Chicken Noodle Soup	1 bucket	110	3.0	970	25	24.5
Country Vegetable Soup	1 bucket	90	1.0	820	0	10.0
Dumplings 'n Chicken	1 bucket	170	3.0	990	-	15.9
Fettucine Marinara	1 bucket	210	2.0	870	-	8.6
Hearty Chicken Soup	1 bucket	120	3.0	950	15	22.25
Lasagna	1 bucket	260	5.0	960	30	17.3
Macaroni 'n Cheese	1 bucket	230	6.0	990	-	23.5
Macaroni 'n Beef	1 bucket	260	5.0	960	30	17.3
Pasta Italiano	1 bucket	280	9.0	910	-	28.9
Ravioli	1 bucket	280	4.0	810	-	12.9
Spaghetti 'n Meat Sauce	1 bucket	260	5.0	960	30	17.3
Split Pea 'n Ham Soup	1 bucket	130	3.0	740	15	20.8
Vegetable Beef Soup	1 bucket	110	2.0	920	15	16.4

PACKAGED ENTREES & SIDE DISHES

PACKAGED ENTREES & SIDE DISHES

☞ My Own Meal	S. S.	CAL	FAT(g)	SOD(mg)	CHL(mg)	%FAT
Chicken, Please	8 oz.	240	6.0	670	-	22.5
My Kind of Chicken	8 oz.	240	8.0	800	-	30.0

☞ Ranch Style	S. S.	CAL	FAT(g)	SOD(mg)	CHL(mg)	%FAT
Beans, Ranch Style	1 bucket	200	4.0	960	10	18.0
Blackeye Peas with Jalapeno	1 bucket	180	2.0	1290	-	10.0
Pintos with Jalapeno	1 bucket	180	2.0	1420	-	10.0
Blackeye Peas	1 bucket	170	2.0	920	-	10.6

PACKAGED ENTREES

☞ Chef Boyardee	S. S.	CAL	FAT(g)	SOD(mg)	CHL(mg)	%FAT
Crust Mix, Quick & Easy	1.5 oz.	150	2.0	300	-	12.0
Lasagna Dinner, Complete	5.9 oz.	280	8.0	900	-	25.7
Pizza Mix, Cheese, Complete	3.84 oz.	230	6.0	740	-	23.5
Pizza Mix, Pepperoni, Complete	3.38 oz.	230	6.0	700	-	23.5
Pizza Mix, Plain	3.50 oz.	180	3.0	640	-	15.0

☞ Kraft	S. S.	CAL	FAT(g)	SOD(mg)	CHL(mg)	%FAT
Macaroni and Cheese Deluxe Dinner	3/4 cup	260	8.0	590	20	27.7
Spaghetti Dinner, Mild American	1 cup	300	7.0	630	0	21.0
Spaghetti Dinner, Tangy Italian Style	1 cup	310	8.0	670	5	23.2
Microwave Entree, Beef Stew	1	230	4.0	970	45	15.7
Microwave Entree, Chicken Cacciatore	1	260	6.0	790	60	20.8
Microwave Entree, Sweet & Sour Chicken	1	290	1.0	730	35	3.1
Microwave Entree, Cheese Tortellini	1	320	8.0	1310	-	22.5

☞Top Shelf Entrees

	S.S.	CAL	FAT(g)	SOD(mg)	CHL(mg)	%FAT
Chicken Cacciatore	10 oz.	200	2.1	690	35	9.5
Glazed Breast Chicken	10 oz.	170	2.0	780	35	10.6
Spaghettini	10 oz.	260	6.0	980	20	20.8
Tender Roast Beef	10 oz.	250	7.0	940	55	25.2
Vegetable Lasagna	10 oz.	280	9.0	970	30	28.9
Chicken Cacciatore	10 oz.	200	1.0	690	35	4.5

PASTA SIDE DISHES

☞Betty Crocker

	S.S.	CAL	FAT(g)	SOD(mg)	CHL(mg)	%FAT
Suddenly Salad*, Creamy Macaroni	1/2 cup	140	4.0	310	-	30.0
Suddenly Salad*, Pasta Primavera	1/2 cup	150	5.0	370	-	30.0
Suddenly Salad*, Ranch and Bacon	1/2 cup	160	5.0	350	-	28.0
*Use low-fat directions only						

☞Kraft

	S.S.	CAL	FAT(g)	SOD(mg)	CHL(mg)	%FAT
Light Italian Pasta Salad and Dressing	1/2 cup	130	3.0	420	0	20.8
Potatoes & Cheese, 2-Cheese	1/2 cup	130	4.0	540	10	27.7
Potatoes & Cheese, Broccoli Au Gratin	1/2 cup	150	5.0	530	40	30.0
Potatoes & Cheese, Scalloped	1/2 cup	150	5.0	510	15	30.0
Potatoes & Cheese, Sour Cream	1/2 cup	150	5.0	610	10	30.0

RICE SIDE DISHES

☞Knorr

	S.S.	CAL	FAT(g)	SOD(mg)	CHL(mg)	%FAT
Pilaf, Harvest Medley	1/2 cup	110	1.0	420	0	8.2
Spicy Cous Cous*	1/2 cup	160	1.1	370	0	6.2
Pilaf, Basmati with Tomato and Fine Herbs*	1/2 cup	200	0.5	420	0	2.3
Pilaf, Lemon Herb Jasmine*	1/2 cup	140	0.9	380	0	5.8

PACKAGED ENTREES & SIDE DISHES

PACKAGED ENTREES & SIDE DISHES

☞ Knorr	S. S.	CAL	FAT(g)	SOD(mg)	CHL(mg)	%FAT
*Prepared without added butter or margarine						

☞ Kraft	S. S.	CAL	FAT(g)	SOD(mg)	CHL(mg)	%FAT
Rice & Cheese, 3-Cheese & Herbs	1/2 cup	150	4.0	600	5	24.0
Rice & Cheese, Cheddar Broccoli	1/2 cup	150	5.0	420	5	30.0
Rice & Cheese, Cheddar Chicken	1/2 cup	150	4.0	590	5	24.0

☞ Lipton	S. S.	CAL	FAT(g)	SOD(mg)	CHL(mg)	%FAT
Rice & Beans	1/2 cup	150	3.0	440	-	18.0
Rice & Beans, Cajun Style	1/2 cup	150	3.0	440	-	18.0
Rice & Sauce, Beef	1/2 cup	150	3.0	610	-	18.0
Rice & Sauce, Cajun	1/2 cup	150	3.0	630	-	18.0
Rice & Sauce, Chicken	1/2 cup	150	4.0	470	-	24.0
Rice & Sauce, Chicken Broccoli	1/2 cup	150	4.0	500	-	24.0
Rice & Sauce, Herbs & Butter	1/2 cup	150	5.0	470	-	30.0
Rice & Sauce, Long Grain & Wild	1/2 cup	150	3.0	560	-	18.0
Rice & Sauce, Long Grain & Wild Rice Mushroom & Herb	1/2 cup	150	3.0	360	-	18.0
Rice & Sauce, Mushroom	1/2 cup	150	3.0	530	-	18.0
Rice & Sauce, Spanish	1/2 cup	140	3.0	560	-	19.3

☞ Minute Rice*	S. S.	CAL	FAT(g)	SOD(mg)	CHL(mg)	%FAT
Minute Boil-in-Bag Rice	1/2 cup	90	0.0	0	0	0.0
Minute Microwave Dishes, Beef Flavored Rice	1/2 cup	140	0.0	530	0	0.0
Minute Microwave Dishes, Cheddar Cheese, Broccoli and Rice	1/2 cup	140	2.0	500	5	12.9
Minute Microwave Dishes, Chicken Flavored Rice	1/2 cup	130	1.0	640	0	6.9
Minute Microwave Dishes, French Style Rice Pilaf	1/2 cup	110	0.0	390	0	0.0

☞**Minute Rice***

	S. S.	CAL	FAT(g)	SOD(mg)	CHL(mg)	%FAT
Minute Premium Long Grain Rice	2/3 cup	120	0.0	0	0	0.0
Minute Rice	2/3 cup	120	0.0	0	0	0.0
Minute Rice Mix, Drumstick	1/2 cup	120	0.0	650	0	0.0
Minute Rice Mix, Fried Rice	1/2 cup	120	0.0	550	0	0.0
Minute Rice Mix, Long Grain & Wild Rice	1/2 cup	120	0.0	530	0	0.0
Minute Rice Mix, Rib Roast	1/2 cup	120	0.0	680	0	0.0
*Prepared without salt or butter						

☞**Near East***

	S. S.	CAL	FAT(g)	SOD(mg)	CHL(mg)	%FAT
Barley Pilaf Mix	1/2 cup	160	4.0	450	-	22.5
Pilaf Mix, Chicken Flavored	1/2 cup	160	4.0	460	-	22.5
Pilaf Mix, Lentil	1/2 cup	180	6.0	480	-	30.0
Rice Mix, Spanish	1/2 cup	180	6.0	690	-	30.0
Rice Pilaf Mix	1/2 cup	160	4.0	490	-	22.5
Rice Pilaf Mix, Brown	1/2 cup	160	5.0	380	-	28.0
Rice, Long Grain and Wild	1/2 cup	160	4.0	470	-	22.5
*Prepared without salt or butter						

☞**Knorr**

	S. S.	CAL	FAT(g)	SOD(mg)	CHL(mg)	%FAT
Pilaf, Spicy Cous Cous	1/2 cup	160	1.0	370	0	5.6
Pilaf, Lemon Herb Jasmine	1/2 cup	140	1.0	380	0	6.4
Pilaf, Harvest Medley	1/2 cup	110	1.0	420	0	8.2
Pilaf, Basmati with Tomato and Fine Herbs	1/2 cup	230	5.0	450	0	19.6

☞**Rice-A-Roni**

	S. S.	CAL	FAT(g)	SOD(mg)	CHL(mg)	%FAT
Beef	1/2 cup	140	4.0	610	-	25.7
Beef & Mushroom	1/2 cup	150	3.0	740	-	18.0
Chicken	1/2 cup	150	4.0	560	-	24.0

PACKAGED ENTREES & SIDE DISHES

👉 Rice-A-Roni

	S. S.	CAL	FAT(g)	SOD(mg)	CHL(mg)	%FAT
Chicken & Broccoli	1/2 cup	150	3.0	710	-	18.0
Chicken & Vegetables	1/2 cup	140	3.0	790	-	19.3
Herb & Butter	1/2 cup	130	4.0	790	-	27.7
Long Grain & Wild Rice Chicken with Almonds	1/2 cup	130	3.0	660	-	20.8
Long Grain & Wild Rice Original	1/2 cup	140	4.0	690	-	25.7
Long Grain & Wild Rice Pilaf	1/2 cup	130	3.0	550	-	20.8
Rice Pilaf	1/2 cup	150	4.0	620	-	24.0
Risotto	1/2 cup	200	6.0	1130	-	27.0
Spanish Rice	1/2 cup	150	4.0	1090	-	24.0
Yellow Rice	1/2 cup	140	4.0	780	-	25.7
Savory Classics, Almond Chicken with Wild Rice	1/2 cup	140	4.0	660	-	25.7
Savory Classics, Chicken & Broccoli Dijon	1/2 cup	160	5.0	610	-	28.2
Savory Classics, Chicken Florentine	1/2 cup	130	4.0	910	-	27.7
Savory Classics, Garden Pilaf	1/2 cup	140	4.0	1000	-	25.7

👉 Success Rice*

	S. S.	CAL	FAT(g)	SOD(mg)	CHL(mg)	%FAT
Au Gratin Herb Rice Mix	1/2 cup	100	0.0	260	-	0.0
Brown and Wild RiceMi	1/2 cup	120	0.0	500	-	0.0
SLE Broccoli and Cheese	1/2 cup	120	<1.0	310	-	<7.5
Success Beef	1/2 cup	100	0.0	370	-	0.0
Success Chicken	1/2 cup	110	2.0	420	-	16.4
Success Pilaf	1/2 cup	120	0.0	410	-	0.0
Success Yellow	1/2 cup	100	0.0	480	-	0.0

*Prepared without added margarine

👉 Uncle Ben's

	S. S.	CAL	FAT(g)	SOD(mg)	CHL(mg)	%FAT
Boil-in-Bag Rice*	1/2 cup	90	<1.0	10	-	<10.0
Converted Rice*	2/3 cup	120	<1.0	0	-	<7.5
Country Inn, Broccoli Almondine	1/2 cup	157	5.0	631	-	28.7
Country Inn, Chicken Stock Rice	1/2 cup	157	4.0	591	-	22.9

☞ Uncle Ben's	S. S.	CAL	FAT(g)	SOD(mg)	CHL(mg)	%FAT
Country Inn, Chicken Rice Royale	1/2 cup	147	4.0	591	-	24.5
Country Inn, Vegetable Pilaf	1/2 cup	147	4.0	311	-	24.5
Long Grain & Wild Rice, Brown & Wild Rice*	1/2 cup	130	1.0	500	-	6.9
Long Grain & Wild Rice, Chicken Stock Sauce*	1/2 cup	140	2.0	650	-	12.9
Long Grain & Wild Rice, Original Fast Cooking Recipe*	1/2 cup	100	<1.0	410	-	<9.0
Long Grain & Wild Rice, Original Recipe*	1/2 cup	100	<1.0	500	-	<9.0
Natural Whole Grain Rice*	2/3 cup	130	1.0	0	-	6.9
Rice In An Instant*	2/3 cup	120	<1.0	10	-	<7.5
*Prepared without added margarine						

PACKAGED ENTREES & SIDE DISHES

PASTA & PASTA SAUCES

PASTA, DRY

☞ **Generic**	S. S.	CAL	FAT(g)	SOD(mg)	CHL(mg)	%FAT
Pasta, Dry, Egg Noodles	3.6 oz.	133	1.5	7	33	9.9
Pasta, Dry, Macaroni	3.6 oz.	141	0.7	1	0	4.3
Pasta, Dry, Spaghetti	3.6 oz.	141	0.7	1	0	4.3
Pasta, Fresh	3.6 oz.	131	1.1	6	33	7.2
Pasta, Fresh, Spinach	3.6 oz.	130	0.9	6	33	6.5

PASTA, FRESH

☞ **Contadina Fresh**	S. S.	CAL	FAT(g)	SOD(mg)	CHL(mg)	%FAT
Agnolotti	4.5 oz.	380	10.0	460	60	23.7
Angel's Hair Fettucini or Linguini	4.5 oz.	390	5.0	45	140	11.5
Angel's Hair Fettucini or Linguini, Spinach	4.5 oz.	360	5.0	75	145	12.5
Italian Sausage Tortelloni	4.5 oz.	370	12.0	460	145	29.2
Ravioli with Beef	4.5 oz.	340	11.0	490	100	29.1
Rigatoni	3.5 oz.	310	4.0	35	110	11.6
Salad Pasta, Rotini	2.25 oz.	190	3.0	25	75	14.2
Salad Pasta, Tricolor Rotini	2.25 oz.	190	3.0	30	65	14.2
Salad Pasta, Tricolor Shells	2 oz.	170	2.0	30	70	10.6
Tortellini with Cheese	4.5 oz.	370	8.0	580	65	19.5
Tortellini with Cheese, Spinach	4.5 oz.	370	8.0	600	65	19.5
Tortellini with Meat	4.5 oz.	380	10.0	660	75	23.7
Tortellini with Meat, Spinach	4.5 oz.	380	10.0	680	75	23.7
Tortelloni with Chicken & Prosciutto	4.5 oz.	340	7.0	750	75	18.5
Tortelloni with Chicken and Prosciutto, Spinach	4.5 oz.	340	7.0	750	75	18.5

☞ **Di Giorno**	S. S.	CAL	FAT(g)	SOD(mg)	CHL(mg)	%FAT
Angel's Hair	3. oz.	250	3.0	140	0	10.8

☞ **Di Giorno**	S. S.	CAL	FAT(g)	SOD(mg)	CHL(mg)	%FAT
Fettuccine	3 oz.	250	3.0	140	0	10.8
Fettuccine, Spinach	3 oz.	250	2.0	115	0	7.0
Lasagna	1 oz.	80	1.0	50	0	11.3
Linguine	3 oz.	250	3.0	140	0	10.8
Linguine, Herb	3 oz.	260	3.0	140	0	10.4
Spaghetti	3 oz.	250	3.0	140	0	10.8

☞ **Romance**	S. S.	CAL	FAT(g)	SOD(mg)	CHL(mg)	%FAT
Fresh Cheese Ravioli	10 oz.	285	6.7	485	-	21.1

☞ **Trio's**	S. S.	CAL	FAT(g)	SOD(mg)	CHL(mg)	%FAT
Linguine, Egg Free	3 oz.	240	<1.0	25	0	<3.8
Pasta, Cut	3 oz.	240	2.0	25	55	7.5
Ravioli, Spinach & Ricotta	2.5 oz.	180	4.0	220	95	20.0
Tortellini, Cheese	2.5 oz.	210	5.0	330	120	21.4
Tortellini, Mushroom	2.5 oz.	180	3.0	270	75	15.0

PASTA SAUCES

☞ **Enrico's**	S. S.	CAL	FAT(g)	SOD(mg)	CHL(mg)	%FAT
Spaghetti Sauce, All Natural	4 oz.	60	1.0	345	0	15.0
Spaghetti Sauce, All Natural, No Salt	4 oz.	60	1.0	30	0	15.0
Spaghetti Sauce, Mushroom	4 oz.	60	1.0	-	0	15.0
Spaghetti Sauce, Mushroom and Green Pepper	4 oz.	60	1.0	345	0	15.0

☞ **Healthy Choice**	S. S.	CAL	FAT(g)	SOD(mg)	CHL(mg)	%FAT
Spaghetti Sauce with Garlic and Herb	4 oz.	40	<1.0	390	0	<22.5
Spaghetti Sauce with Green Peppers	4 oz.	40	<1.0	390	0	<22.5

☞Healthy Choice

☞Healthy Choice	S. S.	CAL	FAT(g)	SOD(mg)	CHL(mg)	%FAT
Spaghetti Sauce with Meat	4 oz.	50	<1.0	380	0	<18.0
Spaghetti Sauce with Mushrooms	4 oz.	40	<1.0	390	0	<22.5
Spaghetti Sauce, Traditional	4 oz.	40	<1.0	380	0	<22.5

☞Hunt

☞Hunt	S. S.	CAL	FAT(g)	SOD(mg)	CHL(mg)	%FAT
Spaghetti Sauce, Chunky	4 oz.	50	<1.0	470	0	<18.0
Spaghetti Sauce, Classic Italian, with Parmesan	4 oz.	60	2.0	550	0	30.0
Spaghetti Sauce, Homestyle	4 oz.	60	2.0	530	0	30.0
Spaghetti Sauce, Homestyle with Meat	1 cup	170	5.0	1150	-	26.5
Spaghetti Sauce, Homestyle with Mushrooms	4 oz.	50	1.0	530	0	18.0
Spaghetti Sauce, Traditional	4 oz.	70	2.0	530	0	25.7
Spaghetti Sauce, with Meat	4 oz.	70	2.0	570	2	25.7
Spaghetti Sauce, with Mushrooms	4 oz.	70	2.0	560	0	25.7

☞Prego

☞Prego	S. S.	CAL	FAT(g)	SOD(mg)	CHL(mg)	%FAT
Spaghetti Sauce, Extra Chunky Garden Combination	4 oz.	80	2.0	420	-	22.5
Spaghetti Sauce, Extra Chunky Mushroom with Extra Spice	4 oz.	100	3.0	450	-	27.0
Spaghetti Sauce, Three Cheese	4 oz.	100	2.0	410	-	18.0
Spaghetti Sauce, Tomato & Basil	4 oz.	100	2.0	370	-	18.0

☞Ragu

☞Ragu	S. S.	CAL	FAT(g)	SOD(mg)	CHL(mg)	%FAT
Fino Italian Pasta Sauce, Parmesan	4 oz.	90	3.0	540	0	30.0
Fino Italian Pasta Sauce, Tomato & Herbs	4 oz.	90	3.0	490	0	30.0
Spaghetti Sauce, Original Style with Mushrooms	4 oz.	80	2.0	740	2	22.5
Spaghetti Sauce, Thick & Hearty	4 oz.	100	3.0	460	0	27.0

☞ Ragu	S. S.	CAL	FAT(g)	SOD(mg)	CHL(mg)	%FAT
Spaghetti Sauce, Thick & Hearty with Mushrooms	4 oz.	100	3.0	460	0	27.0
Today's Recipe Pasta Sauce, Chunky Mushroom	4 oz.	50	1.0	370	0	18.0
Today's Recipe Pasta Sauce, Garden Harvest	4 oz.	50	1.0	370	0	18.0
Today's Recipe Pasta Sauce, Tomato Herb	4 oz.	50	1.0	370	0	18.0

☞ Sensational	S. S.	CAL	FAT(g)	SOD(mg)	CHL(mg)	%FAT
Pasta Sauce, Mushroom	4 oz.	60	1.0	713	-	15.0
Pasta Sauce, Northern Italian Style	4 oz.	60	1.0	722	-	15.0

PASTA SIDE DISHES

☞ Kraft Light	S. S.	CAL	FAT(g)	SOD(mg)	CHL(mg)	%FAT
Italian Pasta Salad and Dressing	1/2 cup	130	3.0	420	0	20.8

PRODUCE SECTION

NUTS

☞Generic	S. S.	CAL	FAT(g)	SOD(mg)	CHL(mg)	%FAT
Chestnuts	1 oz.	60	0.6	1	0	9.0

ORIENTAL PASTA

☞Asumaya	S. S.	CAL	FAT(g)	SOD(mg)	CHL(mg)	%FAT
Won Ton Wraps	14 oz.	285	1.4	628	-	4.3
Egg Roll Wraps	16 oz.	286	1.3	525	-	4.2
Gyoza	12 oz.	282	1.3	577	-	4.0
Chinese Noodles	14 oz.	293	1.3	530	-	4.0
Japanese Noodles	14 oz.	289	1.1	542	-	3.3

◆ Coconut, Avocado, And Other Types Of Nuts Are Greater Than 30% FAT

◆ All Other Fresh Fruits And Vegetables Are Acceptable

PUDDINGS & DESSERT MIXES

DESSERT TOPPING MIXES

☞ **Dream Whip**	S. S.	CAL	FAT(g)	SOD(mg)	CHL(mg)	%FAT
Whipped Topping Mix*	1 Tbsp.	6	0.0	0	0	0.0
*As packaged						

PREPARED PUDDINGS

☞ **Jell-O**	S. S.	CAL	FAT(g)	SOD(mg)	CHL(mg)	%FAT
Pudding Snacks, Butterscotch/Chocolate/Vanilla Swirl	4 oz.	180	6	140	0	30.0
Pudding Snacks, Vanilla/Chocolate Swirl	4 oz.	180	6	140	0	30.0
Light Pudding Snacks, Chocolate	4 oz.	100	2	125	5	18.0
Light Pudding Snacks, Chocolate Fudge	4 oz.	100	1	125	5	9.0
Light Pudding Snacks, Chocolate Vanilla Combo	4 oz.	100	2	125	5	18.0
Light Pudding Snacks, Vanilla	4 oz.	100	2	130	5	18.0

☞ **Swiss Miss***	S. S.	CAL	FAT(g)	SOD(mg)	CHL(mg)	%FAT
Pudding Sundae, Chocolate	4 oz.	220	7	140	1	28.6
Pudding Sundae, Vanilla	4 oz.	220	7	180	1	28.6
Light Pudding, Vanilla	4 oz.	100	1	105	<1	9.0
Light Pudding, Chocolate	4 oz.	100	1	120	1	9.0
Pudding, Chocolate	4 oz.	180	6	160	1	30.0
Pudding, Chocolate Fudge	4 oz.	220	6	180	1	24.5
Parfait, Vanilla	4 oz.	180	6	150	1	30.0
Pudding, Tapioca	4 oz.	160	5	170	1	28.1
Pudding, Butterscotch	4 oz.	180	6	135	1	30.0

PUDDINGS & DESSERT MIXES

☞Swiss Miss*	S. S.	CAL	FAT(g)	SOD(mg)	CHL(mg)	%FAT
Pudding, Custard	4 oz.	190	6	190	5	28.4
*Often in the Refrigerator Section						

☞Hunt	S. S.	CAL	FAT(g)	SOD(mg)	CHL(mg)	%FAT
Snack Pack Pudding, Tapioca, Lite	4 oz.	100	2	105	1	18.0
Snack Pack Pudding, Chocolate, Lite	4 oz.	100	2	120	1	18.0
Snack Pack Pudding, Tapioca	4.25 oz.	150	5	150	1	30.0
Snack Pack Pudding, Lemon	4.25 oz.	150	4	75	0	24.0

☞Del Monte	S. S.	CAL	FAT(g)	SOD(mg)	CHL(mg)	%FAT
Pudding Cup, Banana	5 oz.	180	5	285	-	25.0
Pudding Cup, Butterscotch	5 oz.	180	5	285	-	25.0
Pudding Cup, Chocolate Fudge	5 oz.	190	6	260	-	28.4
Pudding Cup, Chocolate	5 oz.	190	6	280	-	28.4
Pudding Cup, Tapioca	5 oz.	180	4	250	-	20.0
Pudding Cup, Vanilla	5 oz.	180	5	285	-	25.0

PUDDING, GELATIN AND DESSERT MIXES

☞D-Zerta	S. S.	CAL	FAT(g)	SOD(mg)	CHL(mg)	%FAT
Low Calorie Gelatin, All Flavors	1/2 cup	8	0.0	0	0	0.0
Reduced Calorie Pudding, Butterscotch	1/2 cup	70	0.0	65	0	0.0
Reduced Calorie Pudding, Chocolate	1/2 cup	60	0.0	70	0	0.0
Reduced Calorie Pudding, Vanilla	1/2 cup	70	0.0	65	0	0.0

☞Jell-O	S. S.	CAL	FAT(g)	SOD(mg)	CHL(mg)	%FAT
1-2-3 Gelatin, All Flavors	2/3 cup	130	2.0	55	0	13.8
Gelatin, All Flavors	1/2 cup	80	0.0	<75	0	0.0

☞ Jell-O

	S. S.	CAL	FAT(g)	SOD(mg)	CHL(mg)	%FAT
Sugar Free Gelatin, All Flavors	1/2 cup	8	0.0	<80	0	0.0
Sugar Free Instant Pudding and Pie Filling, Banana	1/2 cup	80	2.0	390	10	22.5
Sugar Free Instant Pudding and Pie Filling, Butterscotch	1/2 cup	90	2.0	390	10	20.0
Sugar Free Instant Pudding and Pie Filling, Chocolate	1/2 cup	90	3.0	380	10	30.0
Sugar Free Instant Pudding and Pie Filling, Chocolate Fudge	1/2 cup	100	3.0	330	10	27.0
Sugar Free Instant Pudding and Pie Filling, Pistachio	1/2 cup	90	3.0	390	10	30.0
Sugar Free Instant Pudding and Pie Filling, Vanilla	1/2 cup	90	2.0	390	10	20.0
Sugar Free Pudding and Pie Filling, Chocolate	1/2 cup	90	3.0	160	10	30.0
Sugar Free Pudding and Pie Filling, Vanilla	1/2 cup	80	2.0	200	10	22.5

☞ Royal

	S. S.	CAL	FAT(g)	SOD(mg)	CHL(mg)	%FAT
Gelatin Dessert, All Flavors	1/2 cup	80	0.0	90-130	0	0.0
Sugar Free Gelatin, All Flavors Except Orange	1/2 cup	8	0.0	85-100	0	0.0
Sugar Free Gelatin, Orange	1/2 cup	10	0.0	90	0	0.0

☞ Sans Sucre de Paris

	S. S.	CAL	FAT(g)	SOD(mg)	CHL(mg)	%FAT
Mousse Mix, Cheesecake	1/2 cup	73	1.0	180	1	12.3
Mousse Mix, Chocolate	1/2 cup	75	3.0	77	4	36.0
Mousse Mix, Chocolate Cheesecake	1/2 cup	73	1.0	180	1	12.3
Mousse Mix, Lemon	1/2 cup	70	3.0	49	4	38.6
Mousse Mix, Strawberry	1/2 cup	70	3.0	49	4	38.6

☞Sweet 'n Low	S.S.	CAL	FAT(g)	SOD(mg)	CHL(mg)	%FAT
Custard Mix, Chocolate	1/2 cup	70	0.0	115	5	0.0
Custard Mix, Lemon	1/2 cup	70	0.0	145	5	0.0
Custard Mix, Vanilla	1/2 cup	70	1.0	145	5	12.9

PUDDINGS & DESSERT MIXES

REFRIGERATOR SECTION
(NON-DAIRY)

DOUGHS

☞ **Ballard**	S. S.	CAL	FAT(g)	SOD(mg)	CHL(mg)	%FAT
Extralights Biscuits, Ovenready	1 biscuit	50	<1.0	180	0	<18.0
Extralights Biscuits, Ovenready, Buttermilk	1 biscuit	50	<1.0	180	0	18.0

☞ **Contadina Fresh**	S. S.	CAL	FAT(g)	SOD(mg)	CHL(mg)	%FAT
Agnolotti	4.5 oz.	380	10.0	460	60	23.7
Angel's Hair Fettucini or Linguini	4.5 oz.	390	5.0	45	140	11.5
Angel's Hair Fettucini or Linguini, Spinach	4.5 oz.	360	5.0	75	145	12.5
Italian Sausage Tortelloni	4.5 oz.	370	12.0	460	145	29.2
Ravioli with Beef	4.5 oz.	340	11.0	490	100	29.1
Rigatoni	3.5 oz.	310	4.0	35	110	11.6
Salad Pasta, Rotini	2.25 oz.	190	3.0	25	75	14.2
Salad Pasta, Tricolor Rotini	2.25 oz.	190	3.0	30	65	14.2
Salad Pasta, Tricolor Shells	2 oz.	170	2.0	30	70	10.6
Tortellini with Cheese	4.5 oz.	370	8.0	580	65	19.5
Tortellini with Cheese, Spinach	4.5 oz.	370	8.0	600	65	19.5
Tortellini with Meat	4.5 oz.	380	10.0	660	75	23.7
Tortellini with Meat, Spinach	4.5 oz.	380	10.0	680	75	23.7
Tortelloni with Chicken and Prosciutto	4.5 oz.	340	7.0	750	75	18.5
Tortelloni with Chicken and Prosciutto, Spinach	4.5 oz.	340	7.0	750	75	18.5

☞ **Di Giorno**	S. S.	CAL	FAT(g)	SOD(mg)	CHL(mg)	%FAT
Angel's Hair	3 oz.	250	3.0	140	0	10.8
Fettuccine	3 oz.	250	3.0	140	0	10.8
Fettuccine, Spinach	3 oz.	250	2.0	115	0	7.0

REFRIGERATOR SECTION

☞ Di Giorno	S. S.	CAL	FAT(g)	SOD(mg)	CHL(mg)	%FAT
Lasagna	1 oz.	80	1.0	50	0	11.3
Linguine	3 oz.	250	3.0	140	0	10.8
Linguine, Herb	3 oz.	260	3.0	140	0	10.4
Spaghetti	3 oz.	250	3.0	140	0	10.8

☞ Hearty Grains	S. S.	CAL	FAT(g)	SOD(mg)	CHL(mg)	%FAT
Twists, Country Oatmeal	1 twist	80	2.0	120	0	22.5
Twists, Cracked Wheat & Honey	1 twist	80	2.0	120	0	22.5
Multi-Grain	1 roll	80	2.0	230	0	22.5
Oatmeal Raisin	1 roll	90	2.0	210	0	20.0

☞ Hungry Jack	S. S.	CAL	FAT(g)	SOD(mg)	CHL(mg)	%FAT
Biscuits, Buttermilk, Extra Rich	1 biscuit	50	1.0	180	0	18.0

☞ Merico	S. S.	CAL	FAT(g)	SOD(mg)	CHL(mg)	%FAT
Biscuits, Butter Fluffy	2 biscuits	170	3.0	230	0	15.9
Biscuits, Homestyle	2 biscuits	100	1.0	330	0	9.0
Biscuits, Oat Bran	2 biscuits	180	4.0	460	0	20.0
Biscuits, Texas Style	2 biscuits	190	5.0	510	0	23.7
Biscuits, Weight Watchers Buttermilk	2 biscuits	120	1.0	570	0	7.5
Cinnamon Danish	1 roll	120	4.0	360	2	30.0
Cinnamon Rolls	1 roll	100	3.0	300	5	27.0
English Muffins, Cinnamon Raisin	1 muffin	140	1.0	250	0	6.4
English Muffins, Multi Grain	1 muffin	130	1.0	270	0	6.9
English Muffins, Oat Bran	1 muffin	120	1.0	220	0	7.5
English Muffins, Regular	1 muffin	130	1.0	310	0	6.9
English Muffins, Sun Maid Raisin	1 muffin	160	1.0	210	0	5.6
Muffins, Blueberry Tub	1 muffin	170	5.0	240	15	26.5

☞Pillsbury

	S. S.	CAL	FAT(g)	SOD(mg)	CHL(mg)	%FAT
All Ready Pizza Crust	1/8 pizza	90	1.0	170	0	10.0
Biscuits, Butter	1 biscuit	50	<1.0	180	0	<18.0
Biscuits, Buttermilk	1 biscuit	50	1.0	180	0	18.0
Biscuits, Country	1 biscuit	50	1.0	180	0	18.0
Biscuits, Heat n' Eat Buttermilk	2 biscuits	170	5.0	530	0	26.5
Biscuits, Tender Layer Buttermilk	1 biscuit	50	1.0	170	0	18.0
Cookie Dough, Oatmeal Raisin	1 cookie	60	2.0	55	0	30.0
Crusty French Loaf	1" slice	60	<1.0	120	0	<15.0
Pipin' Hot Wheat Loaf	1" slice	70	2.0	170	0	25.7
Pipin' Hot White Loaf	1"slice	70	2.0	170	0	25.7
Soft Bread Sticks	1 stick	100	2.0	230	0	18.0

☞Roman Meal

	S. S.	CAL	FAT(g)	SOD(mg)	CHL(mg)	%FAT
Biscuits	2 biscuits	180	4.0	460	0	20.0
Bread Loaf	1 oz.	90	3.0	200	0	30.0
Bread Sticks	1 stick	120	4.0	270	0	30.0
English Muffins, Honey Nut Oat Bran	1/2 muffin	80	1.0	115	0	11.3
English Muffins, Regular	1/2 muffin	70	1.0	90	0	12.9

☞Romance

	S. S.	CAL	FAT(g)	SOD(mg)	CHL(mg)	%FAT
Fresh Cheese Ravioli	10 oz.	285	6.7	485	-	21.1

TORTILLAS

☞Generic

	S. S.	CAL	FAT(g)	SOD(mg)	CHL(mg)	%FAT
Tortillas, Corn	1 tortilla	67	1.1	53	-	14.8

REFRIGERATOR SECTION

☞ Azteca

	S. S.	CAL	FAT(g)	SOD(mg)	CHL(mg)	%FAT
Tortillas, Corn	1 tortilla	45	0.0	10	0	0.0
Tortillas, Flour, 7"	1 tortilla	80	2.0	110	0	22.5
Tortillas, Flour, 9"	1 tortilla	130	3.0	180	0	20.8

☞ El Aguila

	S. S.	CAL	FAT(g)	SOD(mg)	CHL(mg)	%FAT
Tortilla, Corn	1.1 oz.	50	1.0	5	<1	18.0
Tortilla, Corn, Blancas	0.8 oz.	210	3.0	10	0	12.9
Tortilla, Flour, Lite	1.4 oz.	110	2.0	250	<1	16.4

☞ Mission

	S. S.	CAL	FAT(g)	SOD(mg)	CHL(mg)	%FAT
Tortillas, Corn, for tacos	1 tortilla	45	1.0	25	-	20.0
Tortillas, Corn, for table use	1 tortilla	50	1.0	30	-	18.0
Tortillas, Flour, Fajita Size	1 tortilla	100	2.0	160	0	18.0

☞ Old El Paso

	S. S.	CAL	FAT(g)	SOD(mg)	CHL(mg)	%FAT
Tortillas, Corn	1 tortilla	60	1.0	170	0	15.0
Tortillas, Flour	1 tortilla	150	3.0	360	0	18.0

☞ Ramirez & Sons

	S. S.	CAL	FAT(g)	SOD(mg)	CHL(mg)	%FAT
Tortillas, Corn	1 tortilla	35	1.0	20	0	25.7
Tortillas, Flour	1 tortilla	150	5.0	280	0	30.0

☞ Tyson

	S. S.	CAL	FAT(g)	SOD(mg)	CHL(mg)	%FAT
Tortillas, Corn, Enchilada Style	1 tortilla	54	0.4	4	0	6.7
Tortillas, Flour, Burrito Style	1 tortilla	173	4.0	40	0	20.8

☞Tyson	S. S.	CAL	FAT(g)	SOD(mg)	CHL(mg)	%FAT
Tortillas, Flour, Fajita Style	1 tortilla	84	2.0	20	0	21.4
Tortillas, Flour, Soft Taco Style	1 tortilla	121	3.0	30	0	22.3

RICE SECTION

RICES

☞**Generic**	S. S.	CAL	FAT(g)	SOD(mg)	CHL(mg)	%FAT
Rice, Brown, Long-Grain	3.6 oz.	111	0.9	5	0	7.3
Rice, White, Long-Grain	3.6 oz.	129	0.3	2	0	2.0
Rice, White, Long-Grain, Parboiled	3.6 oz.	114	0.3	3	0	2.1
Rice, White, Long-Grain, Pre-Cooked or Instant	3.6 oz.	98	0.2	3	0	1.5
Rice, White, Medium-Grain	3.6 oz.	130	0.2	0	0	1.5
Rice, White, Short-Grain	3.6 oz.	130	0.2	0	0	1.3

RICE SIDE DISHES

☞**Kraft**	S. S.	CAL	FAT(g)	SOD(mg)	CHL(mg)	%FAT
Rice & Cheese, 3-Cheese & Herbs	1/2 cup	150	4.0	600	5	24.0
Rice & Cheese, Cheddar Broccoli	1/2 cup	150	5.0	420	5	30.0
Rice & Cheese, Cheddar Chicken	1/2 cup	150	4.0	590	5	24.0

☞**Lipton**	S. S.	CAL	FAT(g)	SOD(mg)	CHL(mg)	%FAT
Beans & Sauce, Cajun	1/2 cup	150	3.0	440	-	18.0
Beans & Sauce, Hearty Chicken	1/2 cup	150	4.0	600	-	24.0
Rice & Beans	1/2 cup	150	3.0	440	-	18.0
Rice & Beans, Cajun Style	1/2 cup	150	3.0	440	-	18.0
Rice & Sauce, Beef	1/2 cup	150	3.0	610	-	18.0
Rice & Sauce, Cajun	1/2 cup	150	3.0	630	-	18.0
Rice & Sauce, Chicken	1/2 cup	150	4.0	470	-	24.0
Rice & Sauce, Chicken Broccoli	1/2 cup	150	4.0	500	-	24.0
Rice & Sauce, Herbs & Butter	1/2 cup	150	5.0	470	-	30.0
Rice & Sauce, Long Grain & Wild	1/2 cup	150	3.0	560	-	18.0
Rice & Sauce, Long Grain & Wild Rice Mushroom & Herb	1/2 cup	150	3.0	360	-	18.0
Rice & Sauce, Mushroom	1/2 cup	150	3.0	530	-	18.0

☞ Lipton	S. S.	CAL	FAT(g)	SOD(mg)	CHL(mg)	%FAT
Rice & Sauce, Spanish	1/2 cup	140	3.0	560	-	19.3

☞ Minute Rice*	S. S.	CAL	FAT(g)	SOD(mg)	CHL(mg)	%FAT
Minute Boil-in-Bag Rice	1/2 cup	90	0.0	0	0	0.0
Minute Microwave Dishes, Beef Flavored Rice	1/2 cup	140	0.0	530	0	0.0
Minute Microwave Dishes, Cheddar Cheese, Broccoli and Rice	1/2 cup	140	2.0	500	5	12.9
Minute Microwave Dishes, Chicken Flavored Rice	1/2 cup	130	1.0	640	0	6.9
Minute Microwave Dishes, French Style Rice Pilaf	1/2 cup	110	0.0	390	0	0.0
Minute Premium Long Grain Rice	2/3 cup	120	0.0	0	0	0.0
Minute Rice	2/3 cup	120	0.0	0	0	0.0
Minute Rice Mix, Drumstick	1/2 cup	120	0.0	650	0	0.0
Minute Rice Mix, Fried Rice	1/2 cup	120	0.0	550	0	0.0
Minute Rice Mix, Long Grain & Wild Rice	1/2 cup	120	0.0	532	0	0.0
Minute Rice Mix, Rib Roast	1/2 cup	120	0.0	680	0	0.0
*Prepared without salt or butter						

☞ Near East*	S. S.	CAL	FAT(g)	SOD(mg)	CHL(mg)	%FAT
Barley Pilaf Mix	1/2 cup	160	4.0	450	-	22.5
Pilaf Mix, Chicken Flavored	1/2 cup	160	4.0	460	-	22.5
Pilaf Mix, Lentil	1/2 cup	180	6.0	480	-	30.0
Rice Mix, Spanish	1/2 cup	180	6.0	690	-	30.0
Rice Pilaf Mix	1/2 cup	160	4.0	490	-	22.5
Rice Pilaf Mix, Brown	1/2 cup	160	5.0	380	-	28.0
Rice, Long Grain and Wild	1/2 cup	160	4.0	470	-	22.5
*Prepared without added margarine						

☞ Rice-A-Roni

	S. S.	CAL	FAT(g)	SOD(mg)	CHL(mg)	%FAT
Beef	1/2 cup	140	4.0	610	-	25.7
Beef & Mushroom	1/2 cup	150	3.0	740	-	18.0
Chicken	1/2 cup	150	4.0	560	-	24.0
Chicken & Broccoli	1/2 cup	150	3.0	710	-	18.0
Chicken & Vegetables	1/2 cup	140	3.0	790	-	19.3
Herb & Butter	1/2 cup	130	4.0	790	-	27.7
Long Grain & Wild Rice Chicken with Almonds	1/2 cup	130	3.0	660	-	20.8
Long Grain & Wild Rice Original	1/2 cup	140	4.0	690	-	25.7
Long Grain & Wild Rice Pilaf	1/2 cup	130	3.0	550	-	20.8
Rice Pilaf	1/2 cup	150	4.0	620	-	24.0
Risotto	1/2 cup	200	6.0	1130	-	27.0
Spanish Rice	1/2 cup	150	4.0	1090	-	24.0
Yellow Rice	1/2 cup	140	4.0	780	-	25.7
Savory Classics, Almond Chicken with Wild Rice	1/2 cup	140	4.0	660	-	25.7
Savory Classics, Chicken & Broccoli Dijon	1/2 cup	160	5.0	610	-	28.2
Savory Classics, Chicken Florentine	1/2 cup	130	4.0	910	-	27.7
Savory Classics, Garden Pilaf	1/2 cup	140	4.0	1000	-	25.7

☞ Success Rice*

	S. S.	CAL	FAT(g)	SOD(mg)	CHL(mg)	%FAT
Au Gratin Herb Success Rice Mix	1/2 cup	100	0.0	260	-	0.0
Brown and Wild Success Rice Mix	1/2 cup	120	0.0	500	-	0.0
SLE Broccoli and Cheese	1/2 cup	120	<1.0	310	-	<7.5
Success Beef	1/2 cup	100	0.0	370	-	0.0
Success Chicken	1/2 cup	110	2.0	420	-	16.4
Success Pilaf	1/2 cup	120	0.0	410	-	0.0
Success Yellow	1/2 cup	100	0.0	480	-	0.0

*Prepared without added margarine

☞ Uncle Ben's

	S. S.	CAL	FAT(g)	SOD(mg)	CHL(mg)	%FAT
Boil-In-Bag Rice*	1/2 cup	90	<1.0	10	-	<10.0

☞ Uncle Ben's	S. S.	CAL	FAT(g)	SOD(mg)	CHL(mg)	%FAT
Converted Rice*	2/3 cup	120	<1.0	0	-	<7.5
Country Inn, Broccoli Almondine	1/2 cup	157	5.0	631	-	28.7
Country Inn, Chicken Stock Rice	1/2 cup	157	4.0	591	-	22.9
Country Inn, Chicken Rice Royale	1/2 cup	147	4.0	591	-	24.5
Country Inn, Vegetable Pilaf	1/2 cup	147	4.0	311	-	24.5
Long Grain & Wild Rice, Brown & Wild Rice*	1/2 cup	130	1.0	500	-	6.9
Long Grain & Wild Rice, Chicken Stock Sauce*	1/2 cup	140	2.0	650	-	12.9
Long Grain & Wild Rice, Original Fast Cooking Recipe*	1/2 cup	100	<1.0	410	-	<9.0
Long Grain & Wild Rice, Original Recipe*	1/2 cup	100	<1.0	500	-	<9.0
Natural Whole Grain Rice*	2/3 cup	130	1.0	0	-	6.9
Rice In An Instant*	2/3 cup	120	<1.0	10	-	<7.5

*Prepared without added margarine

SALAD DRESSINGS & MAYONNAISE

CROUTONS

☞ **Arnold**	S. S.	CAL	FAT(g)	SOD(mg)	CHL(mg)	%FAT
Croutons, Cheese & Garlic	0.5 oz.	60	1.0	135	0	15.0
Croutons, Fine Herb	0.5 oz.	50	<1.0	150	0	<18.0
Croutons, Seasoned	0.5 oz.	60	1.0	160	0	15.0

☞ **Brownberry**	S. S.	CAL	FAT(g)	SOD(mg)	CHL(mg)	%FAT
Croutons, Onion & Garlic	0.5 oz.	60	2.0	190	0	30.0
Croutons, Seasoned	0.5 oz.	60	2.0	160	0	30.0
Croutons, Toasted	0.5 oz.	60	1.0	150	0	15.0
Croutons, Cheese & Garlic	0.5 oz.	60	1.0	90	0	15.0
Croutons, Plain	0.5 oz.	60	1.0	70	0	15.0
Croutons, Seasoned, Unsalted	0.5 oz.	60	1.0	15	0	15.0

☞ **Wonder**	S. S.	CAL	FAT(g)	SOD(mg)	CHL(mg)	%FAT
Croutons, Seasoned	1 oz.	135	1.0	145	0	6.7

MAYONNAISE

☞ **Cains**	S. S.	CAL	FAT(g)	SOD(mg)	CHL(mg)	%FAT
Mayonnaise Dressing, Fat Free	1 Tbsp.	10	0.0	115	0	0.0

☞ **Kraft Free**	S. S.	CAL	FAT(g)	SOD(mg)	CHL(mg)	%FAT
Mayonnaise Dressing, Nonfat	1 Tbsp.	12	0.0	190	0	0.0

SALAD DRESSINGS & MAYONNAISE

☞ **Miracle Whip Free**	S. S.	CAL	FAT(g)	SOD(mg)	CHL(mg)	%FAT
Dressing, Nonfat	1 Tbsp.	20	0.0	210	0	0.0

☞ **Weight Watchers**	S. S.	CAL	FAT(g)	SOD(mg)	CHL(mg)	%FAT
Mayonnaise Dressing, Fat-Free	1 Tbsp.	12	0.0	125	0	0.0
Whipped Dressing, Fat-Free	1 Tbsp.	16	0.0	115	0	0.0

SALAD DRESSINGS

☞ **Cains**	S. S.	CAL	FAT(g)	SOD(mg)	CHL(mg)	%FAT
Light Hearted Dressing, Bell Pepper Italian	1 Tbsp.	16	0.0	260	0	0.0
Light Hearted Dressing, Orange Dijon	1 Tbsp.	18	0.0	90	0	0.0
Light Hearted Dressing, Raspberry Vinaigrette	1 Tbsp.	20	0.0	135	0	0.0
Light Hearted Dressing, Red Tomato French	1 Tbsp.	18	0.0	120	0	0.0

☞ **Estee**	S. S.	CAL	FAT(g)	SOD(mg)	CHL(mg)	%FAT
Reduced Calorie Dressing, Blue Cheese	1 Tbsp.	8	<1.0	50	0	-
Reduced Calorie Dressing, Creamy Italian	1 Tbsp.	4	0.0	15	0	0.0
Reduced Calorie Dressing, French	1 Tbsp.	4	0.0	10	0	0.0
Reduced Calorie Dressing, Italian	1 Tbsp.	4	0.0	10	0	0.0

☞ **Healthy Sensation**	S. S.	CAL	FAT(g)	SOD(mg)	CHL(mg)	%FAT
Ranch	0.5 oz.	15	0.4	138	0	24.0
Blue Cheese	0.5 oz.	19	0.5	144	1	23.7
Thousand Island	0.5 oz.	20	0.4	134	0	18.0
French	0.5 oz.	21	0.5	121	0	21.4
Honey Dijon	0.5 oz.	26	0.5	142	0	17.3

☞ Hidden Valley Ranch	S. S.	CAL	FAT(g)	SOD(mg)	CHL(mg)	%FAT
Low Fat Blue Cheese	1 Tbsp.	12	0.0	140	0	0.0
Low Fat French	1 Tbsp.	20	0.0	115	0	0.0
Low Fat Italian	1 Tbsp.	16	0.0	140	0	0.0
Low Fat Italian Parmesan	1 Tbsp.	16	0.0	140	0	0.0
Low Fat Thousand Island	1 Tbsp.	20	0.0	140	0	0.0

☞ Kraft	S. S.	CAL	FAT(g)	SOD(mg)	CHL(mg)	%FAT
Blue Cheese Fat Free	1 Tbsp.	16	0.0	120	0	0.0
Catalina Fat Free	1 Tbsp.	16	0.0	120	0	0.0
French Fat Free	1 Tbsp.	20	0.0	120	0	0.0
Italian Fat Free	1 Tbsp.	6	0.0	210	0	0.0
Oil Free Italian	1 Tbsp.	4	0.0	220	0	0.0
Ranch Fat Free	1 Tbsp.	16	0.0	150	0	0.0
Thousand Island Fat Free	1 Tbsp.	20	0.0	135	0	0.0

☞ Luzianne Blue Plate	S. S.	CAL	FAT(g)	SOD(mg)	CHL(mg)	%FAT
Herb Magic, Creamy Cucumber	1 Tbsp.	8	0.0	100	0	0.0
Herb Magic, Herb Basket	1 Tbsp.	6	0.0	170	0	0.0
Herb Magic, Italian	1 Tbsp.	4	0.0	125	0	0.0
Herb Magic, Ranch	1 Tbsp.	6	0.0	110	0	0.0
Herb Magic, Sweet & Sour	1 Tbsp.	18	0.0	80	0	0.0
Herb Magic, Thousand Island	1 Tbsp.	8	0.0	45	0	0.0
Herb Magic, Vinaigrette	1 Tbsp.	6	0.0	170	0	0.0
Herb Magic, Zesty Tomato	1 Tbsp.	14	0.0	70	0	0.0

☞ Magic Mountain	S. S.	CAL	FAT(g)	SOD(mg)	CHL(mg)	%FAT
Non-fat Dressing, Bleu Cheese	1 Tbsp.	14	0.0	125	1	0.0
Non-fat Dressing, French	1 Tbsp.	14	0.0	120	0	0.0
Non-fat Dressing, Greek	1 Tbsp.	6	0.0	165	0	0.0

☞ **Magic Mountain**	S. S.	CAL	FAT(g)	SOD(mg)	CHL(mg)	%FAT
Non-fat Dressing, Herb & Spice	1 Tbsp.	7	0.0	90	0	0.0
Non-fat Dressing, Italian	1 Tbsp.	6	0.0	160	0	0.0
Non-fat Dressing, Spanish	1 Tbsp.	8	0.0	75	0	0.0

☞ **Medford Farms Lite Dressing**	S. S.	CAL	FAT(g)	SOD(mg)	CHL(mg)	%FAT
Blue Cheese	1 Tbsp.	8	<1.0	130	-	-
Italian	1 Tbsp.	4	<1.0	130	-	-
Thousand Island	1 Tbsp.	9	0.0	130	-	0.0
Vinaigrette	1 Tbsp.	5	<1.0	130	-	-

☞ **Pritikin**	S. S.	CAL	FAT(g)	SOD(mg)	CHL(mg)	%FAT
French	1 Tbsp.	10	0.0	0	0	0.0
Italian	1 Tbsp.	8	0.0	0	0	0.0
Ranch	1 Tbsp.	16	0.0	0	0	0.0
Vinaigrette	1 Tbsp.	8	0.0	0	0	0.0
Sweet Spicy	1 Tbsp.	18	0.0	0	0	0.0
Garlic & Herb	1 Tbsp.	6	0.0	0	0	0.0

☞ **Richard Simmons Salad Spray**	S. S.	CAL	FAT(g)	SOD(mg)	CHL(mg)	%FAT
Dijon Vinaigrette	1 Tbsp.	14	<1.0	160	0	-
French	1 Tbsp.	14	<1.0	130	0	-
Ranch	1 Tbsp.	17	<1.0	190	1	-
Roma Cheese	1 Tbsp.	14	<1.0	190	1	-

☞ **Walden Farms**	S. S.	CAL	FAT(g)	SOD(mg)	CHL(mg)	%FAT
Reduced Calorie Dressing, Italian	1 Tbsp.	9	0.0	300	0	0.0

☞ Weight Watchers	S. S.	CAL	FAT(g)	SOD(mg)	CHL(mg)	%FAT
Caesar Salad	1 Tbsp.	4	0.0	200	-	0.0
Caesar Salad, Individual Packets	1 pouch	6	0.0	280	-	0.0
Creamy Cucumber	1 Tbsp.	18	0.0	85	-	0.0
Creamy Italian	1 Tbsp.	12	0.0	85	-	0.0
Creamy Peppercorn	1 Tbsp.	8	0.0	85	-	0.0
Creamy Ranch, Individual Packets	1 pouch	35	<1.0	130	-	<25.7

☞ Wish Bone	S. S.	CAL	FAT(g)	SOD(mg)	CHL(mg)	%FAT
Italian, Lite	1 Tbsp.	6	0.0	210	0	0.0
Red French, Lite	1 Tbsp.	17	0.0	155	0	0.0
Sweet 'N Spicy, Lite	1 Tbsp.	17	0.0	134	0	0.0
Russian, Lite	1 Tbsp.	21	0.0	142	0	0.0
French, Fat-Free	1 Tbsp.	6	0.0	279	0	0.0

SAUCES & CONDIMENTS

BARBECUE SAUCES

☞ **Chris's & Pitt's**	S. S.	CAL	FAT(g)	SOD(mg)	CHL(mg)	%FAT
Barbecue Sauce	1 Tbsp.	15	0.1	141	-	6.0

☞ **French's**	S. S.	CAL	FAT(g)	SOD(mg)	CHL(mg)	%FAT
Cattleman's BBQ Sauce, Milk	1 Tbsp.	25	0.0	260	-	0.0
Cattleman's BBQ Sauce, Smoky	1 Tbsp.	25	0.0	300	-	0.0

☞ **Hunt**	S. S.	CAL	FAT(g)	SOD(mg)	CHL(mg)	%FAT
Barbecue Sauce, Country Style	0.5 oz.	20	<1.0	140	0	-
Barbecue Sauce, Hickory	0.5 oz.	20	<1.0	160	0	-
Barbecue Sauce, Homestyle	0.5 oz.	20	<1.0	170	0	-
Barbecue Sauce, Kansas	0.5 oz.	20	<1.0	85	0	-
Barbecue Sauce, New Orleans	0.5 oz.	20	<1.0	150	0	-
Barbecue Sauce, Original	0.5 oz.	20	<1.0	160	0	-
Barbecue Sauce, Southern Style	0.5 oz.	20	<1.0	170	0	-
Barbecue Sauce, Texas	0.5 oz.	25	<1.0	150	0	-
Barbecue Sauce, Western	0.5 oz.	20	<1.0	170	0	-

☞ **Kraft**	S. S.	CAL	FAT(g)	SOD(mg)	CHL(mg)	%FAT
Barbecue Sauce	2 Tbsp.	40	1.0	490	0	22.5
Barbecue Sauce, Garlic	2 Tbsp.	40	0.0	530	0	0.0
Barbecue Sauce, Hickory Smoke	2 Tbsp.	40	1.0	490	0	22.5
Barbecue Sauce, Hickory Smoke Onion Bits	2 Tbsp.	50	1.0	420	0	18.0
Barbecue Sauce, Hot	2 Tbsp.	40	1.0	510	0	22.5
Barbecue Sauce, Hot Hickory Smoke	2 Tbsp.	40	1.0	500	0	22.5

SAUCES & CONDIMENTS

☞ Kraft

	S. S.	CAL	FAT(g)	SOD(mg)	CHL(mg)	%FAT
Barbecue Sauce, Italian Seasonings	2 Tbsp.	50	1.0	280	0	18.0
Barbecue Sauce, Kansas City Style	2 Tbsp.	50	1.0	290	0	18.0
Barbecue Sauce, Mesquite Smoke	2 Tbsp.	40	1.0	420	0	22.5
Barbecue Sauce, Onion Bits	2 Tbsp.	50	1.0	420	0	18.0
Barbecue Sauce, Thick 'n Spicy Chunky	2 Tbsp.	60	1.0	450	0	15.0
Barbecue Sauce, Thick 'n Spicy Hickory Smoke	2 Tbsp.	50	1.0	510	0	18.0
Barbecue Sauce, Thick 'n Spicy Kansas City Style	2 Tbsp.	60	1.0	300	0	15.0
Barbecue Sauce, Thick 'n Spicy Original	2 Tbsp.	50	1.0	490	0	18.0
Barbecue Sauce, Thick 'n Spicy with Honey	2 Tbsp.	60	1.0	350	0	15.0

☞ Lawry's

	S. S.	CAL	FAT(g)	SOD(mg)	CHL(mg)	%FAT
Dijon & Honey BBQ Sauce	1/4 cup	203	1.2	1768	-	5.3

CATSUP

☞ Hain

	S. S.	CAL	FAT(g)	SOD(mg)	CHL(mg)	%FAT
Natural Catsup	1 Tbsp.	16	0.0	155	0	0.0
Natural Catsup, No Salt Added	1 Tbsp.	16	0.0	15	0	0.0

☞ Heinz

	S. S.	CAL	FAT(g)	SOD(mg)	CHL(mg)	%FAT
Ketchup, Hot	1 Tbsp.	16	0.0	195	-	0.0
Ketchup, Lite	1 Tbsp.	8	0.0	115	-	0.0
Ketchup, Regular	1 Tbsp.	16	0.0	213	-	0.0

☞ Hunt

	S. S.	CAL	FAT(g)	SOD(mg)	CHL(mg)	%FAT
Ketchup, No Added Salt	0.5 oz.	20	<1.0	0	0	-

☞ **Hunt**	S. S.	CAL	FAT(g)	SOD(mg)	CHL(mg)	%FAT
Ketchup, Tomato	0.5 oz.	15	<1.0	160	0	-

HORSERADISH

☞ **Kraft**	S. S.	CAL	FAT(g)	SOD(mg)	CHL(mg)	%FAT
Horseradish, Creamy Style, Prepared	1 Tbsp.	10	0.0	85	0	0.0
Horseradish, Prepared	1 Tbsp.	10	0.0	140	0	0.0

MUSTARDS

☞ **French's**	S. S.	CAL	FAT(g)	SOD(mg)	CHL(mg)	%FAT
Mustard, Bold 'n Spicy	1 tsp.	6	0.0	50	-	0.0
Mustard, with Onion	1 tsp.	8	0.0	70	-	0.0

☞ **Grey Poupon**	S. S.	CAL	FAT(g)	SOD(mg)	CHL(mg)	%FAT
Mustard, Country Dijon	1 tsp.	6	0.0	120	0	0.0
Mustard, Dijon	1 tsp.	6	0.0	120	0	0.0
Mustard, Parisian	1 tsp.	6	0.0	55	0	0.0

☞ **Gulden's**	S. S.	CAL	FAT(g)	SOD(mg)	CHL(mg)	%FAT
Mustard, Creamy Mild	.25 oz.	6	0.0	60	-	0.0
Mustard, Diablo	.25 oz.	8	0.0	55	-	0.0
Mustard, Spicy Brown	.25 oz.	8	0.0	45	-	0.0

RELISH

☞ **Vlasic**	S. S.	CAL	FAT(g)	SOD(mg)	CHL(mg)	%FAT
Relish, Dill Relish	1 oz.	2	0.0	415	0	0.0
Relish, Hamburger	1 oz.	40	0.0	255	0	0.0

SAUCES & CONDIMENTS

☞ **Vlasic**	S. S.	CAL	FAT(g)	SOD(mg)	CHL(mg)	%FAT
Relish, Hot Dog	1 oz.	40	1.0	255	0	22.5
Relish, Hot Piccalilli	1 oz.	35	0.0	165	0	0.0
Relish, India	1 oz.	30	0.0	205	0	0.0
Relish, Sweet	1 oz.	30	0.0	220	0	0.0

ORIENTAL SAUCES

☞ **Kikkoman**	S. S.	CAL	FAT(g)	SOD(mg)	CHL(mg)	%FAT
Soy Sauce	1 Tbsp.	12	0.0	938	0	0.0
Soy Sauce, Lite	1 Tbsp.	13	0.0	564	0	0.0
Stir-Fry Sauce	1 Tbsp.	16	0.0	369	1	1.1
Sweet & Sour Sauce	1 Tbsp.	19	0.0	97	0	1.4
Teriyaki Baste & Glaze	1 Tbsp.	24	0.0	310	0	1.1
Teriyaki Sauce	1 Tbsp.	15	0.0	626	0	0.0
Teriyaki Sauce, Lite	1 Tbsp.	14	0.1	298	trace	3.2

☞ **Kraft**	S. S.	CAL	FAT(g)	SOD(mg)	CHL(mg)	%FAT
Sauceworks Sweet and Sour Sauce	1 Tbsp.	25	0.0	50	0	0.0

☞ **La Choy**	S. S.	CAL	FAT(g)	SOD(mg)	CHL(mg)	%FAT
Brown Gravy	1.2 tsp.	15	<1.0	15	0	-
Hot & Spicy Szechwan Sauce	1 Tbsp.	25	<1.0	70	0	-
Mandarin Orange Sauce	1 Tbsp.	25	<1.0	40	0	-
Soy Sauce	1/2 tsp.	2	<1.0	230	0	-
Soy Sauce, Lite	1/2 tsp.	1	<1.0	110	0	-
Sweet & Sour Duck Sauce	1 Tbsp.	25	<1.0	40	0	-
Sweet & Sour Sauce	1 Tbsp.	25	<1.0	190	0	-
Tangy Plum Sauce	1 Tbsp.	25	<1.0	10	0	-
Teriyaki Sauce	1/2 tsp.	5	<1.0	290	0	-
Teriyaki Sauce, Basting	1/2 tsp.	2	<1.0	110	0	-
Teriyaki Sauce, Lite	1/2 tsp.	5	<1.0	85	0	-

☞ La Choy	S. S.	CAL	FAT(g)	SOD(mg)	CHL(mg)	%FAT
Thick & Rich Teriyaki Sauce	1 Tbsp.	25	<1.0	300	0	-

☞ Lawry's	S. S.	CAL	FAT(g)	SOD(mg)	CHL(mg)	%FAT
Stir Fry	1/4 cup	120	3.8	1128	-	28.5
Sweet 'n Sour Liquid Sauce	1/4 cup	549	7.5	4056	-	12.3
Teriyaki Barbecue Marinade	1/4 cup	164	2.3	12330	-	12.6
Teriyaki with Pineapple Juice	1/4 cup	72	0.4	7100	-	5.0

PASTA SAUCES

☞ Enrico's	S. S.	CAL	FAT(g)	SOD(mg)	CHL(mg)	%FAT
Spaghetti Sauce, All Natural	4 oz.	60	1.0	345	0	15.0
Spaghetti Sauce, All Natural, No Salt	4 oz.	60	1.0	30	0	15.0
Spaghetti Sauce, Mushroom	4 oz.	60	1.0	-	0	15.0
Spaghetti Sauce, Mushroom and Green Pepper	4 oz.	60	1.0	345	0	15.0

☞ Healthy Choice	S. S.	CAL	FAT(g)	SOD(mg)	CHL(mg)	%FAT
Spaghetti Sauce with Garlic and Herb	4 oz.	40	<1.0	390	0	<22.5
Spaghetti Sauce with Green Peppers	4 oz.	40	<1.0	390	0	<22.5
Spaghetti Sauce with Meat	4 oz.	50	<1.0	380	0	<18.0
Spaghetti Sauce with Mushrooms	4 oz.	40	<1.0	390	0	<22.5
Spaghetti Sauce, Traditional	4 oz.	40	<1.0	380	0	<22.5

☞ Hunt	S. S.	CAL	FAT(g)	SOD(mg)	CHL(mg)	%FAT
Spaghetti Sauce, Chunky	4 oz.	50	<1.0	470	0	<18.0
Spaghetti Sauce, Classic Italian, with Parmesan	4 oz.	60	2.0	550	0	30.0
Spaghetti Sauce, Homestyle	4 oz.	60	2.0	530	0	30.0

SAUCES & CONDIMENTS

SAUCES & CONDIMENTS

☞ Hunt	S. S.	CAL	FAT(g)	SOD(mg)	CHL(mg)	%FAT
Spaghetti Sauce, Homestyle with Meat	1 cup	170	5.0	1150	-	26.5
Spaghetti Sauce, Homestyle with Mushrooms	4 oz.	50	1.0	530	0	18.0
Spaghetti Sauce, Traditional	4 oz.	70	2.0	530	0	25.7
Spaghetti Sauce, with Meat	4 oz.	70	2.0	570	2	25.7
Spaghetti Sauce, with Mushrooms	4 oz.	70	2.0	560	0	25.7

☞ Prego	S. S.	CAL	FAT(g)	SOD(mg)	CHL(mg)	%FAT
Spaghetti Sauce, Extra Chunky Garden Combination	4 oz.	80	2.0	420	-	22.5
Spaghetti Sauce, Extra Chunky Mushroom with Extra Spice	4 oz.	100	3.0	450	-	27.0
Spaghetti Sauce, Three Cheese	4 oz.	100	2.0	410	-	18.0
Spaghetti Sauce, Tomato & Basil	4 oz.	100	2.0	370	-	18.0

☞ Ragu	S. S.	CAL	FAT(g)	SOD(mg)	CHL(mg)	%FAT
Fino Italian Pasta Sauce, Parmesan	4 oz.	90	3.0	540	0	30.0
Fino Italian Pasta Sauce, Tomato & Herbs	4 oz.	90	3.0	490	0	30.0
Spaghetti Sauce, Original Style with Mushrooms	4 oz.	80	2.0	740	2	22.5
Spaghetti Sauce, Thick & Hearty	4 oz.	100	3.0	460	0	27.0
Spaghetti Sauce, Thick & Hearty with Mushrooms	4 oz.	100	3.0	460	0	27.0
Today's Recipe Pasta Sauce, Chunky Mushroom	4 oz.	50	1.0	370	0	18.0
Today's Recipe Pasta Sauce, Garden Harvest	4 oz.	50	1.0	370	0	18.0
Today's Recipe Pasta Sauce, Tomato Herb	4 oz.	50	1.0	370	0	18.0

☞ Sensational	S. S.	CAL	FAT(g)	SOD(mg)	CHL(mg)	%FAT
Pasta Sauce, Mushroom	4 oz.	60	1.0	713	-	15.0

☞ Sensational	S. S.	CAL	FAT(g)	SOD(mg)	CHL(mg)	%FAT
Pasta Sauce, Northern Italian Style	4 oz.	60	1.0	722	-	15.0

PICANTE SAUCES

☞ Chi Chi's	S. S.	CAL	FAT(g)	SOD(mg)	CHL(mg)	%FAT
Salsa, Hot	1 oz.	8	0.04	138	0	4.5
Salsa, Medium	1 oz.	8	0.0	130	2.5	0.0
Salsa, Mild	1 oz.	9	0.04	96	0	4.0
Taco Sauce, Hot	1 oz.	17	0.12	247	0	6.4
Taco Sauce, Mild	1 oz.	18	0.07	165	0	3.5
Picante Sauce, Hot	1 oz.	11	0.06	236	0	4.9
Picante Sauce, Mild	1 oz.	11	0.02	191	0	1.6

☞ Hain	S. S.	CAL	FAT(g)	SOD(mg)	CHL(mg)	%FAT
Salsa, Hot	1/4 cup	22	0.0	480	0	0.0
Salsa, Mild	1/4 cup	20	0.0	410	-	0.0

☞ La Victoria	S. S.	CAL	FAT(g)	SOD(mg)	CHL(mg)	%FAT
Chili Dip	1 Tbsp.	6	<1.0	90	-	-
Nacho Jalapenos	1 Tbsp.	2	<1.0	335	-	-
Salsa Brava	1 Tbsp.	6	<1.0	100	-	-
Salsa Casera	1 Tbsp.	4	<1.0	80	-	-
Salsa Jalapena, Green	1 Tbsp.	4	<1.0	105	-	-
Salsa Jalapena, Red	1 Tbsp.	6	<1.0	95	-	-
Salsa Picante	1 Tbsp.	4	<1.0	80	-	-
Salsa Ranchera	1 Tbsp.	6	<1.0	85	-	-
Salsa Suprema	1 Tbsp.	4	<1.0	95	-	-
Salsa Victoria	1 Tbsp.	4	<1.0	80	-	-
Salsa, Green Chili	1 Tbsp.	3	<1.0	44	-	-
Salsa, Omlette	1 Tbsp.	6	<1.0	95	-	-
Taco Sauce, Green	1 Tbsp.	4	<1.0	85	-	-

SAUCES & CONDIMENTS

☞ La Victoria	S. S.	CAL	FAT(g)	SOD(mg)	CHL(mg)	%FAT
Taco Sauce, Red	1 Tbsp.	6	<1.0	85	-	-
Tomatillo Entero	1 Tbsp.	4	<1.0	102	-	-

☞ Pace	S. S.	CAL	FAT(g)	SOD(mg)	CHL(mg)	%FAT
Picante Sauce	3 tsp.	3	0.1	111	0	23.8

☞ Rosarita	S. S.	CAL	FAT(g)	SOD(mg)	CHL(mg)	%FAT
Picante Sauce, Hot Chunky	3 Tbsp.	18	<1.0	515	0	-
Picante Sauce, Medium Chunky	3 Tbsp.	16	<1.0	650	0	-
Picante Sauce, Mild Chunky	3 Tbsp.	25	<1.0	630	0	-

MISCELLANEOUS SAUCES

☞ French's	S. S.	CAL	FAT(g)	SOD(mg)	CHL(mg)	%FAT
Worcestershire Sauce, Regular and Smoky	1 Tbsp.	10	0.0	160	-	0.0

☞ Heinz	S. S.	CAL	FAT(g)	SOD(mg)	CHL(mg)	%FAT
Chili Sauce	1 Tbsp.	16	0.0	225	-	0.0
Seafood Cocktail Sauce	1 Tbsp.	17	0.1	180	-	5.3
Worcestershire Sauce	1 Tbsp.	5	0.0	165	-	0.0

☞ Holland House	S. S.	CAL	FAT(g)	SOD(mg)	CHL(mg)	%FAT
Wine Marinade, Garden Herb	1 oz.	36	<1.0	536	<1	-
Wine Marinade, Hot & Spicy	1 oz.	19	<1.0	384	<1	-
Wine Marinade, Lemon & Herb	1 oz.	16	<1.0	382	<1	-
Wine Marinade, Red Wine & Herb	1 oz.	27	<1.0	352	<1	-

☞ Holland House	S. S.	CAL	FAT(g)	SOD(mg)	CHL(mg)	%FAT
Wine Marinade, Teriyaki	1 oz.	29	<1.0	397	<1	-

☞ Knorr's	S. S.	CAL	FAT(g)	SOD(mg)	CHL(mg)	%FAT
Cooking Sauce, Chasseur	1/4 jar	130	3.2	810	-	22.2
Cooking Sauce, Five Spice	1/4 jar	70	1.8	880	-	23.1
Cooking Sauce, Tomato Provencale	1/4 jar	60	1.9	530	-	28.5
Grilling and Broiling Sauce, Spicy Plum	1/4 jar	80	1.1	770	-	12.4

☞ Kraft	S. S.	CAL	FAT(g)	SOD(mg)	CHL(mg)	%FAT
Sauceworks Cocktail Sauce	1 Tbsp.	12	0.0	170	0	0.0

☞ Lawry's	S. S.	CAL	FAT(g)	SOD(mg)	CHL(mg)	%FAT
Citrus Grill	1 Tbsp.	17	0.4	1675	-	21.2
Herb & Garlic with Lemon Juice	1/4 cup	36	0.4	3688	-	10.0
Mesquite with Lime Juice	1/4 cup	24	0.4	4142	-	15.0

☞ Lea & Perrins	S. S.	CAL	FAT(g)	SOD(mg)	CHL(mg)	%FAT
White Wine Worcestershire Sauce	1 tsp.	3	<1.0	42	-	-
Worcestershire Sauce	1 tsp.	5	<1.0	55	-	-

☞ Nabisco	S. S.	CAL	FAT(g)	SOD(mg)	CHL(mg)	%FAT
Escoffier Sauce	1 Tbsp.	20	0.0	160	-	0.0

SAUCES & CONDIMENTS

☞ **Ragu**	S. S.	CAL	FAT(g)	SOD(mg)	CHL(mg)	%FAT
Chicken Tonight, Chicken Cacciatore	4 oz.	70	2.0	490	0	25.7
Chicken Tonight, Oriental Chicken	4 oz.	70	10	580	0	12.9
Chicken Tonight, Salsa Chicken	4 oz.	35	0.0	680	0	0.0

STEAK SAUCES

☞ **A-1**	S. S.	CAL	FAT(g)	SOD(mg)	CHL(mg)	%FAT
Steak Sauce	1 Tbsp.	12	0.0	280	0	0.0

☞ **French's**	S. S.	CAL	FAT(g)	SOD(mg)	CHL(mg)	%FAT
Steak Sauce	1 Tbsp.	25	0.0	150	-	0.0

☞ **Heinz**	S. S.	CAL	FAT(g)	SOD(mg)	CHL(mg)	%FAT
57 Sauce	1 Tbsp.	17	0.2	199	-	10.6
Traditional Steak Sauce	1 Tbsp.	12	0.0	200	-	0.0

☞ **Kikkoman**	S. S.	CAL	FAT(g)	SOD(mg)	CHL(mg)	%FAT
Steak Sauce	1 Tbsp.	20	0.0	234	0	1.4

☞ **Lea & Perrins**	S. S.	CAL	FAT(g)	SOD(mg)	CHL(mg)	%FAT
Steak Sauce	1 oz.	40	<1.0	220	-	<22.5

SEAFOOD

☞ALL TYPES	S. S.	CAL	FAT(g)	SOD(mg)	CHL(mg)	%FAT
Abalone	3 oz.	89	0.6	255	72	6.1
Barracuda	3.5 oz.	113	2.6	-	-	20.7
Bass, Black	3.5 oz.	93	1.2	68	-	11.6
Bass, Freshwater	3 oz.	97	3.1	59	58	28.8
Bass, Striped	3 oz.	82	2.0	59	68	22.0
Bullhead, Black	3.5 oz.	84	1.6	-	-	17.1
Burbot	3 oz.	76	0.7	82	51	8.3
Cisco	3 oz.	84	1.6	47	-	17.1
Clams	3 oz.	63	0.8	47	29	11.4
Cod, Atlantic	3 oz.	70	0.6	46	37	7.7
Cod, Pacific	3 oz.	70	0.5	60	31	6.4
Crab, Alaskan King	3 oz.	71	0.5	711	35	6.3
Crab, Blue	3 oz.	74	0.9	249	66	10.9
Crab, Dungeness	3 oz.	73	0.8	251	50	9.9
Crab, Queen	3 oz.	76	1.0	458	47	11.8
Crayfish	3 oz.	76	0.9	45	118	10.7
Croaker, Atlantic	3 oz.	89	2.7	47	52	27.3
Cusk	3 oz.	74	0.6	27	35	7.3
Cuttlefish	3 oz.	67	0.6	316	95	8.1
Dolphinfish	3 oa.	73	0.6	74	62	7.4
Flatfish	3 oz.	78	1.0	69	41	11.5
Flounder	3 oz.	68	0.5	56	-	6.6
Groper	3 oz.	78	0.9	45	31	10.4
Haddock	3 oz.	74	0.6	58	49	7.3
Halibut	3 oz.	93	2.0	46	27	19.4
Kingfish	3.5 oz.	105	3.0	83	-	25.7
Ling	3 oz.	74	0.5	115	-	6.1
Lingcod	3 oz.	72	0.9	50	44	11.3
Lobster, Northern	3 oz.	77	0.8	-	81	9.4
Lobster, Spiny	3 oz.	95	1.3	150	60	12.3
Mackerel, King	3 oz.	89	1.7	134	45	17.2
Monkfish	3 oz.	64	1.3	16	21	18.3

SEAFOOD

☞ ALL TYPES	S. S.	CAL	FAT(g)	SOD(mg)	CHL(mg)	%FAT
Mullet	3 oz.	99	3.2	55	42	29.1
Mussels	3 oz.	76	1.9	243	24	22.5
Oysters, Pacific	3 oz.	69	2.0	90	-	26.1
Perch	3 oz.	77	0.8	52	76	9.4
Perch, Ocean	3 oz.	80	1.4	64	36	15.8
Pike, Northern	3 oz.	75	0.6	33	33	7.2
Pike, Pickerel	3.5 oz.	84	0.5	-	-	5.4
Pike, Walleye	3 oz.	79	1.0	43	73	11.4
Pollock, Atlantic	3 oz.	78	0.8	73	60	9.2
Pollock, Walleye	3 oz.	68	0.7	84	61	9.3
Porgy	3.5 oz.	112	3.4	63	-	27.3
Pout	3 oz.	67	0.8	52	44	10.7
Rockfish	3 oz.	80	1.3	51	29	14.6
Salmon, Chum	3 oz.	102	3.2	42	63	28.2
Salmon, Pink	3 oz.	99	2.9	57	44	26.4
Scallops	3 oz.	75	0.6	137	28	7.2
Scup	3 oz.	89	2.3	36	-	23.3
Sea Bass	3 oz.	82	1.7	58	35	18.7
Sheepshead	3 oz.	92	2.1	61	-	20.5
Shrimp	3 oz.	90	1.5	126	130	15.0
Skate	3.5 oz.	98	0.7	-	-	6.4
Smelt, Atlantic	4-5 med.	98	0.0	-	-	0.0
Smelt, Rainbow	3 oz.	83	2.1	51	60	22.8
Snapper	3 oz.	85	1.1	54	31	11.6
Sole	3.5 oz.	68	0.5	56	-	6.6
Sucker, White	3 oz.	79	2.0	34	35	22.8
Sunfish, Pumpkinseed	3 oz.	76	0.6	68	57	7.1
Surimi	3 oz.	84	0.8	122	25	8.6
Swordfish	3 oz.	103	3.4	76	33	29.7
Tautog (Blackfish)	3.5 oz.	89	1.1	-	-	11.1
Tilfish	3 oz.	81	2.0	45	-	22.2
Tomcod	3.5 oz.	77	0.4	-	-	4.7
Trout, Rainbow	3 oz.	100	2.9	23	48	26.1
Tuna, Skipjack	3 oz.	88	0.9	31	40	9.2
Tuna, Yellowfin	3 oz.	92	0.8	31	38	7.8
Turbot, European	3 oz.	81	2.5	127	-	27.8

☞ ALL TYPES	S. S.	CAL	FAT(g)	SOD(mg)	CHL(mg)	%FAT
Whelk	3 oz.	117	0.3	175	55	2.3
Whiting	3 oz.	77	1.1	61	57	12.9
Wolffish	3 oz.	82	2.0	72	39	22.0

SNACKS

BREADSTICKS

☞ **Angonoa's**	S. S.	CAL	FAT(g)	SOD(mg)	CHL(mg)	%FAT
Breadsticks, Cheese	1 oz.	110	2.0	210	-	16.4
Breadsticks, Garlic	1 oz.	120	2.0	160	-	15.0
Breadsticks, Italian	1 oz.	120	2.0	240	-	15.0
Breadsticks, Low Sodium	1 oz.	120	4.0	15	-	30.0
Breadsticks, Onion	1 oz.	120	3.0	150	-	22.5
Breadsticks, Sesame Royale	1 oz.	120	4.0	200	-	30.0
Mini Breadsticks, Cheese	1 oz.	110	2.0	160	-	16.4
Mini Breadsticks, Pizza	1 oz.	120	2.0	220	-	15.0
Mini Breadsticks, Sesame	1 oz.	120	4.0	200	-	30.0
Mini Breadsticks, Whole Wheat	1 oz.	120	4.0	170	-	30.0

☞ **Barbara's Bakery**	S. S.	CAL	FAT(g)	SOD(mg)	CHL(mg)	%FAT
Bread Sticks, Italian Style	1 oz.	120	3.0	-	0	22.5
Bread Sticks, Regular	1 oz.	120	3.0	-	0	22.5
Sesame Sticks	1 oz.	130	4.0	-	-	27.7

☞ **Fattorie & Pandea**	S. S.	CAL	FAT(g)	SOD(mg)	CHL(mg)	%FAT
Breadsticks, Sesame Seeds	3	65	2.0	100	-	27.7
Breadsticks, Traditional	3	60	1.0	100	-	15.0
Breadsticks, Whole Wheat	3	57	1.0	100	-	15.8

☞ **International**	S. S.	CAL	FAT(g)	SOD(mg)	CHL(mg)	%FAT
Bialys Bread Sticks, All Varieties	1 stick	110	<1.0	210	0	<8.2

SNACKS

☞ Oroweat	S. S.	CAL	FAT(g)	SOD(mg)	CHL(mg)	%FAT
Breadsticks, Plain	1 oz.	110	1.0	240	-	8.2
Breadsticks, Sesame	1 oz.	120	3.0	180	-	22.5

☞ Stella D'Oro	S. S.	CAL	FAT(g)	SOD(mg)	CHL(mg)	%FAT
Breadsticks, Onion	1	40	1.0	-	0	22.5
Breadsticks, Pizza	1	45	1.0	-	0	20.0
Breadsticks, Regular	1	40	1.0	55	0	22.5
Breadsticks, Sesame	1	50	2.0	43	0	36.0
Breadsticks, Wheat	1	40	1.0	-	0	22.5

CHIPS

☞ Barbara's Bakery	S. S.	CAL	FAT(g)	SOD(mg)	CHL(mg)	%FAT
Tortilla Chips, Organic Yellow Corn	1 oz.	140	0.7	120	0	4.5
Tortilla Chips, Organic Yellow Corn, No Salt Added	1 oz.	140	0.7	15	0	4.5

☞ Doritos	S. S.	CAL	FAT(g)	SOD(mg)	CHL(mg)	%FAT
Tortilla Chips, Light Cool Ranch	16 chips	130	4.0	220	0	27.7
Tortilla Chips, Light Nacho Cheese	16 chips	120	4.0	230	0	30.0

☞ Elgalindo	S. S.	CAL	FAT(g)	SOD(mg)	CHL(mg)	%FAT
Tortilla Chips, Blue Corn, Baked	1 oz.	100	<1.0	60	0	<9.0

☞ Guiltless Gourmet	S. S.	CAL	FAT(g)	SOD(mg)	CHL(mg)	%FAT
Tortilla Chips, Baked	1 oz.	110	1.4	119	0	11.5

FRUIT SNACKS

☞ **Betty Crocker**	S. S.	CAL	FAT(g)	SOD(mg)	CHL(mg)	%FAT
Fruit Corners Fruit Roll–Ups, All Flavors	1 roll	50	<1.0	40	-	<18.0
Fruit Wrinkles, All Flavors	1 pouch	100	1.0	55	-	9.0
Garfield and Friends, 1-2 Punch	1 pouch	100	2.0	70	-	18.0
Garfield and Friends, Fruit Party	1 roll	50	<1.0	40	-	<18.0
Garfield and Friends, Very Strawberry	1 pouch	90	1.0	60	-	10.0
Garfield and Friends, Wild Blue	1 roll	50	<1.0	20	-	<18.0
Shark Bites & Berry Bears, All Flavors	1 pouch	100	<1.0	20	-	<9.0
Squeezit, Apple	6.75 oz.	110	<1.0	5	-	<8.2
Squeezit, Cherry	6.75 oz.	110	<1.0	30	-	<8.2
Squeezit, Grape	6.75 oz.	110	<1.0	30	-	<8.2
Squeezit, Orange	6.75 oz.	110	<1.0	5	-	<8.2
Squeezit, Red Punch	6.75 oz.	110	<1.0	5	-	<8.2
Squeezit, Wild Berry	6.75 oz.	110	<1.0	5	-	<8.2
Thunder Jets, All Flavors	1 pouch	100	1.0	30	-	9.0

☞ **Sunkist**	S. S.	CAL	FAT(g)	SOD(mg)	CHL(mg)	%FAT
F.S. Sunkist Strawberry Fruit Roll	1 roll	48	0.1	13	0	1.9
Fruit Roll, Apple	1 roll	75	0.0	17	0	0.0
Fruit Roll, Apricot	1 roll	76	0.5	11	0	5.9
Fruit Roll, Cherry	1 roll	75	0.1	18	0	1.2
Fruit Roll, Fruit Punch	1 roll	74	0.0	12	0	0.0
Fruit Roll, Grape	1 roll	76	0.1	13	0	1.2
Fruit Roll, Raspberry	1 roll	75	0.1	20	0	1.2
Fruit Roll, Strawberry	1 roll	74	0.1	17	0	1.2
Fun Fruit Alphabets	0.9 oz.	100	1.4	10	0	12.6
Fun Fruit Animals	0.9 oz.	100	1.4	10	0	12.6
Fun Fruit Dinosaurs	0.9 oz.	100	1.4	10	0	12.6
Fun Fruit Funny Feet	0.9 oz.	100	1.4	10	0	12.6
Fun Fruit Link Nintendo	0.9 oz.	100	1.4	10	0	12.6
Fun Fruit Mario Nintendo	0.9 oz.	100	1.4	10	0	12.6
Fun Fruit Numbers	0.9 oz.	100	1.4	10	0	12.6

SNACKS

☞ Sunkist	S. S.	CAL	FAT(g)	SOD(mg)	CHL(mg)	%FAT
Fun Fruit Rock and Roll Shapes	0.9 oz.	100	1.4	10	0	12.6
Fun Fruit Space Shapes	0.9 oz.	100	1.4	10	0	12.6
Fun Fruit Spooky Fruit	0.9 oz.	100	1.4	10	0	12.6
Fun Fruit Wacky Players	0.9 oz.	100	1.4	10	0	12.6
Fun Fruit Wild Safari	0.9 oz.	100	1.4	10	0	12.6
Fun Fruits	0.9 oz.	100	1.4	10	0	12.6

POPCORN

☞ Boston	S. S.	CAL	FAT(g)	SOD(mg)	CHL(mg)	%FAT
Lite Caramel Gourmet Popcorn	1 0z.	120	2.0	100	0	15.0

☞ Jiffy Pop	S. S.	CAL	FAT(g)	SOD(mg)	CHL(mg)	%FAT
Bag-But-Lite Popping Corn	3 cups	80	2.0	70	0	22.5

☞ Nature's Choice	S. S.	CAL	FAT(g)	SOD(mg)	CHL(mg)	%FAT
Carmel Corn with Peanuts	1.67 oz.	190	2.0	-	-	9.5
Carmel Corn, Original	1.67 oz.	180	1.0	-	-	5.0

☞ Orville Redenbacher's	S. S.	CAL	FAT(g)	SOD(mg)	CHL(mg)	%FAT
Popping Corn, Gourmet Hot Air	3 cups	40	<1.0	0	0	<22.5
Popping Corn, Light Butter Microwave	3 cups	60	2.0	180	0	30.0
Popping Corn, Lite Natural Microwave	3 cups	60	2.0	210	0	30.0

☞ TV Time	S. S.	CAL	FAT(g)	SOD(mg)	CHL(mg)	%FAT
Merry Poppin "Light" Microwave Popping Corn, Butter Flavor	4 cups	120	3.0	225	0	22.5
Merry Poppin "Light" Microwave Popping Corn, Natural Flavor	4 cups	120	3.0	225	0	22.5

☞ Ultra Slim Fast	S. S.	CAL	FAT(g)	SOD(mg)	CHL(mg)	%FAT
Lite 'N Tasty Popcorn	1/2 oz.	60	2.0	150	0	30.0

☞ Weaver's	S. S.	CAL	FAT(g)	SOD(mg)	CHL(mg)	%FAT
Light Gourmet Popcorn, Light Butter Flavor	3 cups	70	1.0	85	0	12.9

PRETZELS

☞ Barbara's Bakery	S. S.	CAL	FAT(g)	SOD(mg)	CHL(mg)	%FAT
Pretzels, Honey Sweet	1 oz.	127	3.0	-	0	21.3
Pretzels, Nine Grain	1 oz.	112	2.0	-	0	16.1
Pretzels, Oat Bran	1 oz.	120	2.0	-	0	15.0
Pretzels, Pumpernickel	1 oz.	111	2.0	-	0	16.2
Pretzels, Rice Bran	1 oz.	120	3.0	160	0	22.5
Pretzels, Rice Bran, No Salt Added	1 oz.	120	3.0	10	0	22.5
Pretzels, Whole Wheat	1 oz.	120	3.0	-	0	22.5

☞ Keebler	S. S.	CAL	FAT(g)	SOD(mg)	CHL(mg)	%FAT
Butter Pretzel Knots	1 oz.	110	1.0	530	0	8.2

☞ Mr. Salty	S. S.	CAL	FAT(g)	SOD(mg)	CHL(mg)	%FAT
Pretzel Sticks, Fat Free	1 oz.	100	0.0	380	0	0.0

☞ Mr. Salty	S. S.	CAL	FAT(g)	SOD(mg)	CHL(mg)	%FAT
Pretzel Sticks, Very Thin	1 oz.	110	1.0	600	0	8.2
Pretzel Twists	1 oz.	110	2.0	580	0	16.4
Pretzel Twists, Fat Free	1 oz.	100	0.0	380	0	0.0

☞ Rold Gold	S. S.	CAL	FAT(g)	SOD(mg)	CHL(mg)	%FAT
Pretzels, Bavarian	3	120	2.0	430	0	15.0
Pretzels, Pretzel Twist	10	110	1.0	510	0	8.2
Pretzels, Rods	3	110	2.0	410	0	16.4
Pretzels, Sticks	50	110	2.0	490	0	16.4
Pretzels, Tiny Twist	15	110	1.0	420	0	8.2
Pretzels, Unsalted	1 oz.	110	1.0	115	0	8.2

☞ Seyfert's	S. S.	CAL	FAT(g)	SOD(mg)	CHL(mg)	%FAT
Pretzels, Butter, Rods	1 oz.	110	1.0	530	40	8.2

RICE/GRAIN CAKES

☞ Crispy Cakes	S. S.	CAL	FAT(g)	SOD(mg)	CHL(mg)	%FAT
Brown Rice 'N Sesame Square Rice Cakes, Italian Spices	1	20	0.2	30	0	9.0
Brown Rice 'N Sesame Square Rice Cakes, Chili 'N Spices	1	20	0.2	60	0	6.8
Brown Rice 'N Sesame Square Rice Cakes, Raisins 'N Spice	1	20	0.2	1	0	9.0
Brown Rice 'N Sesame Square Rice Cakes, Apple Cinnamon	1	20	0.2	1	0	9.0

☞ Hain	S. S.	CAL	FAT(g)	SOD(mg)	CHL(mg)	%FAT
Mini Rice Cakes, Apple Cinnamon	0.5 oz.	50	<1.0	5	0	<18.0
Mini Rice Cakes, Cheese	0.5 oz.	60	2.0	80	0	30.0

☞ Hain	S. S.	CAL	FAT(g)	SOD(mg)	CHL(mg)	%FAT
Mini Rice Cakes, Honey Nut	0.5 oz.	60	1.0	15	0	15.0
Mini Rice Cakes, Nacho Cheese	0.5 oz.	70	2.0	90	0	25.7
Mini Rice Cakes, Plain	0.5 oz.	50	<1.0	75	-	<18.0
Mini Rice Cakes, Plain, No Added Salt	0.5 oz.	50	<1.0	5	-	<18.0
Mini Rice Cakes, Teriyaki	0.5 oz.	50	<1.0	80	-	<18.0
Rice Cakes, 5-Grain	1	40	<1.0	10	-	<22.5
Rice Cakes, Plain	1	40	<1.0	1	-	<22.5
Rice Cakes, Plain, No Added Salt	1	40	<1.0	<5	-	<22.5
Rice Cakes, Sesame	1	40	<1.0	10	-	<22.5
Rice Cakes, Sesame, No Salt	1	40	<1.0	<5	-	<22.5

☞ Mother's	S. S.	CAL	FAT(g)	SOD(mg)	CHL(mg)	%FAT
Popped Corn Cakes, Butter Flavored	1	35	0.0	55	0	0.0
Popped Corn Cakes, Mild White Cheddar	1	40	0.0	110	0	0.0
Popped Corn Cakes, Plain	1	35	0.0	30	0	0.0
Rice Cakes, Barley & Oats	1	35	0.0	35	0	0.0
Rice Cakes, Buckwheat	1	35	0.0	35	0	0.0
Rice Cakes, Corn	1	35	0.0	35	0	0.0
Rice Cakes, Multigrain	1	35	0.0	35	0	0.0
Rice Cakes, Plain	1	35	0.0	0	0	0.0
Rice Cakes, Sesame	1	35	0.0	35	0	0.0

☞ Quaker	S. S.	CAL	FAT(g)	SOD(mg)	CHL(mg)	%FAT
Fat Free, Apple Cinnamon	1	40	0.0	0	0	0.0
Fat Free, Butter Popped Corn	1	35	0.0	55	0	0.0
Fat Free, Caramel Corn	1	50	0.0	30	0	0.0
Fat Free, Nacho Corn	1	40	0.0	80	0	0.0
Fat Free, Popped Corn	1	35	0.0	55	0	0.0
Grain Cakes, Corn	1	35	0.2	53	-	5.1
Grain Cakes, Rye	1	35	0.3	52	0	7.7
Grain Cakes, Wheat	1	34	0.3	52	0	7.9

☞ **Quaker**	S. S.	CAL	FAT(g)	SOD(mg)	CHL(mg)	%FAT
Rice Cakes, Corn	1	35	0.3	31	0	7.7
Rice Cakes, Multi Grain	1	34	0.4	29	-	10.6
Rice Cakes, Plain	1	35	0.3	36	0	7.7
Rice Cakes, Plain, Salt Free	1	35	0.3	0	0	7.7
Rice Cakes, Sesame	1	35	0.3	36	0	7.7
Rice Cakes, Sesame Salt Free	1	35	0.3	1	0	7.7

MICELLANEOUS SNACKS

☞ **Cracker Jack**	S. S.	CAL	FAT(g)	SOD(mg)	CHL(mg)	%FAT
Caramel Coated Popcorn and Peanuts	1 oz.	120	3.0	85	-	22.5

☞ **Frito-Lay**	S. S.	CAL	FAT(g)	SOD(mg)	CHL(mg)	%FAT
Corn Nuts, Toasted	1.38 oz.	170	5.0	265	0	26.5
Dip, Jalapeño Bean	1 oz.	30	1.0	180	0	30.0
Dip, Picante	1 oz.	10	0.0	160	0	0.0

☞ **Guiltless Gourmet**	S. S.	CAL	FAT(g)	SOD(mg)	CHL(mg)	%FAT
Dip, Black Bean and Pinto Bean, Mild & Spicy	1 oz.	25	0.0	80	0	0.0
Dip, Cheddar Queso, Mild & Spicy	1 oz.	22	0.3	150	<1	12.3
Dip, Picante Sauce, All varieties	1 oz.	6	0.0	133	0	0.0

☞ **Jacobsen's**	S. S.	CAL	FAT(g)	SOD(mg)	CHL(mg)	%FAT
Snack Toast, Cinnamon	1 slice	60	1.0	65	0	15.0
Snack Toast, Cinnamon & Raisin	1 slice	60	1.0	65	0	15.0
Snack Toast, Original	1 slice	45	1.0	65	0	20.0

SNACKS

STUFFINGS & STUFFING MIXES

☞ Arnold	S. S.	CAL	FAT(g)	SOD(mg)	CHL(mg)	%FAT
Bread Crumbs, Italian	0.5 oz.	50	<1.0	200	0	<18.0
Bread Crumbs, Plain	0.5 oz.	50	<1.0	80	0	<18.0
Stuffing, All Purpose Seasoned	0.5 oz.	50	<1.0	200	0	<18.0
Stuffing, Bread Cube	0.5 oz.	50	1.0	110	0	18.0
Stuffing, Corn	0.5 oz.	50	1.0	140	0	18.0
Stuffing, Herb Seasoned	0.5 oz.	50	<1.0	150	0	<18.0
Stuffing, Sage & Onion	0.5 oz.	50	<1.0	230	0	<18.0

☞ Contadina	S. S.	CAL	FAT(g)	SOD(mg)	CHL(mg)	%FAT
Seasoned Bread Crumbs	1 Tbsp.	35	<1.0	250	-	<25.7

☞ Devonsheer	S. S.	CAL	FAT(g)	SOD(mg)	CHL(mg)	%FAT
Bread Crumbs, Italian Style	1 oz.	104	1.3	408	0	11.3
Bread Crumbs, Plain	1 oz.	108	1.4	272	0	11.7

☞ Gold Medal	S. S.	CAL	FAT(g)	SOD(mg)	CHL(mg)	%FAT
Flour, Better for Bread	1 cup	400	1.0	0	0	2.3

☞ Golden Grain*	S. S.	CAL	FAT(g)	SOD(mg)	CHL(mg)	%FAT
Bread Stuffing Mix, Chicken Flavor	1/2 cup	106	1.2	637	0	10.2
Bread Stuffing Mix, Cornbread	1/2 cup	105	1.0	774	0	8.6
Bread Stuffing Mix, Herb & Butter	1/2 cup	104	1.1	713	0	9.5

STUFFINGS & STUFFING MIXES

☞ Golden Grain*

	S. S.	CAL	FAT(g)	SOD(mg)	CHL(mg)	%FAT
Bread Stuffing Mix. with Wild Rice	1/2 cup	108	1.1	611	0	9.2
*Prepared without butter, margarine or salt						

☞ Kellogg's

	S. S.	CAL	FAT(g)	SOD(mg)	CHL(mg)	%FAT
Corn Flake Crumbs	1 oz.	100	0.0	290	0	0.0
Croutettes	0.7 oz.	70	0.0	260	-	0.0

☞ Nabisco

	S. S.	CAL	FAT(g)	SOD(mg)	CHL(mg)	%FAT
Cracker Meal	1/4 cup	110	0.0	10	0	0.0

☞ Pepperidge Farm

	S. S.	CAL	FAT(g)	SOD(mg)	CHL(mg)	%FAT
Distinctive Stuffings, Apple & Raisin	1 oz.	110	1.0	410	-	8.2
Distinctive Stuffings, Classic Chicken	1 oz.	110	1.0	410	-	8.2
Distinctive Stuffings, Country Garden Herb	1 oz.	120	4.0	300	-	30.0
Distinctive Stuffings, Harvest Vegetables & Almond	1 oz.	110	3.0	250	-	24.5
Stuffing, Corn Bread	1 oz.	110	1.0	320	-	8.2
Stuffing, Country Style	1 oz.	100	1.0	400	-	9.0
Stuffing, Cube	1 oz.	110	1.0	400	-	8.2
Stuffing, Herb Seasoned	1 oz.	110	1.0	380	-	8.2

☞ Progresso

	S. S.	CAL	FAT(g)	SOD(mg)	CHL(mg)	%FAT
Bread Crumbs, Italian Style	2 Tbsp.	60	<1.0	240	0	<15.0
Bread Crumbs, Onion	2 Tbsp.	55	<1.0	320	0	<16.4
Bread Crumbs,. Plain	2 Tbsp.	60	<1.0	100	0	<15.0

☞ **Stove Top**	**S. S.**	**CAL**	**FAT(g)**	**SOD(mg)**	**CHL(mg)**	**%FAT**
Flexible Serving Stuffing Mix, Chicken Flavor	1/2 cup	120	3.0	520	0	22.5
Flexible Serving Stuffing Mix, Cornbread	1/2 cup	130	30	540	0	20.8
Flexible Serving Stuffing Mix, Homestyle Herb	1/2 cup	120	3.0	460	0	22.5
Flexible Serving Stuffing Mix, Pork	1/2 cup	120	3.0	580	0	22.5
Microwave Stuffing Mix*, Chicken Flavor	1/2 cup	130	4.0	440	0	27.7
Microwave Stuffing Mix*, Homestyle Cornbread	1/2 cup	120	3.0	410	0	22.5
Microwave Stuffing Mix*, Mushroom and Onion	1/2 cup	130	3.0	470	0	20.8
Stuffing Mix, Americana	1/2 cup	100	1.0	570	0	9.0
Stuffing Mix, Beef	1/2 cup	110	1.0	520	0	8.2
Stuffing Mix, Chicken Flavor	1/2 cup	110	1.0	490	0	8.2
Stuffing Mix, Cornbread	1/2 cup	110	1.0	490	0	8.2
Stuffing Mix, Long Grain and Wild Rice	1/2 cup	110	1.0	480	0	8.2
Stuffing Mix, Mushroom and Onion	1/2 cup	110	1.0	410	0	8.2
Stuffing Mix, Pork	1/2 cup	110	1.0	490	0	8.2
Stuffing Mix, Savory Herbs	1/2 cup	110	1.0	510	0	8.2
Stuffing Mix, Turkey	1/2 cup	110	1.0	560	0	8.2
Stuffing Mix, with Rice	1/2 cup	110	1.0	490	0	8.2
*Prepared without margarine or salt						

COOKING LOW-FAT DELICIOUSLY
CHAPTER 4

Cooking without added fat is easier and tastier than you would imagine. Since fatty ingredients such as oil, margarine, butter, and cream add flavor, texture, and moisture, the trick to fat-free cooking is to add flavor, texture, and moisture using other ingredients. This chapter is not intended to be a cookbook, but rather to provide food for thought. Use these ideas, and add your own creative touch.

Defatting the Meat. Choosing the right ingredients is essential to successful low-fat cooking. See the introduction to the Shopping Guide for details about choosing quality low-fat meat, poultry and seafood. In preparing meat for cooking, be sure to trim as much excess fat as possible. In addition, removing the skin from chicken or turkey is extremely important, since up to 50% of the fat in poultry is contained in the skin. After cooking, drain *all* of the excess fat and squeeze the meat dry between several layers of paper towels. This is important even when using leaner items such as ground turkey breast or ground top round.

Marinate. Add flavor and moisture to skinless poultry, fish, and lean meat by marinating with one or a combination of the following items: wine, dry wine, flavored seltzer, flavored vinegar (balsamic, cider, herb-flavored, raspberry, rice, tarragon, or wine-flavored), fruit juice (apple cider, grape, lime, lemon, orange, etc.) store-bought nonfat Italian dressing, low-salt soy sauce, Worcestershire sauce, white wine Worcestershire sauce, salsa, horseradish, tomato sauce, or non-fat plain yogurt. One tasty combination includes pineapple juice, nonfat Italian dressing, soy sauce, ginger and garlic. The nonfat Italian dressing can be replaced with red wine vinegar to make an excellent red meat marinade. Holland House has recently introduced five flavors of oil-free marinades: teriyaki, red wine and herb, lemon and herb, hot and spicy, and garden herb.

Stocks: The Secret to Fine Low-Fat Cooking. Stocks are critical components of low-fat cooking since they add body and flavor to sauces, salad dressings, and soups that canned broth or boullion cubes can't add. Once you prepare your stock, remove the fat by refrigerating and skimming off the fat or by pouring hot stock through a fat-straining cup. Freezing stock in ice cube trays and storing in plastic bags makes it available at a moment's notice for quick sautéing. Pre-prepared frozen stock is available at some gourmet stores and large supermarkets. The health section of your supermarket or health food store often carries "natural" low-salt canned broths which tend to be a more acceptable substitute than regular low-salt canned broth. Keep the can in the refrigerator so you can skim off the fat before use.

Sauté Without Fat. Nonfat liquids can be used to sauté and can add a variety of flavors to your food. Avoiding oil, butter, and margarine is easy by sautéing with nonfat ingredients such as clam juice, fish, chicken or beef stock, liquid Butter Buds, nonfat Italian dressing, low-salt bouillon, refrigerated low-salt canned broth, flavored vinegars, low-salt soy sauce, lime juice, lemon juice, orange juice, pineapple juice, fresh lemon slices, Worcestershire sauce, tomato sauce, salsa, V-8 juice, white grape juice, wine, vermouth or any other nonfat liquid.

Seasoning Without Fat. If sautéing is not required or additional flavor is desired, season with a variety of low-fat items. Any of the items suggested in the sautéing section above are terrific seasoners. In addition, barbecue sauce, chili sauce, cocktail sauce, fancy mustards, horseradish sauce, one of Knorr's low-fat cooking sauces, chutney, Lawry's Dijon & Honey barbecue sauce, or Ocean Spray Cran-Fruit can add flavor to foods in seconds.

Furthermore, don't underestimate the flavoring value of herbs and spices.

Poaching. Poaching fish or chicken is a great way to prepare a moist and delicious entrée. Use nonfat ingredients such as tomato, lemon, or lime juice, low-salt broth, wine and herbs to make a liquid for poaching. Place the fish or chicken in enough liquid to barely cover it and simmer with the pan covered. Poach shellfish for two to three minutes and chicken for about twenty. Be careful not to poach fish or chicken too long, since overcooking will make it dry.

Poaching in the microwave is a delicious and fast way to cook poultry. Pour about 1/2 cup low-salt chicken broth, stock, water or water/wine mixture over one pound of chicken breasts in a microwave-safe dish. Cover and microwave on high seven minutes or until tender without overcooking. (Cook twice as much chicken by doubling both the amount of liquid and the cooking time). Onions, celery, and spices can be added before cooking, if desired. In addition to fish and poultry, try poaching pears, apples, or peaches in red wine, fruit juice, and cinnamon or cloves.

Stir-Frying. Although often equated with low-fat cooking, this method can be dangerously high in fat. However, when less than one tablespoon of oil is used, this is a terrific, fast way to cook food. Using a very hot pan or wok, stir-fry with nonfat liquid such as stock, low-salt soy sauce, wine, or marinade used for meat. The vegetables can be steamed by these liquids when a lid is used and thus reduce the need for oil.

Broiling and Grilling. By placing meat on a rack that allows the fat to drip away, broiling and grilling allow some of the fat contained in food to drain off. This is not, however, a justification to use higher fat meats. As always, begin with the leaner items mentioned above and coat the broiler or grill with non-stick cooking spray. Marinating and basting frequently with the marinades described above will keep meats from becoming dry.

Roasting and Baking. Since both roasting and baking are dry-heat cooking methods, lean meats, poultry and seafood require basting with any of the nonfat liquids mentioned. Another option is to use oven bags which also help keep lean meat and poultry from drying out during cooking. A cooking rack placed in the roasting pan or baking dish is again important to help fat drain off. Try this method instead of frying.

Microwaving. Microwaving fish is another low-fat method that is fast and easy. Season with nonfat low-salt seasoning such as lemon pepper. Using salt before cooking or overcooking will make fish tough and dry. Cover and cook on high power for three to six minutes per pound. Fish is ready when it becomes flaky and opaque. For recipes that need browning or crisping, broil briefly after microwaving.

The microwave can be a great way to prepare vegetables, too. It's not only quick, but it preserves and enhances the color, texture, nutrition, and flavor of vegetables. In addition, sautéing chopped fresh vegetables in the microwave is convenient and can save on dirty dishes. Use two teaspoons of water or any nonfat liquid to sauté chopped fresh vegetables such as onions, celery, and peppers. Cook in a covered, microwave-safe dish on high for two or three minutes per cup of vegetables.

Avoid the problems of scorching and stirring by preparing low-fat sauces in the microwave. Using any low-fat sauce recipe, blend the cornstarch, flour or other thickener and the liquid in a two quart dish until smooth, then add the remaining ingredients. Microwave on high until hot and bubbly, stirring once or twice (usually 2 to 5 minutes). If the sauce contains yogurt, cheese, or sour cream, microwave them on medium high to prevent curdling. See the sauce section below for specific recipes.

On The Side. Nonfat side dishes can be delicious, too. Potatoes, rice, pasta, and beans are very low in fat and can be cooked and seasoned in a variety of simple ways without adding fat. Boiling new potatoes, pasta, rice, or vegetables in stock or low-salt chicken broth adds lots of flavor. Rice and vegetables can also be boiled in low-salt V-8 juice. Low-salt soy sauce, flavored vinegars, white wine Worcestershire, non-fat salad dressings, or the low-fat sauce recipes from the sauce section combined with sautéed onions, peppers or other vegetables add flavor and variety. Make mashed and baked potatoes richer by adding non-fat sour cream or blenderized cottage cheese mixed with chives, onions, or garlic. Sliced or cubed top round, pork tenderloin, poultry, or seafood added to any of these sauce mixtures makes pasta, rice and potatoes into a terrific main dish.

Fresh, Fast and Fat-Reduced. The hectic pace of life can leave us with less time to prepare great homestyle meals. Below are a few tips to get the great taste of fresh food in less time and with less fat.

Fresh herbs and spices can really enhance the taste of your meals. Since it isn't always practical to take the time and effort to buy and grind fresh herbs, a good alternative is bottled herbs found in the produce section. These are just as easy to use as dried spices, but have a much fresher flavor.

Another valuable enhancement is fresh salsa, found in the refrigerator section of your supermarket. This allows you to add the fresh taste of tomatoes, onions, herbs, and spices without the work of making your own salsa. It is often no more expensive then bottled salsa or picante sauce and tastes terrific on a variety of foods from fish to potatoes.

Although parmesan and romano cheese are quite high in fat, their strong flavor when freshly grated can add a robust flavor to your salads, pastas, breads, vegetables and other dishes. Since only a small amount is necessary, the additional fat is minimal. Pregrated cheeses have lost much of their flavor before they reach the supermarket, so more cheese (and more fat) are required to get the same result as with freshly grated cheese.

Low-Fat Secrets in your Supermarket. You probably walk by some of the best and easiest-to-prepare low-fat products without even noticing them. Try some of them for interesting new dishes.

Egg roll wrappers and won ton wraps are found in the produce section of most supermarkets. They are very low-fat and don't have to be fried to be good. Steam, boil or bake these pasta wraps after filling with any of a variety of foods such as vegetables, skim milk ricotta cheese, low-fat beef, pork, poultry, or seafood. To get the best results, brush egg white or a very small amount of oil on the wraps before baking.

Fillo dough leaves are another fat free product that is often overlooked. Filled and rolled into one large strudel, individual filled rolls, shells, or crusts, they make attractive hors d'oeuvres, main courses and desserts. Rather than using butter between each layer, lightly coat the outer layer with nonstick cooking spray or brush the outer layer with a lower calorie margarine melted and diluted with water.

Fresh pizza dough, available at many supermarket bakeries, can be a great way to start quick recipes. Using low-fat spaghetti sauce, part skim mozzarella cheese, and a variety of vegetables, you can have a pizza ready to pop in the oven in five minutes. If you must have meat on your pizza, Canadian bacon is a relatively low-fat choice. From bread sticks to calzones this dough can make cooking just a little easier. If your supermarket doesn't have fresh pizza dough, try frozen bread dough or bread shells instead.

Nabisco Crackermeal is a great item to use in cooking. It has no fat or salt and makes a great coating for poultry and fish. Dip poultry, scallops or fish in nonfat Italian dressing or nonfat mayonnaise and then in Crackermeal seasoned with herbs and spices.

Fresh or frozen tortellini and ravioli can be the perfect answer for a quick low-fat meal. Several brands found in the shopping guide are low-fat. Add the tortellini to soups, green salads and pasta salads, or make it into a main dish by whipping up a low-fat sauce.

Low-Fat Baking. While yeast breads are usually low-fat, other baked goods such as muffins, corn bread, banana bread, and coffee cake are often high in fat. Using the following fat-reducing techniques can help make your favorite baked goods low-fat yet delicious.

- **Begin** with recipes calling for no more than one-half cup (eight tablespoons) of oil, butter, or margarine. Replace at least half, but ideally three-fourths of the amount called for with nonfat plain yogurt on an equal basis cup for cup. Apple-sauce, apple butter, pumpkin, ripe bananas, mashed zucchini, or fruit purées can also be used as replacements, either alone or in combination with nonfat plain yogurt. In this way, you should be able to reduce the added fat to no more than two tablespoons or one-eighth cup. When using applesauce or apple butter all of the fat can be replaced.

- **Use** nonfat egg substitutes such as Fleishmann's Egg Beaters instead of eggs or limit the number of egg yolks to one per recipe using only the egg white for each additional egg.

- **Use** 1% milk, skim milk, buttermilk or evaporated skim milk in recipes calling for whole milk. If more than 1/4 cup of marga-rine, butter or other fat has been replaced by another moistening ingredient, it is usually a good idea to add an additional tablespoon of milk.

- **Use** nonstick cooking spray to coat your baking pans rather than margarine or shortening.

- **Use** three tablespoons of baking cocoa plus one tablespoon of oil in place of one ounce of baking chocolate. The Choco-late Syrups listed in the Shopping Guide can also make low-fat chocolate desserts.

- **Avoid** recipes calling for coconut.

- **Use** Dream Whip whipped topping mix to give some desserts a lift, along with a lighter, creamier texture.

- **Limit** nuts to one-fourth to one-third cup per recipe, or use Grape-Nuts Cereal to replace the nuts.

- **Make** pie and dessert crusts by combining no-added-sugar preserves with graham cracker crumbs or replace the margarine or butter in any graham cracker crust recipe with liquid Butter Buds.

Substitute for High-Fat Items

Butter and Margarine. Nonfat butter substitutes such as Molly McButter or Butter Buds can be used on hot, moist foods such as potatoes, pasta, rice, fish, and vegetables. On toast, bagels, English muffins and bread, use no-sugar-added fruit spreads, apple butter or cream cheese substitute.

Cream and Half and Half. Given the heavy body of evaporated canned skim milk, using it as a substitute for cream, half and half, or whole milk provides a delicious creamy taste without the fat.

Cooking Oil. Instead of using cooking oil in your frying pan or skillet, keep food from sticking using either non-stick spray, olive oil non-stick spray or any of the ingredients in the sautéing section above.

Salad Dressing. Most major brands have excellent nonfat salad dressings in a variety of flavors. Be sure the label specifically indicates there is no fat. These dressings can also be used as a quick and tasty nonfat seasoning item for many different foods. Specific brands can be found in the shopping guide.

Flavored vinegars can add a real accent to salads. Balsamic vinegar adds a sweet flavor, while champagne, rice, and tarragon vinegars have milder flavors. By adding a milder flavor than regular vinegars, a smaller quantity of oil is needed to give the salad dressing the proper balance. With the stronger flavored oils like hazelnut, walnut, sesame and olive oils, even less oil can be used. Choose the better quality vinegars in the gourmet section of your supermarket or at a specialty store to avoid the harsh taste of cheaper vinegars.

Alternative bases for homemade salad dressings include frozen juice concentrates, fresh squeezed juice, buttermilk, blenderized tofu, and blenderized skim milk ricotta. A small amount of flavored mustard or hot sauce can add a tangy flavor.

Cream Cheese. Try utilizing one of the new fat free cream cheese substitutes recently put on the market or make your own. Allow low-fat or even whole milk plain yogurt to drain through cheesecloth for about twenty-four hours until it has the consistency of regular cream cheese. Avoid nonfat yogurt since it produces an acidic, overly tart cheese. Each tablespoon of yogurt cheese made with whole milk still has 1 gram of fat. This is considerably lower in fat than regular or "light" cream cheese, but you should still go easy on the serving sizes. Use it as a cream cheese substitute in your favorite recipes, as a sandwich spread, or on bagels and low-fat crackers. Pot cheese also makes a good cream cheese substitute.

Sour Cream. If a nonfat sour cream substitute is not available in your area, use blenderized nonfat or 1% cottage cheese to make a delicious sour cream substitute. This makes a terrific sauce and salad dressing base. Add two tablespoons of nonfat ranch dressing and some chopped green onions to make an appetizing potato topping.

Mayonnaise. Use one of the new brands of fat-free mayonnaise or salad dressing.

Sauce/Canned Soup Substitute. Low-fat sauces can be a terrific way to add flavor and moisture to foods without adding fat. Puréed vegetables make flavorful sauces without the addition of fat. Since frozen vegetables don't compromise the quality of purées, these already cleaned, cut and blanched vegetables can be put in a blender along with herbs and seasonings. The addition of nonfat mayonnaise, low-fat ricotta cheese or a teaspoon of oil may also be added to these puréed sauces to provide optimal texture. Buttermilk thickened with cornstarch or cream of rice cereal blenderized make excellent cream sauce bases. Unfortunately, sauces can make cooking more laborious. The following low-fat sauce base recipes are simple to make in a microwave. Simply season to taste with herbs, seasoning or even puréed vegetables.

White Sauce Base
    1/4 cup flour
    1/4 cup nonfat powdered milk
    2 cups cold skim milk
    Seasonings

Mix flour and powdered milk in a two quart microwave-safe bowl. Add milk gradually while stirring with a wire whisk. Microwave on high for about four minutes or until thickened, stirring once. Season to taste.

Creamy Sauce Base
    1 cup nonfat or 1% low-fat cottage cheese
    1/4 cup nonfat mayonnaise
    1/4 cup skim milk or 1/4 cup buttermilk
    Dash of fresh lemon juice
    Seasoning

Combine all ingredients in blender until smooth. Microwave on medium high about four minutes until hot and bubbly. Season to taste.

Basic Wine Sauce
    1/2 cup defatted chicken stock or 1 tsp. low salt chicken
        bouillon dissolved in 1/2 cup hot water
    1 Tbsp. white wine or white grape juice
    2 tsp. cornstarch
    1/3 cup cold skim milk
    Dash of onion powder
    Salt and pepper

In a microwave-safe bowl, add stock or broth, wine and onion powder. Blend cornstarch and milk until smooth, then stir into broth mixture. Microwave on high about three minutes until hot and bubbly. Add salt and pepper to taste.

Low-Fat Gravy

1/2 cup flour
Defatted meat drippings or 3 cups canned broth

Spray skillet with nonstick cooking spray. Place flour in skillet and brown over medium-high heat stirring continuously with wire whisk until peanut butter-colored. Add broth or drippings and stir briskly until smooth. Pan drippings or stock can be defatted without waiting for fat to congeal in the refrigerator by pouring hot liquid through a fat-straining cup. Season to taste.

Canned Cream Soup Substitute

1 1/2 Tbsp. cornstarch
1/8 cup nonfat powdered milk
2 tsp. low sodium chicken bouillon granules
1/8 teaspoon dried Italian seasoning
1/4 teaspoon onion powder
1/8 teaspoon poultry seasoning
1/4 teaspoon celery salt
Ground pepper
1 1/4 cup cold water

Mix all dry ingredients in a one quart microwave-safe bowl. Add water and blend until smooth. Microwave for about three minutes on high until thickened, stirring twice. Add pepper to taste. Makes the equivalent of one 10.5 oz. can of cream soup. Substitute this for canned soup in any recipe or add an extra 1/4 cup water to use it as a sauce. **Make this recipe in bulk and store in an airtight container.**

Campbell Soup Company does have a low-fat cream of mushroom and a cream of chicken soup on the market which can also be used. These soups contain between 25 to 30 percent of their calories from fat while our recipe contains only 7 percent of its calories from fat. Made in bulk our recipe can be just as easy and much cheaper.

Changing Manufacturers' Directions from High-Fat to Low-Fat. Even those not in the habit of using convenience foods resort to them on occasion. Although not known for being particularly healthful, many convenience products' fat content can be lowered by changing the manufacturers' directions. Some packaged foods are of themselves low-fat but call for higher fat ingredients in their preparation. The following simple substitutions can convert the prepared item into a lower fat food. Don't forget to check the package to be sure too much fat hasn't already been added. Even those products low enough in fat to be placed in the shopping guide can be made lower in fat by using these guidelines. Don't assume that these modifications will significantly change the taste of products: in fact, most will taste essentially the same.

Guidelines for Reducing Fat in Prepared Foods

1. Eliminate any butter, margarine, or oil regardless of the amount. Liquid Butter Buds can be used as a substitute for butter or margarine.
2. Use nonfat milk rather than whole milk.
3. Use ground eye of round, top round beef, or ground turkey breast rather than regular ground beef.
4. Use nonfat mayonnaise rather than regular mayonnaise.
5. For pasta salads, use fat free Italian dressing in place of oil.
6. In baked goods calling for oil, substitute an equal quantity of nonfat plain yogurt or nonfat sour cream.
7. Use frozen egg substitutes such as Egg Beaters.

The following list shows a few examples of how much fat can be eliminated by using these types of substitutions. Packaged convenience products, unfortunately, tend to be high in sodium and sometimes cholesterol. Compare and try to choose products lower in sodium and omit salt if called for in the directions. The cholesterol content often is decreased with the reduction of fat when preparing the product.

BETTY CROCKER

☞ Suddenly Salad Caesar	S. S.	CAL	FAT(g)	SOD(mg)	CHL(mg)	%FAT
Prepared as directed	1/2 cup	170	8.0	450	-	42.4
Eliminate oil and use 3 Tbsp. nonfat Italian salad dressing	1/2 cup	113	1.0	550	-	8.0

KRAFT

☞ Macaroni & Cheese Dinner	S. S.	CAL	FAT(g)	SOD(mg)	CHL(mg)	%FAT
Prepared as directed	3/4 cup	290	13	530	5.0	40.3
Eliminate 1/4 cup margarine & use 1/4 cup skim milk	3/4 cup	195	2.0	428	3.0	9.2

LIPTON

☞ Golden Saute Beef Rice Mix	S. S.	CAL	FAT(g)	SOD(mg)	CHL(mg)	%FAT
Prepared as directed	1/2 cup	170	7.0	570	-	37.1
Prepared using modified directions	1/2 cup	140	4.0	550	-	25.7
Eliminate 2 Tbsp. margarine or butter	1/2 cup	120	1.0	520	-	7.5

PILLSBURY

☞ Cheddar & Bacon Potatoes	S. S.	CAL	FAT(g)	SOD(mg)	CHL(mg)	%FAT
Prepared as directed	1/2 cup	140	6.0	480	-	38.6
Eliminate 2 Tbsp. margarine/ butter & use 2/3 cup skim milk	1/2 cup	101	1.0	496	-	8.9

STOVE TOP

☞ Flexible Serving Stuffing Mix, Chicken	S. S.	CAL	FAT(g)	SOD(mg)	CHL(mg)	%FAT
Prepared as directed	1/2 cup	170	9.0	580	15	47.7
No margarine/butter added	1/2 cup	120	3.0	520	0	22.5

LOW-FAT FAST FOODS
CHAPTER 5

♦ Eating in the Fast Lane:
A Guide to Low-Fat Eating at Fast Food Restaurants

In general, fast food is very high in fat. With all of the recent attention on cholesterol, however, fast food restaurants have been trying to change their unhealthy image. Unfortunately, much of their emphasis has been centered on changing the type of fat used rather than decreasing the total amount of fat. Nevertheless, some items are available that are lower in fat. Since fast food has become an integral part of our fast-paced lifestyle, finding lower fat items offered at these restaurants is essential. So when you're in a hurry or are too tired to do anything but go through the drive-up window, be sure to choose items from the low-fat list below.

☞ **Arby's**	S. S.	CAL	FAT(g)	SOD(mg)	CHL(mg)	%FAT
Cookie, Chocolate Chip	1 oz.	130	4.0	95	0	27.7
Danish, Cinnamon Nut	3.5 oz.	340	9.5	230	0	25.1
Muffin, Blueberry	2.5 oz.	200	5.6	269	22	25.2
Potato, Baked, Plain	1	240	1.9	58	0	7.1
Salad, Side	1	25	0.0	30	0	0.0
Shake, Chocolate	12 oz.	451	11.6	341	32	23.1
Shake, Jamocha	11.5	368	10.5	262	35	25.7
Soup, Beef with Vegetable	8 oz.	96	2.8	996	10	26.3
Soup, Old Fashion Chicken Noodle	8 oz.	99	1.8	929	25	16.4
Soup, Tomato Florentine	8 oz.	84	1.5	910	2	16.1

LOW-FAT FAST FOODS

☞ Baskin-Robbins

	S. S.	CAL	FAT(g)	SOD(mg)	CHL(mg)	%FAT
Frozen Yogurt, Lowfat	1 fl. oz.	<352	1.0	10	1	<30.0
Frozen Yogurt, Nonfat	1 fl. oz.	<25	0.0	10	0	0.0
Ice Cream, Sugar Free, All Flavors	4 fl. oz.	<100	<2.0	<100	<4	<18.0
On The Light Side, Nonfat Dairy Dessert	4 fl. oz.	100	0.0	0	0	0.0
Sorbet Fruit Whip	1 fl. oz.	20	0.0	5	0	0.0

☞ Burger King

	S. S.	CAL	FAT(g)	SOD(mg)	CHL(mg)	%FAT
Bagel	1	272	6.0	438	29	19.9
Salad, Chunky Chicken	1	142	4.0	443	49	25.4
Sandwich, BK Broiler Chicken	1	267	8.0	728	45	27.0
Sandwich, Ocean Catch without Tartar Sauce	1	361	11.0	781	46	27.4
Shake, Chocolate	1	326	10.0	198	31	27.6
Shake, Strawberry	1	394	10.0	230	33	22.8
Shake, Vanilla	1	334	10.0	213	33	26.9
Side Salad	1	25	0.0	27	0	0.0

☞ Carl's Jr.

	S. S.	CAL	FAT(g)	SOD(mg)	CHL(mg)	%FAT
Muffin, Blueberry	1	340	9.0	300	45	23.8
Muffin, Bran	1	310	7.0	370	60	20.3
Muffin, English, with Margarine	1	190	5.0	280	0	23.7
Potato, Lite Menu Lite	1	290	1.0	60	0	3.1
Sandwich, Charbroiler BBQ Chicken, Lite Menu	1	310	6.0	680	30	17.4
Sandwich, Santa Fe Chicken	1	540	130	1180	40	21.7
Shake, All Flavors	1	350	7.0	230	15	18.0

☞ Chick-Fil-A

	S. S.	CAL	FAT(g)	SOD(mg)	CHL(mg)	%FAT
Chicken	1 piece	219	6.8	801	42	27.9
Chicken, Chargrilled	1 piece	128	2.5	698	32	17.4

☞ Chick-Fil-A	S. S.	CAL	FAT(g)	SOD(mg)	CHL(mg)	%FAT
Pie, Lemon	1 slice	329	5.1	300	7	13.9
Salad, Garden, Chargrilled Chicken	1	126	2.1	567	28	15.2
Salad, Tossed	1	21	0.3	19	0	10.7
Sandwich, Chargrilled Chicken	1	258	4.8	1121	40	16.8
Sandwich, Chargrilled Chicken, Deluxe	1	266	4.9	1125	40	16.7
Sandwich, Chick-n-Q	1	206	6.8	660	26	29.7
Sandwich, Chicken	1	360	8.5	1174	66	21.3
Sandwich, Chicken, Deluxe	1	368	8.6	1178	66	21.0
Soup, Hearty Breast of Chicken	1	152	2.7	530	46	15.8

☞ Dairy Queen	S. S.	CAL	FAT(g)	SOD(mg)	CHL(mg)	%FAT
Banana Split	1	510	11.0	250	30	19.4
Blizzard, Strawberry, Regular	1	740	16.0	230	50	19.5
Breeze, Heath, Regular	1	680	21.0	360	15.0	27.8
Breeze, Strawberry, Regular	1	590	1.0	170	5	1.5
Cone, Chocolate, Regular	1	230	7.0	115	20	27.4
Cone, Vanilla, Regular	1	230	7.0	95	20	27.4
Cone, Yogurt, Regular	1	180	<1.0	80	<5	<5.0
Malt, Vanilla	1	610	14.0	230	45	20.7
Mr. Misty	1	250	0.0	0	0	0.0
Sandwich, DQ	1	140	4.0	135	5	25.7
Shake, Chocolate, Regular	1	540	14.0	290	45	23.3
Shake, Vanilla, Regular	1	520	14.0	230	45	24.2
Sundae, Chocolate	1	300	7.0	140	20	21.0
Sundae, Yogurt, Strawberry	1	200	<1.0	80	<5	<4.5
Yogurt Cup, Regular	1	170	<1.0	70	<5	<5.3

☞ Haagen-Dazs	S. S.	CAL	FAT(g)	SOD(mg)	CHL(mg)	%FAT
Sorbet, Lemon	4 fl. oz.	140	0.0	5	-	0.0
Sorbet, Orange	4 fl. oz.	113	0.0	7	-	0.0
Sorbet, Raspberry	4 fl. oz.	93	0.0	7	-	0.0

☞ Haagen-Dazs

	S. S.	CAL	FAT(g)	SOD(mg)	CHL(mg)	%FAT
Yogurt, Frozen, Chocolate	3 fl. oz.	130	3.0	40	25	20.8
Yogurt, Frozen, Peach	3 fl. oz.	120	3.0	30	31	20.8
Yogurt, Frozen, Strawberry	3 fl. oz.	120	3.0	30	29	22.5
Yogurt, Frozen, Vanilla	3 fl. oz.	130	3.0	40	36	20.8
Yogurt, Frozen, Vanilla Almond Crunch	3 fl. oz.	150	5.0	65	33	30.0
Yogurt, Non-Fat Soft, Banana	1 fl. oz.	25	0.0	15	0	0.0
Yogurt, Non-Fat Soft, Chocolate	1 fl. oz.	30	0.0	20	0	0.0
Yogurt, Non-Fat Soft, Strawberry	1 fl. oz.	25	0.0	10	0	0.0
Yogurt, Soft, Chocolate	1 fl. oz.	30	1.0	13	3	30.0
Yogurt, Soft, Raspberry	1 fl. oz.	30	1.0	15	3	30.0

☞ Hardee's

	S. S.	CAL	FAT(g)	SOD(mg)	CHL(mg)	%FAT
Pancakes	3	280	2.0	890	15	6.4
Pancakes with Bacon	3/2	350	9.0	1110	25	23.1
Salad, Chicken 'N' Pasta	1	230	3.0	380	55	11.7
Salad, Side	1	20	<1.0	15	0	-
Sandwich, Grilled Chicken	1	310	9.0	890	60	26.1
Shake, Chocolate	1	460	8.0	340	45	15.7
Shake, Strawberry	1	440	8.0	300	40	16.4
Shake, Vanilla	1	400	9.0	320	50	20.3
Sundae, Cool Twist, Carmel	1	330	10.0	290	20	27.3
Sundae, Cool Twist, Strawberry	1	260	8.0	115	15	27.7

☞ Jack in the Box

	S. S.	CAL	FAT(g)	SOD(mg)	CHL(mg)	%FAT
Breadsticks, Sesame	0.6 oz.	70	2.0	110	-	25.7
Cake, Double Fudge	1 slice	288	9.0	259	20	28.1
Pita, Chicken Fajita, with Cheese	1	292	8.0	703	34	24.7
Pita, Chicken Fajita, without Cheese	1	233	3.3	479	22	12.7
Shake, Chocolate	1	330	7.0	270	25	19.1
Shake, Strawberry	1	320	7.0	240	25	19.7
Shake, Vanilla	1	320	6.0	230	25	16.9

☞ KFC	S. S.	CAL	FAT(g)	SOD(mg)	CHL(mg)	%FAT
Corn-on-the-Cob	2.6 oz.	90	2.0	11	<1	20.0
Mashed Potatoes & Gravy	3.5 oz.	71	1.6	339	<1	20.3

☞ McDonald's	S. S.	CAL	FAT(g)	SOD(mg)	CHL(mg)	%FAT
Cereal, Cheerios	1	80	1.1	210	0	12.4
Cereal, Wheaties	1	90	0.3	220	0	3.0
Dressing, Lite Vinaigrette	0.5 oz.	12	0.5	75	0	30.0
Hotcakes with Margarine & Syrup	1 serving	440	12.0	685	8	24.5
Cone, Vanilla Low-fat Frozen Yogurt	1	105	1.0	80	1	8.6
Sundae, Strawberry Low-Fat Frozen Yogurt	1	210	1.0	95	5	4.3
Sundae, Hot Fudge Low-Fat Frozen Yogurt	1	240	3.0	170	6	11.3
Sundae, Hot Caramel Low-Fat Frozen Yogurt	1	270	3.0	180	13	10.0
Milk, 1% Lowfat	1	110	2.0	130	9	16.4
Muffin, Apple Bran, Fat-Free	1	180	0.0	200	0	0.0
Muffin, English, with Spread	1	170	4.0	285	9	21.2
Salad, Chunky Chicken	1	150	4.0	230	78	24.0
Sandwich, McLean Deluxe	1	320	10.0	670	60	28.1
Sauce, Barbecue	1 packet	50	0.5	340	0	9.0
Sauce, Sweet & Sour	1 packet	60	0.2	190	0	3.0
Shake, Lowfat, Chocolate	1	320	1.7	240	10	4.8
Shake, Lowfat, Strawberry	1	320	1.3	170	10	3.7
Shake, Lowfat, Vanilla	1	290	1.3	170	10	4.0

☞ TCBY	S. S.	CAL	FAT(g)	SOD(mg)	CHL(mg)	%FAT
Frozen Yogurt, Nonfat, All Flavors	1/2 cup	110	<1	45	<5	<8.2
Frozen Yogurt, Regular, All Flavors	1/2 cup	130	3.0	60	10	20.8
Frozen Yogurt, Sugar Free, All Flavors	1/2 cup	80	<1	40	<5	<11.3

LOW-FAT FAST FOODS

LOW-FAT FAST FOODS

☞ Wendy's	S. S.	CAL	FAT(g)	SOD(mg)	CHL(mg)	%FAT
Chicken Filet, Grilled	1	100	3.0	330	55	27.0
Chili, Regular	9 oz.	220	7.0	750	45	28.6
Garden Salad, Prepared	1	70	2.0	60	0	25.7
Potato, Baked, Plain	1	270	1.0	20	0	3.3

☞ Wendy's Garden Spot Salad Bar	S. S.	CAL	FAT(g)	SOD(mg)	CHL(mg)	%FAT
Alfalfa Sprouts	1 oz.	8	0.0	<1	0	0.0
Apple Sauce, Chunky	1 oz.	22	<1	<1	0	-
Bananas	1 oz.	26	<1	<1	0	-
Breadsticks	0.3 oz.	30	1.0	30	0	30.0
Broccoli	1.5 oz.	12	0.0	10	0	0.0
Cantaloupe	2 oz.	20	0.0	5	0	0.0
Carrots	1 oz.	12	0.0	10	0	0.0
Cauliflower	2 oz.	14	0.0	10	0	0.0
Chives	1 oz.	71	1.0	20	0	12.7
Cucumbers	0.5 oz.	2	0.0	<1	0	0.0
Garbanzo Beans	1 oz.	46	1.0	5	0	19.6
Green Peas	1 oz.	21	0.0	30	0	0.0
Green Peppers	1.3 oz.	10	0.0	<1	0	0.0
Honeydew Melon	2 oz.	20	0.0	5	0	0.0
Jalapeño Peppers	0.5 oz.	2	0.0	190	0	0.0
Lettuce, Iceburg	2 oz.	8	0.0	5	0	0.0
Lettuce, Romaine	2 oz.	9	0.0	5	0	0.0
Mushrooms	0.6 oz.	4	0.0	<1	0	0.0
Onions, Red	0.3 oz.	2	0.0	<1	0	0.0
Oranges	2 oz.	26	0.0	0	0	0.0
Pasta Salad	2 oz.	35	<1	120	0	<25.7
Peaches	2 oz.	31	0.0	5	0	0.0
Pineapple Chunks	3.6 oz.	60	0.0	<1	0	0.0
Strawberries	2 oz.	17	0.0	<1	0	0.0
Three Bean Salad	2 oz.	60	<1	15	-	<15.0
Tomatoes	1 oz.	6	0.0	5	0	0.0
Turkey Ham	1 oz.	35	1.0	275	15	25.7
Watermelon	2 oz.	18	0.0	<1	0	0.0

☞Wendy's Garden Spot Salad Bar	S. S.	CAL	FAT(g)	SOD(mg)	CHL(mg)	%FAT
Wine Vinegar	0.5 oz.	2	<1	5	0	-

☞Wendy's Superbar- Mexican Fiesta	S. S.	CAL	FAT(g)	SOD(mg)	CHL(mg)	%FAT
Flour Tortillas	1.3 oz.	110	3.0	220	-	24.5
Picante Sauce	2 oz.	18	<1	5	-	-
Spanish Rice	2 oz.	70	1.0	440	<1	12.9
Taco Sauce	1 oz.	16	<1	140	<1	-

☞Wendy's Superbar- Pasta	S. S.	CAL	FAT(g)	SOD(mg)	CHL(mg)	%FAT
Alfredo Sauce	2 oz.	35	1.0	300	<1	25.7
Cheese Ravioli	2 oz.	45	1.0	290	5	20.0
Cheese Tortellini	2 oz.	60	1.0	280	5	15.0
Fettucini	2 oz.	190	3.0	3	10	14.2
Pasta Medley	2 oz.	60	2.0	5	<1	30.0
Rotini	2 oz.	90	2.0	<1	<1	20.0
Spaghetti Meat Sauce	2 oz.	60	2.0	315	10	30.0
Spaghetti Sauce	2 oz.	28	0.0	345	<1	1.3

◆ FAST FOOD TIPS

In addition to choosing foods from the low-fat list above, the following tips will help you minimize the fat in your fast food meal.

Sinister Salads and Their Dangerous Dressings. Believe it or not, salads at fast food restaurants are not always the best choice. This may be a surprise to those who have forgone something tastier for a "healthier" salad. The truth is that the average prepared salad from ten popular fast food chains is an astonishing

41% fat, *not including the dressing!* Fortunately, there are a few salads that do fit into our low-fat category of less that 30% fat. (See specific listings below).

Even if you choose one of the few salads that is low-fat, nearly all fast food salad dressings are notoriously high in fat and will probably make your salad as high in fat as a hamburger or french fries. Even those dressings billed as "light" or "reduced-calorie" are frequently too high in fat. In fact, of all the "reduced-calorie" dressings surveyed, not a single one was 30% fat or less. Considering all of the tasty, nonfat salad dressings available at the grocery store, even this "light" salad dressing is unacceptable.

LOW-FAT FAST FOODS

FAST FOOD SALADS

☞ **Arby's**	S. S.	CAL	FAT(g)	SOD(mg)	CHL(mg)	%FAT
Garden Salad	1	149	8.6	-	—	51.9
Light Italian Dressing	2 oz.	23	1.1	-	-	43.0
Salad, Cashew Chicken	1	590	37.0	-	-	56.4
Salad, Chef	1	210	11.0	-	-	47.1
Salad, Side	1	25	0.0	-	-	0.0

☞ **Burger King**	S. S.	CAL	FAT(g)	SOD(mg)	CHL(mg)	%FAT
Salad Dressing, Light Italian, Reduced Calorie	2.1 oz.	170	18.0	-	-	95.3
Salad, Chef	1	178	9.0	-	-	45.5
Salad, Chunky	1	142	4.0	-	-	25.4
Salad, Garden	1	95	5.0	-	-	47.4
Salad, Side	1	25	0.0	-	-	0.0

☞ **Carl's Jr.**	S. S.	CAL	FAT(g)	SOD(mg)	CHL(mg)	%FAT
Reduced Calorie French Dressing	1 oz.	40	2.0	-	-	45.0
Salad, Taco	1	310	19.0	-	-	55.2

☞ Carl's Jr.

	S. S.	CAL	FAT(g)	SOD(mg)	CHL(mg)	%FAT
Salad-To-Go, Lite Menu Chicken	1	200	8.0	-	-	36.0
Salad-To-Go, Lite Menu Small Garden	1	50	3.0	-	-	54.0

☞ Chick-Fil-A

	S. S.	CAL	FAT(g)	SOD(mg)	CHL(mg)	%FAT
Chargrilled Chicken Garden Salad	1	126	2.1	-	-	15.2
Chicken Salad Plate	1	579	44.9	-	-	69.8
Chicken Salad-Cup	1	309	28.2	-	-	82.1
Lite Italian Dressing	1.5 oz.	25	1.8	-	-	63.7
Tossed Salad	1	21	0.3	-	-	10.7

☞ Hardee's

	S. S.	CAL	FAT(g)	SOD(mg)	CHL(mg)	%FAT
Chef Salad	1	240	15.0	-	-	56.3
Chicken 'N' Pasta Salad	1	230	3.0	-	-	11.7
Garden Salad	1	210	14.0	-	-	60.0
Salad Dressing, French, Reduced Calorie	2 oz.	130	5.0	-	-	34.6
Salad Dressing, Italian, Reduced Calorie	2 oz.	90	8.0	-	-	80.0
Side Salad	1	20	<1.0	-	-	<45.0

☞ Jack In The Box

	S. S.	CAL	FAT(g)	SOD(mg)	CHL(mg)	%FAT
Salad Dressing, French, Reduced-Calorie	2.5 oz.	176	8.0	-	-	40.9
Salad, Chef	1	325	18.0	-	-	49.8
Salad, Side	1	51	3.0	-	-	52.9
Salad, Taco	1	503	31.0	-	-	55.5

☞ McDonald's

	S. S.	CAL	FAT(g)	SOD(mg)	CHL(mg)	%FAT
Chef Salad	1	170	9.0	-	-	47.6

LOW-FAT FAST FOODS

☞ McDonald's	S. S.	CAL	FAT(g)	SOD(mg)	CHL(mg)	%FAT
Chunky Chicken Salad	1	150	4.0	-	-	24.0
Garden Salad	1	50	2.0	-	-	36.0
Lite Vinaigrette	0.5 oz.	12	0.5	-	-	37.5
Red French Reduced Calorie Dressing	0.5 oz.	40	1.9	-	-	42.8
Side Salad	1	30	1.0	-	-	30.0

☞ Taco Bell	S. S.	CAL	FAT(g)	SOD(mg)	CHL(mg)	%FAT
Taco Salad	1	905	61.0	-	-	60.7
Taco Salad with out Shell	1	484	31.0	-	-	57.6

☞ Wendy's	S. S.	CAL	FAT(g)	SOD(mg)	CHL(mg)	%FAT
Chef Salad	1	130	5.0	-	-	34.6
Garden Salad	1	70	2.0	-	-	25.7
Reduced Calorie Bacon & Tomato	15 g.	45	4.0	-	-	80.0
Reduced Calorie Italian	15 g.	25	2.0	-	-	72.0
Taco Salad	1	530	23.0	-	-	39.1

Have it Your Way: Skip the Special Sauce. Skipping special sauces, mayonnaise and tartar sauce will significantly reduce the fat content of a particular fast food item. For example, Burger King's BK Broiler Sandwich, which has 8 grams of fat and is 27% fat by calories, can be significantly reduced to 4 grams and 16% fat by simply eliminating the BK Sauce. Although eliminating the sauce or mayonnaise is always helpful, many sandwiches are still too high in fat to be reduced below 30%.

Fighting Fat: Hold the Cheese. Avoiding cheese is always a good rule of thumb when eating out. Since one slice (1 oz.) of

American cheese contains about 106 calories and 9 grams of fat, a Hardee's cheeseburger is 40% fat by calories while a Hardee's hamburger without cheese is only 33% fat. (Although at 33% the hamburger cannot be considered low-fat, it is significantly lower than the cheeseburger). Eliminating cheese from items that are already low-fat can also make a big difference. The Chicken Fajita Pita from Jack In The Box is only 25% fat, but can be decreased to a mere 14% fat be holding the cheese.

French Fries: Fast Food but Fat Food. Don't be tempted to order fries with your low-fat entrée. A medium order of fries at Burger King adds a whopping 20 grams of fat to your meal and 48% of its calories come from fat. At McDonald's, the new McLean Deluxe derives 29% of its calories from fat and thus qualifies as a low-fat item. Ironically, it has also been offered in a McLean Deluxe Meal Package which includes an order of fries, negating its lower-fat qualities.

Poultry Ploys: "Lite" Lies. Don't fall into the trap of assuming that a food made from poultry is lower in fat than a beef item. While it is true that skinless white meat cooked without added fat is usually lower in fat than beef, these conditions are almost never met at fast food and other restaurants. The ever-popular McDonald's Chicken McNuggets and Burger King's Chicken Sandwich are 50% fat or more. KFC has recently introduced a new product line called Lite 'n Crispy Chicken. While this product eliminates the skin and gives you the option of selecting white meat, it is still prepared with added fat. As a result, a center breast Lite 'n Crispy derives almost half (49%) of its calories from fat with the other cuts being even higher.

Books by Starburst Publishers
(Partial listing—full list available on request)

The Low-Fat Supermarket —Judith & Scott Smith

A comprehensive reference of over 4,500 brand name products that derive less than 30% of their calories form fat. Information provided includes total calories, fat, cholesterol and sodium content. Organized according to the the sections of a supermarket. Your answer to a healthier you.

(trade paper)   ISBN 0914984438   **$10.95**

Allergy Cooking With Ease —Nicolette M. Dumke

A book designed to provide a wide variety of recipes to meet many different types of dietary and social needs, and, whenever possible, save you time in food preparation. Includes: Recipes for those special foods that most food allergy patients think they will never eat again; Timesaving tricks; and Allergen Avoidance Index.

(trade paper-opens flat)   ISBN 091498442X   **$12.95**

Off The Floor. . . and Into Your Soup? —Charles Christmas, Jr.

A shocking account of what goes on behind the scenes at many retaurants–high class or not. Author looks at the restaurant itself, its employees, and the food that is served to the customer. He also reveals the practical jokes, and more, that kitchen employees do to each other, and the not-so-kind things they do to patrons.

(trade paper)   ISBN 0914984381   **$7.95**

The New American Family —Artlip, Artlip, & Saltzman

American men and women are remarrying at an astounding rate, and nearly 60% of the remarriages involve children under the age of eighteen. Unfortunately, over half of these remarriages also end in divorce, with half of the "redivorces" occuring within five years. The New American Family tells it like it is. It gives examples and personal experiences that help you to see that the second time around is no picnic. It provides practical, good sense suggestions and guidelines for making your new American family the one you always dreamed of.

(trade paper)   ISBN 0914984446   **$10.95**

Dragon Slaying For Parents —Tom Prinz

Subtitled: Removing The Excess Baggage So You Can Be The Parent You Want To Be. Shows how Dragons such as Codependency, Low Self-Esteem and other hidden factors interfere with effective parenting. This book by a marriage, family, and child counselor, is for all parents—to assist them with the difficult task of raising responsible and confident children in the 1990's. It is written especially for parents who believe they have "tried everything!"

(trade paper) ISBN 0914984357 **$9.95**

Man And Wife For Life —Joseph Kanzlemar

A penetrating and often humorous look into real life situations of married people. Helps the reader get a new understanding of the problems and relationships within marriage.

(trade paper) ISBN 0914984233 **$7.95**

Alzheimer's—Does "The System" Care? —Ted & Paula Valenti

Experts consider Alzheimer's disease to be the "disease of the century." More than half the one million elderly people residing in American nursing homes have "senile dementia." This book reveals a unique observation as to the cause of Alzheimer's and the care of its victims.

(hard cover) ISBN 0914984179 **$14.95**

What To Do When The Bill Collector Calls! —David L. Kelcher, Jr.

Reveals the unfair debt collection practices that some agencies use and how this has led to the invasion of privacy, bankruptcy, marital instability, and the loss of jobs. This is a ready reference guide that tells the reader what he can do about the problem.

(trade paper) ISBN 0914984322 **$9.95**

You Can Eliminate Stress From The I.R.S. —Fulton N. Dobson

Almost everyone can expect to undergo a tax audit at least once or twice in their lifetime. This book gives common sense actions to take that will make the audit easier to face. Answers questions like: What are my rights as a taxpayer? What can I expect from my tax accountant? How can I prove to the IRS my ability (or inability) to pay back taxes? . . . and much more.

(trade paper) ISBN 0914984403 **$7.95**

Like A Bulging Wall
—Robert Borrud
Will you survive the 1990's economic crash? This book shows how debt, greed, and covetousness, along with a lifestyle beyond our means, has brought about an explosive situation in this country. Gives "call" from God to prepare for judgement in America. Also lists TOP-RATED U.S. BANKS and SAVINGS & LOANS.

(trade paper) ISBN 0914984284 **$8.95**

The Quick Job Hunt Guide
—Robert D. Siedle
Gives techniques to use when looking for a job. Networking, Following the Ten-Day Plan, and Avoiding the Personnel Department, are some of the ways to "land that job!"

(trade paper) ISBN 0914984330 **$7.95**

Get Rich Slowly . . . But Surely!
—Randy L. Thurman
The only get-rich-quick guide you'll ever need. Achieving financial independence is important to young and old. Anyone who wants to be financially free will discover the way to financial independence easier by applying these long-term, time-tested principles. This book can be read in one sitting!

(trade paper) ISBN 0914984365 **$7.95**

Purchasing Information

<u>Listed books are available from your favorite Bookstore,</u> either from current stock or special order. To assist bookstore in locating your selection be sure to give title, author, and ISBN #. If unable to purchase from the bookstore you may order direct from STARBURST PUBLISHERS. When ordering enclose full payment plus $2.00* for shipping and handling ($2.50* if Canada or Overseas). Payment in US Funds only. Please allow two to three weeks minimum (longer overseas) for delivery. Make checks payable to and mail to STARBURST PUBLISHERS, P.O. Box 4123, LANCASTER, PA 17604. **Prices subject to change without notice.** Catalog available upon request.

*We reserve the right to ship your order the least expensive way. If you desire first class (domestic) or air shipment (overseas) please enclose shpping funds as follows: First Class within the USA enclose $4.00, Airmail Canada enclose $5.00, and Overseas enclose 30% (minimum $5.00) of total order. All remittance must be in US Funds.   11-92